Asian Septorhinoplasty

Eun-Sang Dhong • Min-Wha Na

Asian Septorhinoplasty

Conundrums and Solutions

Springer

Eun-Sang Dhong
Department of Plastic and Reconstructive Surgery
Guro Hospital, College of Medicine
Korea University
Seoul
Korea (Republic of)

Min-Wha Na
Yerom Plastic Surgery Clinic
Seoul
Korea (Republic of)

ISBN 978-981-16-0541-3 ISBN 978-981-16-0542-0 (eBook)
https://doi.org/10.1007/978-981-16-0542-0

This Springer imprint is published by the registered company Springer Nature Singapore Pte Ltd.
The registered company address is: 152 Beach Road, #21-01/04 Gateway East, Singapore 189721, Singapore

Preface

The snow leopard in the Himalayas of India has leather that can withstand −29 °C and it hunts by starving for more than a week within a hunting range of 200 km. Still, hunting blue sheep on a high cliff at an altitude of 4800 m would fail dozens of times. It looks dangerous, as if falling down a cliff, but it challenges again and hunts for life. Winter is harder. When the temperature drops and the ibex descend from the snow-covered peak to the valley, the snow leopard runs through the thick snow and throws itself off the cliff to hunt. Ibex is quick and challenging to hunt. It needs food to get through the winter. It eventually throws itself in the rugged terrain by throwing all the remaining force, biting the neck of a Tibetan blue sheep and rolling down the cliff 60 m dozens of times, and descending. It seems to be lost for a moment but eventually wakes up, and the snow leopard fills the stomach. However, success comes at a tremendous cost. It is badly injured. However, the wild thing will never be sorry for itself. Still, it gets up again and goes on the way it was going. It is a scene of emotion. Indomitable determination is the life itself to live. I remember this video of "Bear Grylls' hostile planet-mountains" on the plane going back from one conference.

"Asian rhinoplasty is challenging." Which is more demanding, tissue reduction or tissue recruitment? No matter how low the dorsum and flat the tip, I think the unoperated nose is the most comfortable. Comforts and beauty are different in the rhinoplasty. The beauty is the emotional-social prejudice to be determined by the public, but the rhinoplasty surgeons should determine the beautiful nose.

After becoming a plastic surgeon, I studied through journals and attended academic conferences to learn. Rhinoplasty needs a long learning curve. I was fortunate. I learned the sincerity for the patients from my father, Dr. Young-song Dhong, a general surgeon, and septoplasty from my brother, Dr. Hun-jong Dhong, an ENT professor.

I don't think I am doing the rhinoplasty perfectly. Perhaps, by the day my practice ends, I would provide the fellow surgeons a more comfortable way to achieve agreeable results. Rhinoplasty requires a lot of time investment to get the best results. It is a surgery that involves a lot of thought before surgery and during the surgery. The nose is the prettiest just after the flap closure. Moreover, Asian rhinoplasty surgeon's hard work to overcome the alloplastic-implant-sequelae and autograft-resorption deserves praise from other plastic surgeons. If I don't look back, I probably do not have time to organize myself.

Now, as I clear it up, I want to share my knowledge and experience to move forward.

Nobody can attend the conference for a year now, but I hope that it will end soon.

I wish all those who read this book a meaningful accomplishment.

Seoul, Korea Eun-Sang Dhong

Contents

1 The Longevity of Alloplastic Implants

Pearls

- Bone resorption under the alloplastic implant is determined by (1) the implant's hardness, (2) the retention period, (3) implant location, and (4) the tension of the soft tissue envelope.
- Not only the tissue defects caused by the removal of the capsule, but the concavity induced by bone resorption should be considered when determining the dorsal on laying volume of the secondary surgery.
- The rhinion weakened by bone resorption makes the spreader graft very difficult and requires a long length.
- Unstable rhinion can induce saddle nose deformity after septorhinoplasty using autologous grafts.
- When correcting the mild hump nose, it is better to carve the implant than the bony dorsum by cutting the implants under part rather than resecting the bony dorsum.
- Putting an implant after medial and lateral osteotomies causes instability, which can cause long-term implant deviation.
- Dorsal implanting is not recommended after osteotomy. However, if necessary, the modification of leaving a broad platform in the rhinion area should be considered.
- Minor differences between the bony axis and the septal axis may be emphasized when the dorsum is projected, so care should be taken when implanting.
- In the secondary operation to solve complications caused by an implant, autografts should resolve the dorsum.

1.1 Bony Resorption Under Alloplastic Implants

Apart from the primary and secondary operation, there is no substitute as convenient and easy as the alloplastic implant in Asian rhinoplasty. As a way to increase the bony dorsum and cartilaginous dorsum at once, the surgeon only needs to pay attention to the tip plasty. Many Asian rhinoplasty surgeons' presentations at conferences focus exclusively on tip surgery and tend to overlook dorsum. The bony dorsum is rigid and immobile, but the cartilaginous dorsum provides a large amount of mobility. The mechanical effect of the rigid alloplastic implant on the underlying tissue is very different at each location. There are a myriad of alloplastic implants, but clinically, for dorsal projection, it is limited to three materials: boat-shaped Silicone, Gore-tex, and Alloderm. There are so many other hybrid products that are too diverse, so the author will not discuss them in this chapter. In general, it is widely used in this order, and among them, the use of Silicone solves the low nasion, which is the most used in Korea.

Bone resorption under the silicone implant applied to chin augmentation or malar augmenta-

E.-S. Dhong, M.-W. Na, *Asian Septorhinoplasty*, https://doi.org/10.1007/978-981-16-0542-0_1

tion has been reported. Methyl methacrylate and silicone are known to cause thinning of the skin on the top with bone resorption on the bottom. The bone under the polyfluoroethylene may also be resorbed [1]. It should be noted that both silicone and Gore-Tex, which are most commonly used in Asian rhinoplasty, may result in resorption of the underlying bone.

- The factors determining bone resorption degree are implant hardness, retention period, and implant location. Here, the pressure of the soft tissue envelope and the external physical force of the facial mimetic muscle play an essential role.
- Implantation through subperiosteal dissection of the nasal bone may decrease the implant's mobility but also a factor that promotes bone resorption.
- Concavity induced by removing capsules around the implant and bone resorption causes a vast amount of dorsal skin depression in secondary rhinoplasty. When preparing the autograft, surgeons should prepare a larger dorsal onlaying graft volume than the actual implant volume (Fig. 1.1).

The extensive bony resorption of the most critical rhinion can be observed in a long-lasting implant (Fig. 1.2).

1.2 Silicone Implant over Osteotomized Nasal Bone

Dorsal to tip projection is sometimes required after humpectomy and correcting a deviated nose. The method of using implants after the humpectomy is not recommended. Also, there is no evidence that it is safe to insert an alloplastic implant in the dorsum after the left or right lateral osteotomy [2]. The alloplastic implant tends to tilt to one side when inserted on the nasal bone in the patient who underwent medial and lateral osteotomy. This phenomenon is found in almost all patients who visited my clinic for the reoperation.

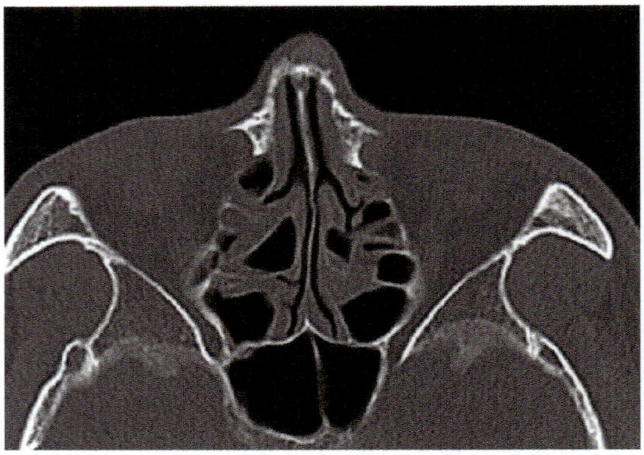

Fig. 1.2 Bone resorption under silicone implant: axial CT scan. Bone resorption with bone erosion

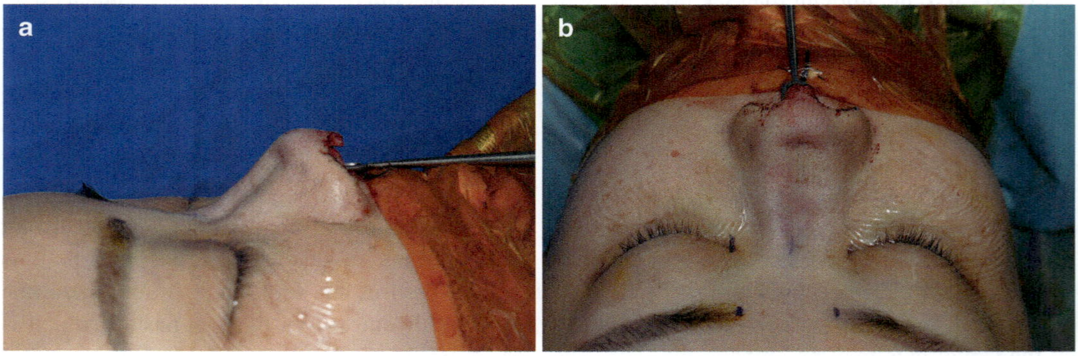

Fig. 1.1 Skin flap remaining after removing the silicone capsule. It created a massive concavity with bone resorption. (**a**) Lateral view, (**b**) frontal view

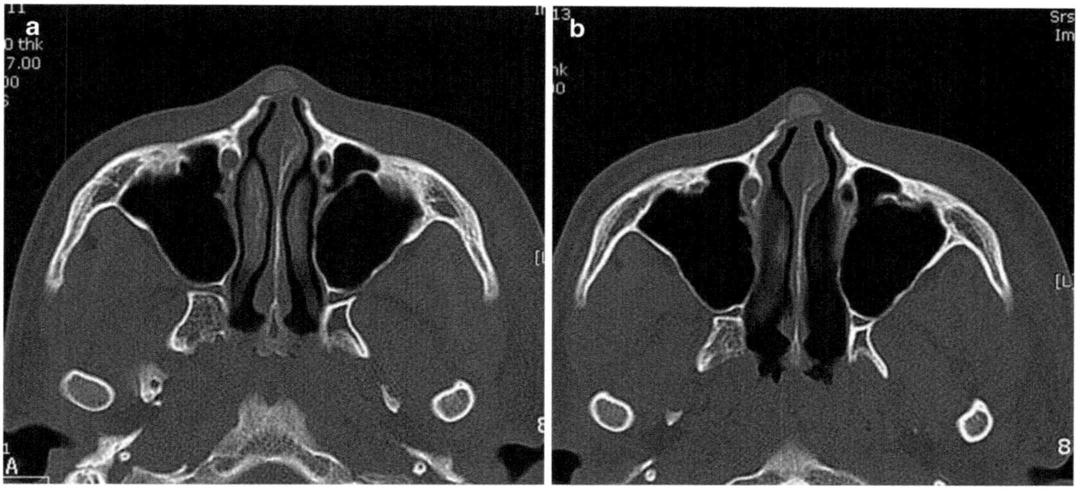

Fig. 1.3 Rhinion: destroyed by a silicone implant. (**a**) A rhinion destroyed by a 5 mm-thick silicone implant. (**b**) The base on the right side is pressing the nasal mucosa. This patient is presumed to be performed medial and lateral osteotomy

If you flatten the rhinion under the implant, as shown in the following picture, you can find that the rhinion is already weakened, and the bottom is severely destroyed. Also, the osteotomized lateral wall cannot be a safe platform for the dorsal implant (Fig. 1.3).

The weakened rhinion acts as an obstacle to reconstruction after implant removal.

However, in many Asian rhinoplasties, there is a tendency to correct the discrepancy by using an alloplastic implant after bony dorsum reduction. Even now, rather than excessive humpectomy, efforts should be made to fit the profile by carving the implant's undersurface.

The destruction of the rhinion makes the spreader graft very difficult. When applying the spreader graft, the length must be long enough; otherwise, anterior (high) septal instability may occur after surgery.

- When correcting the hump nose, the author focuses on the projection of the cartilaginous dorsum rather than reducing the hump excessively.
- Destruction of rhinion and nasal mucosa by the implant is believed to cause late-onset inflammation in the long term (Chap. 2).
- Unstable rhinion can induce saddle nose deformity after septorhinoplasty using autologous tissue. So the instability can later cause inverted V deformity.
- Do not use dorsal implants to cover any open roof deformity after humpectomy.

Medial oblique osteotomy is advantageous for implant support during corrective osteotomies. The Nasal bone can act as a platform on which an implant can be placed (Fig. 1.4). In the lateral osteotomy with medial osteotomy, a greenstick osteotomy is advantageous for the nasal pyramid's stability (Fig. 1.5).

The nasal platform above the rhinion can be preserved using the medial oblique osteotomy line for support.

- The lateral bone instability is often generated; the implant is sinking to the weak side. It can cause long-term implant deviation (Fig. 1.6).

It is difficult to find an implant that is located exactly in the midline on the nasal bone. Therefore, bone rasping may be more advantageous than osteotomy, but it cannot be applied in all cases. Ensuring a stable platform for implant placement is the most crucial key when projecting while reducing the wide nasal bone width. It is better to apply autograft to the dorsum when osteotome is accompanied.

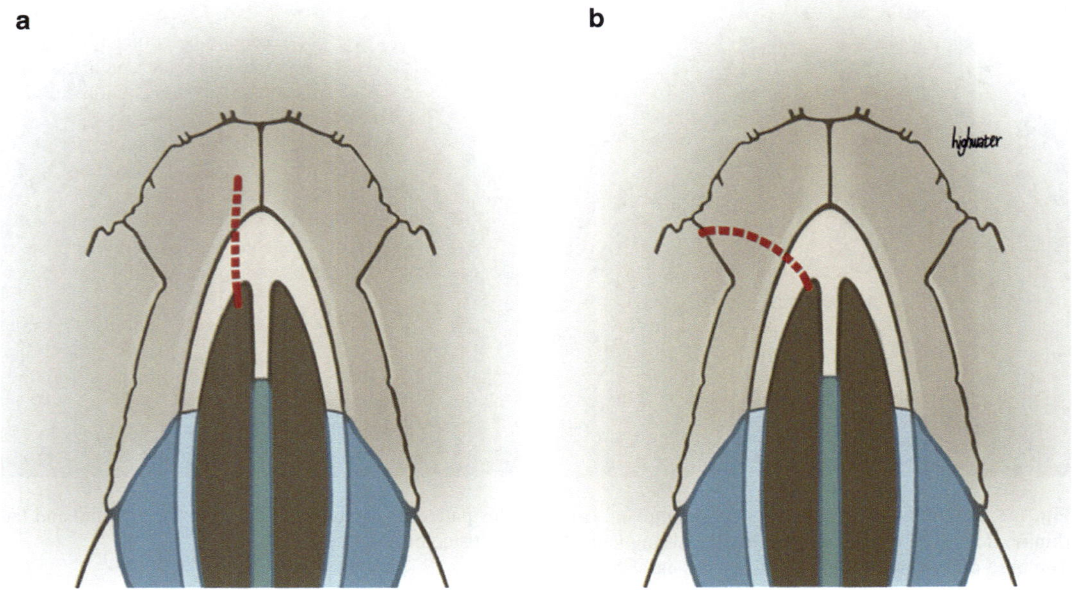

Fig. 1.4 Medial oblique osteotomy can preserve more bones for the stable implant platform. (**a**) Paramedian osteotomy. (**b**) Medial oblique osteotomy

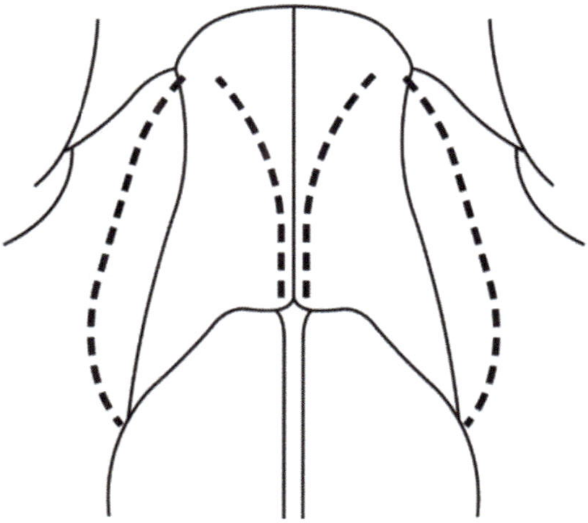

Fig. 1.5 Design of the greenstick fracture between medial oblique osteotomy and lateral low-high osteotomy

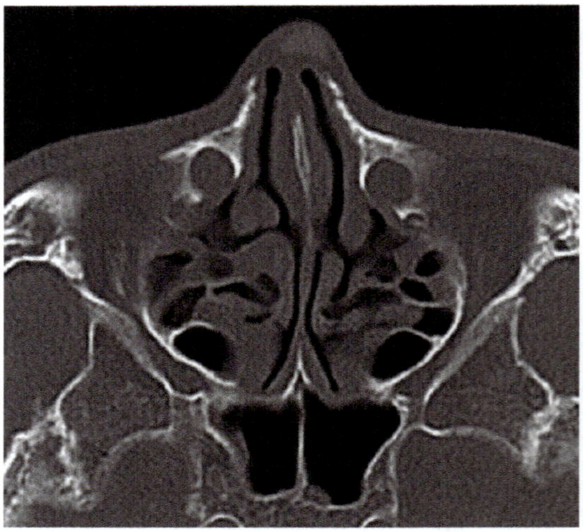

Fig. 1.6 Silicone implant dislocated to the left side with malunion of the lateral nasal bone

1.3 Implant Deviation

Longer Implant than the Pocket

The most significant cause of the deviation is the tension in the implant's longitudinal direction, generated by a longer implant than the pocket size. In this case, lateral capsulotomy is attempted as a closed technique, but this method is not very helpful unless the implant's length is shortened. Any means to reduce tension should be used. With the introduction of very soft silicone, implant deviation occurs even with less longitudinal pressure. Make sure to make enough soft tissue envelopes and use implants that are not too long. Note that implant mobility occurs when excessive dissection is performed.

Bony Axis Vs. Septal Axis

No matter how low the nose, the bony axis, and the axis of the cartilaginous dorsum are often different. If this is overlooked, the implant tilts according to the slope of the platform. Light axis discrepancy can be camouflaged with an appropriate implant-carving, but deviations are often seen again after swelling disappears.

Even patients with very low nasion can find that the cartilaginous dorsum is directed to one side from the rhinion. In this case, although silicone was inserted, there may be a discrepancy between the upper one-third and lower two-third postoperatively, resulting in cosmetic dissatisfaction (Fig. 1.7).

On the other hand, when the deviation of the septum is resolved with a spreader graft, a dorsal autograft yields a more stable result (Fig. 1.8).

However, applying the spreader graft under an implant to correct the deviation is a waste of cartilage. Although the spreader graft is functional and invisible, if covered by the dorsal implant, applying septal cartilage underneath the implant is ineffective. A dorsal implant may camouflage the deviation.

When the spreader graft is adopted, an autologous material is recommended at the dorsum. After the ULC and the septum are separated, an alloplastic implant is not recommended on it. Micromucosal damage after complete dissection between ULC from anterior septum can cause late-onset inflammation.

- There are many cases in augmenting very low nasion, in which alloplastic implants have to be used. In this situation, dissect the pocket more widely.
- Prepare a platform as flat as possible with a rasping. Bring the implant to the midline by sculpting the undersurface asymmetrically.
- It is advantageous not to perform septal dissection when implants must be used on the dorsum. In other words, without dissecting the ULC and anterior septum, the axis deviation of the lower two-third can be corrected by connecting the implant to the tip by appropriate suture rather than the spreader graft.
- Minor differences between the bony axis and the septal axis may be emphasized when the

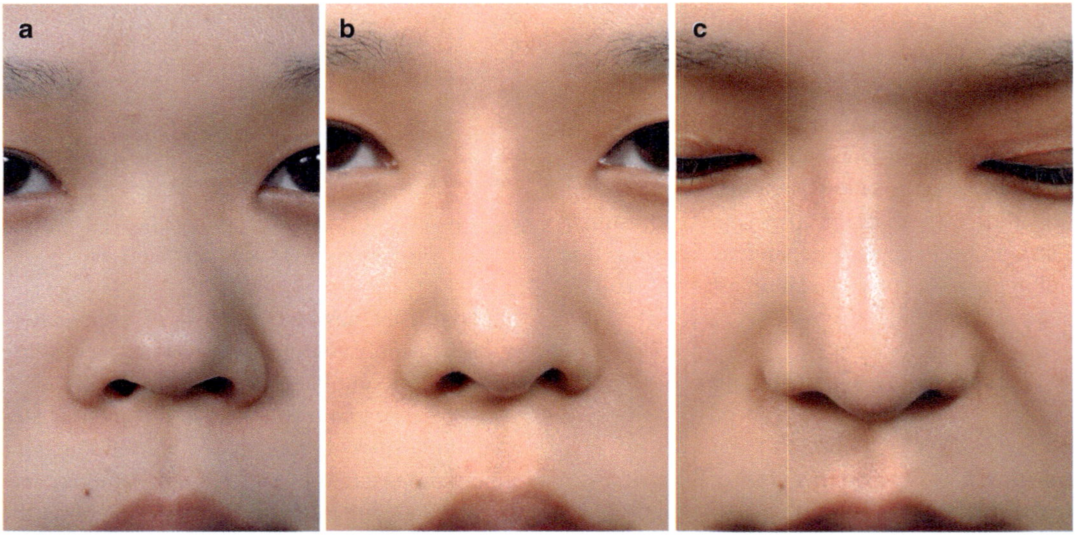

Fig. 1.7 Silicone deviation. (**a**) Very low nasion with axis discrepancy between the bony axis and the axis of the cartilaginous dorsum. (**b**) Frontal view. (**c**) Distinct deviation by the dorsal highlights

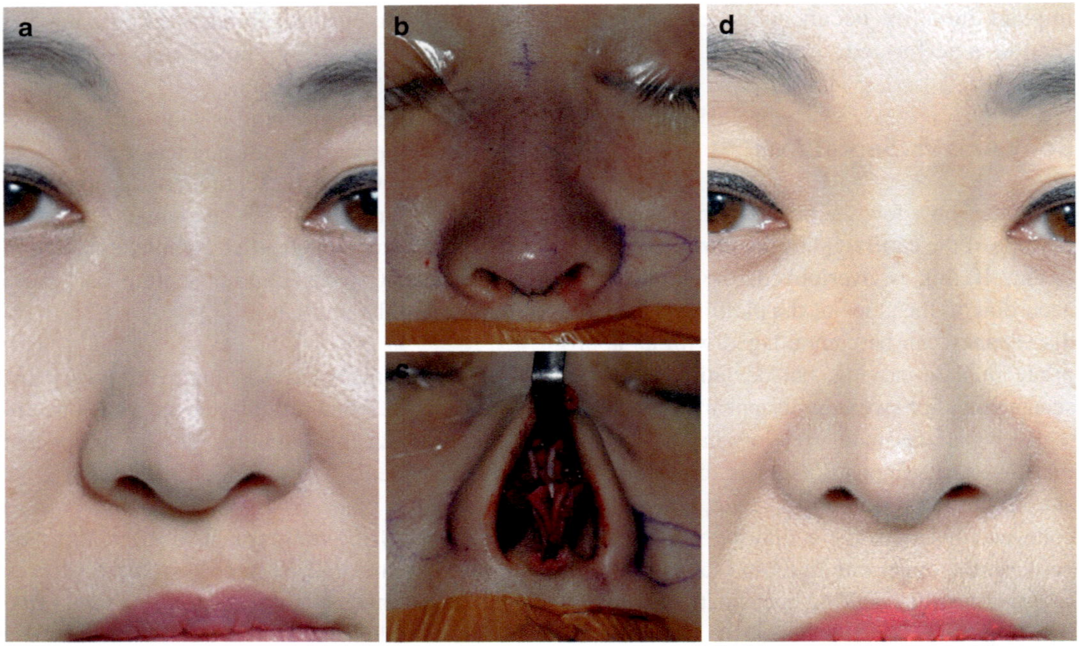

Fig. 1.8 Correction of deviation by autograft only. (**a**) Preoperative view. (**b**) After the spreader graft: correction of the high septum. (**c**) Dorsal highlight was focused on the Lt. side spreader graft. (**d**) Postoperative view

dorsum is projected, so care should be taken when applying a dorsal implant.

Implant-Dependent Dorsum

In Asian rhinoplasties, the techniques have been evolved on the premise that alloplastic materials augment the dorsum. The main methods have focused on tip projection and extension.

The severe deviation cannot achieve a straight dorsal line without proper septal adjustment. Furthermore, implant-dependent dorsum does not apply to secondary rhinoplasty with soft tissue problems.

- As the septum goes, the implant goes.

Secondary Operation Using Silicone Implant (Re-insertion)

In secondary operation, it is unavoidable to remove the silicone and re-insert the silicone implant. If the nasion is too low, or if the patient refuses to apply autograft, the last option is to use an alloplastic implant again.

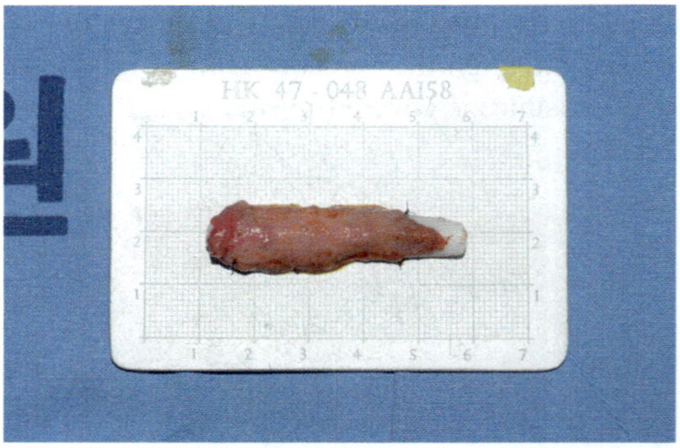

Fig. 1.9 The anterior surface of the silicone implant was covered with flattened superficial mastoid fascia

Soft tissue can be applied to the anterior surface of the silicone implant as a barrier. Placing a superficial mastoid fascia [3] on the anterior side implant fades the demarcation and supports the thin anterior skin (Fig. 1.9).

The indications of applying anterior soft tissue are:

1. After removing all capsules, if the anterior skin envelope remains very thin.
2. Surgery to correct implant demarcation.
3. In secondary operation, when the silicone must be re-inserted after removing the silicone.

1.4 Clinical Features of Complications

Silicone Implants

Capsule: Contracture

Silicone inevitably forms a capsule. If five silicone surgeries are performed, five different capsules are formed. If the capsules are not removed, those are not resorbed naturally (Fig. 1.10). The scar band of myofibroblast or fibroblast formed around the capsule is consistent with the inflammatory reaction. Some capsules are healthy and very thin; these can be used as soft tissues in secondary surgery. Nonhealthy capsules that are made up of very thick scars cause contractures that should be removed. In Chap. 2, the author will discuss the late-onset inflammation of nonhealthy capsules.

Calcification

Calcification is a characteristic feature on the surface of old silicone. It can be easily diagnosed on an X-ray, and in older cases, it may cause skin lesions.

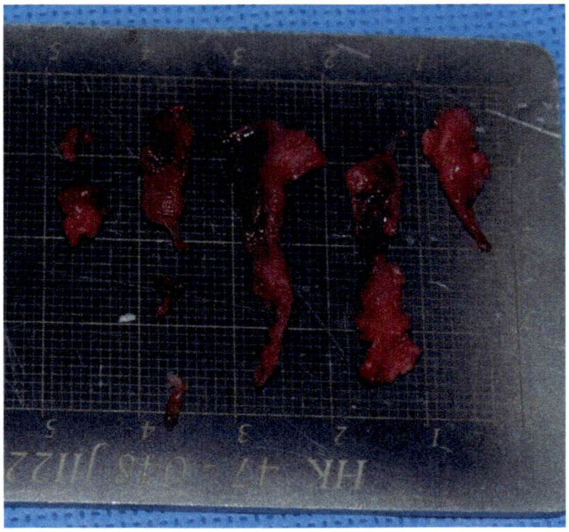

Fig. 1.10 Multilayers of silicone capsules were removed from a secondary surgery

It is essential to remove both the anterior and posterior capsules. When removing the anterior capsule, be careful of skin necrosis (Fig. 1.11).

Demarcation, Transparency

In patients with too low nasion, demarcation around the implant can be found. Also, in thin-skinned patients, the silicone is seen through the sunlight, making it appear transparent. The above method of applying the soft tissue to the anterior surface effectively controls demarcation and transparency (Fig. 1.12).

Gore-tex

Since Gore-tex has micropore, it has a high infection rate along with Medpor among alloplastic implants. In a proportion of 3% or more, implant removal is required due to infection. Surgeons might think that there is no contracture because it doesn't make a capsule, but the bigger problem is the use of silicone and Gore-tex alternately due to multiple surgeries.

- Contracture occurs even in Gore-tex inserted into a capsule made of silicone, and the late-onset inflammation that happens in this situation shows a very complex clinical feature.

Shrinkage and Demarcation

Shrinkage and demarcation of the implant is a phenomenon peculiar to Gore-tex that occurs when the micropore is reduced. It is characterized by a very hard leather-like degeneration when removed. Since it does not make a capsule, it is sometimes more difficult to remove. It should be noted that there is no such opportunity as the capsule can be used as some soft tissue in the case of a patient who has undergone multiple surgeries using a silicone implant. When removing Gore-tex, it also should be noted that the dorsal skin on the affected area is very thin. Such thin skin takes a very long time to regain its elasticity and return to its original shape (Fig. 1.13).

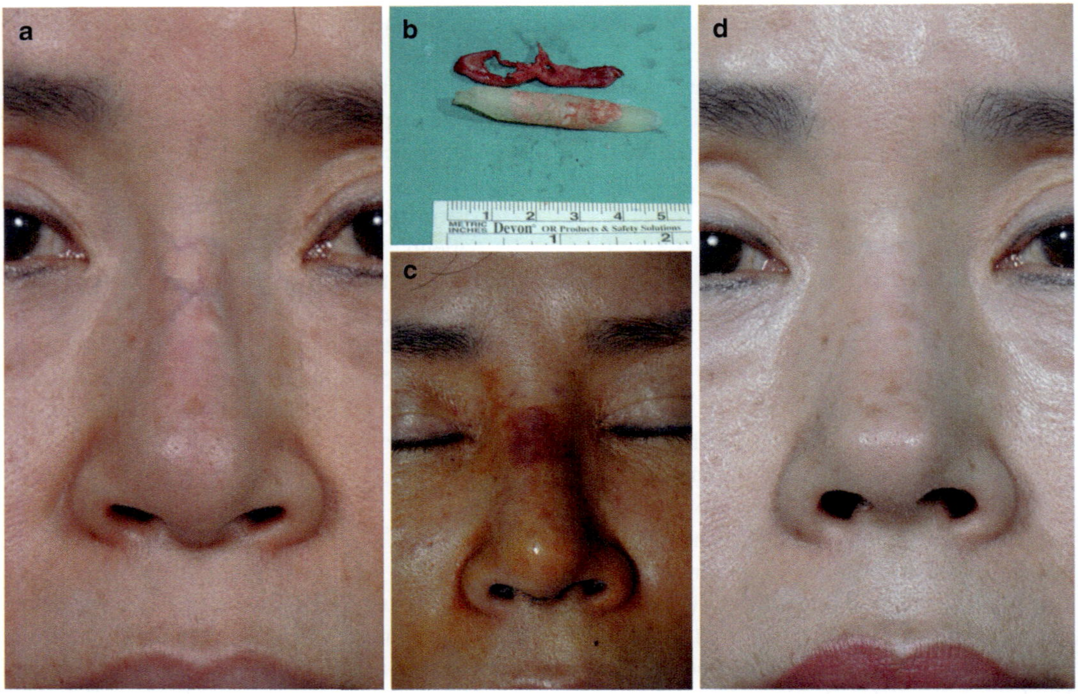

Fig. 1.11 Calcification of old silicone implant. (**a**) Preoperative view; skin thinning with venous engorgement. (**b**) Silicone and the capsule; the anterior surface of the silicone was covered with stone-like calcification. (**c**) Skin problem: the thin skin is in danger of necrosis, hyperbaric O^2 treatment is recommended. (**d**) Postoperative view

Along with demarcation, many patients complain of unknown pain due to this thin skin (Fig. 1.14).

Demarcation around the implant, accompanied by shrinkage, is also commonly found in silicone implants with healthy capsules (Fig. 1.15). In other words, demarcation around the implant may occur in both silicone and Gore-tex. Even too superficially inserted dermofat graft may be demarcated, so care should be taken to handle the thick dermis margin.

IHCC (Irradiated Homologous Cartilage)

Resorption: Fracture

The resorption was found to be the most problematic in the long-term follow-up of IHCC. The resorption rate of autologous costal cartilage is 3%, and that of IHCC is 30% [4]. There had been a problem with fracture-resorption, so the author no longer uses it [5]. Conclusively IHCC is not free from surgical site infection (SSI) and late-onset inflammation (LOI) other than resorption and fracture.

- When used for the nasal framework, many shape problems can occur due to resorption in the long term.
- It is not recommended to use as columellar struts, caudal septal extension grafts, lateral crural strut grafts, or alar rim grafts.
- It is relatively advantageous to use dorsal onlay graft, but there is also a problem of resorption.
- As it is a non-viable cartilage graft, it is not free from inflammation caused by long-term trauma [6]
- It has a complication rate of about 3%, and the frequency of resorption with or without infection is about 2% [7]

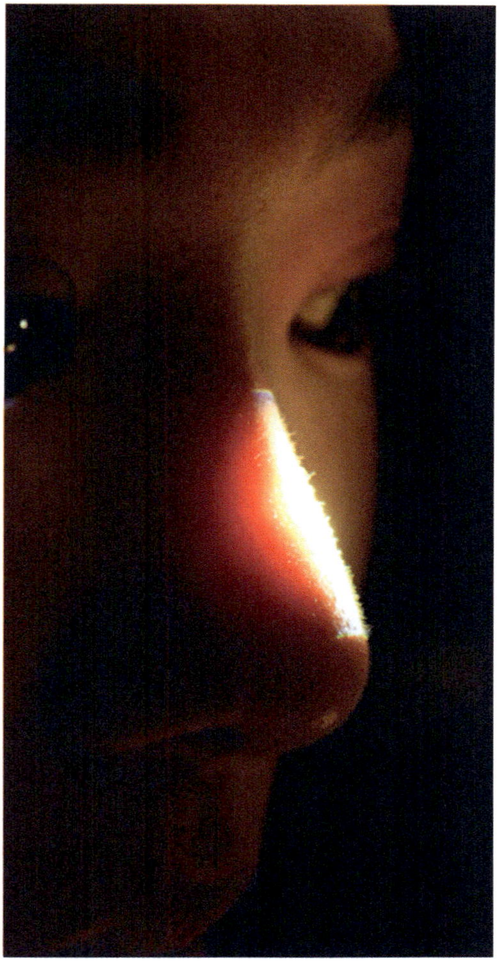

Fig. 1.12 Transparent silicone implant in thin skin

There are many situations in which IHCC has to be used because the amount of autologous cartilage that remains after multiple reoperations is insufficient. However, IHCC use in primary rhinoplasty is increasing enormously due to the convenience. Therefore, the complications of IHCC increase rapidly.

Alloderm

Alloderm is a suitable material that can be used conveniently without sacrificing the donor site, but it is not free from absorption [8]. It is reported that the relationship between multilayered application and absorption is trivial. Still, in Asian rhinoplasty, more than two layers are often used, and the hardness due to scar formation is more problematic than absorption clinically.

- Absorption of alloderm on the bony dorsum is more significant due to insufficient circulation during engraftment.
- Multiple layers of application create an intermediate avascular layer and remain as a stone-like scar.

Central Avascular Scar: Contracture Inside the Preexisting Capsule

An avascular layer or scar is formed in the center where several layers are applied, and a scar lump with a hardness that does not allow the scalpel to enter. An alloderm-contracture may occur when inserted in the capsule that has not been removed [9].

1.5 Surgical Site Infection Vs. Late-Onset Inflammation

The most significant complication of alloplastic implants is infection. According to the meta-analysis report, the infection rate of Gore-tex and Silicone was 4%, and the infection rate of Medpor was 6%, but it was not statistically significant. Relatively, the Mepor and Gore-tex were half as low [10].

Due to empirical antibiotics and the surgical environment's improvement, the infection rate will show very different patterns, so there will be errors in generalization. However, SSI (surgical site infection) and late-onset inflammation seen after wound healing should be distinguished (Chap. 2).

Above is the most crucial perspective of Asian rhinoplasty because most of the contractures come from inflammation.

Fig. 1.13 Demarcated Gore-tex. (**a**) Preoperative quarter view, (**b**) postoperative view

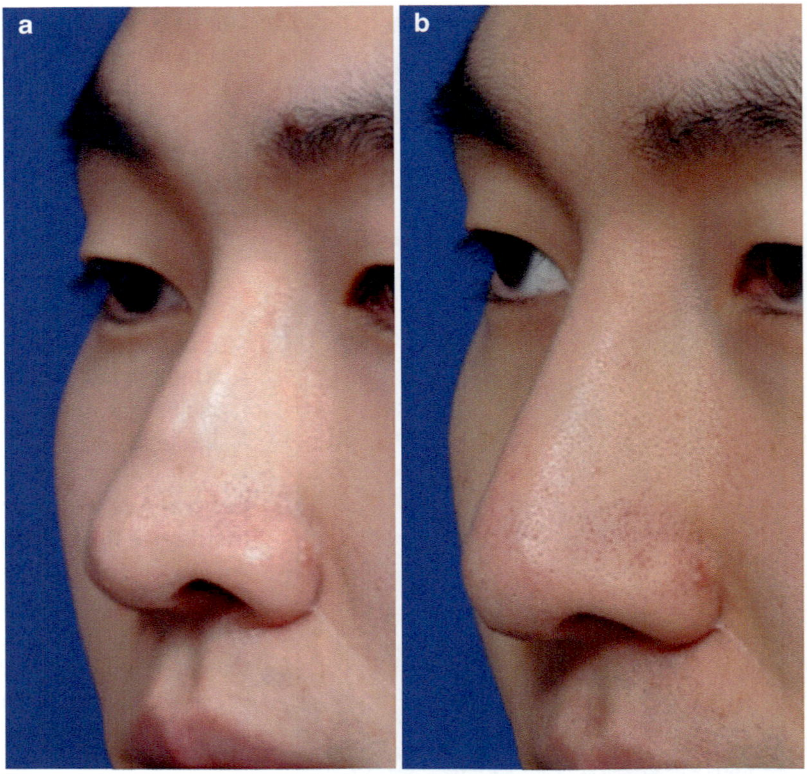

Fig. 1.14 A patient who suffered from unknown nasal pain. (**a**) Preoperative view, (**b**) Pain disappeared after removing dorsal Gore-tex and replaced with autologous dermis graft

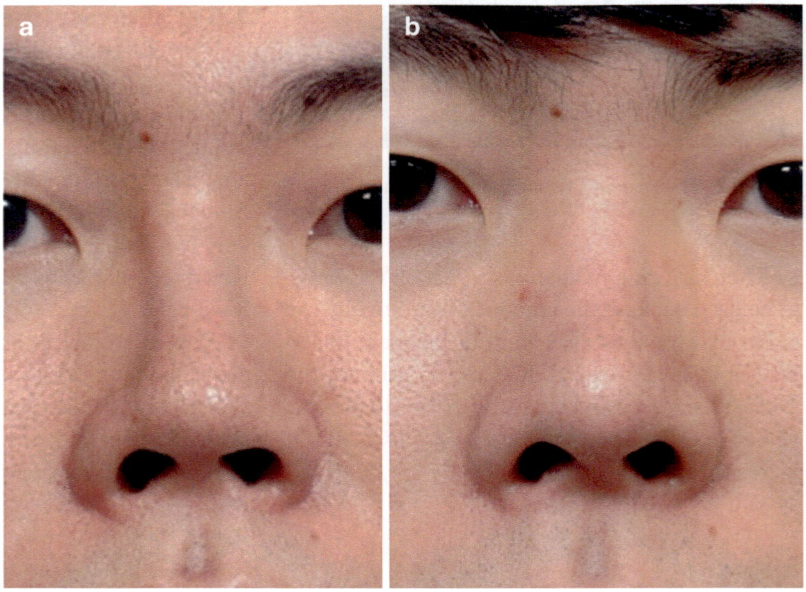

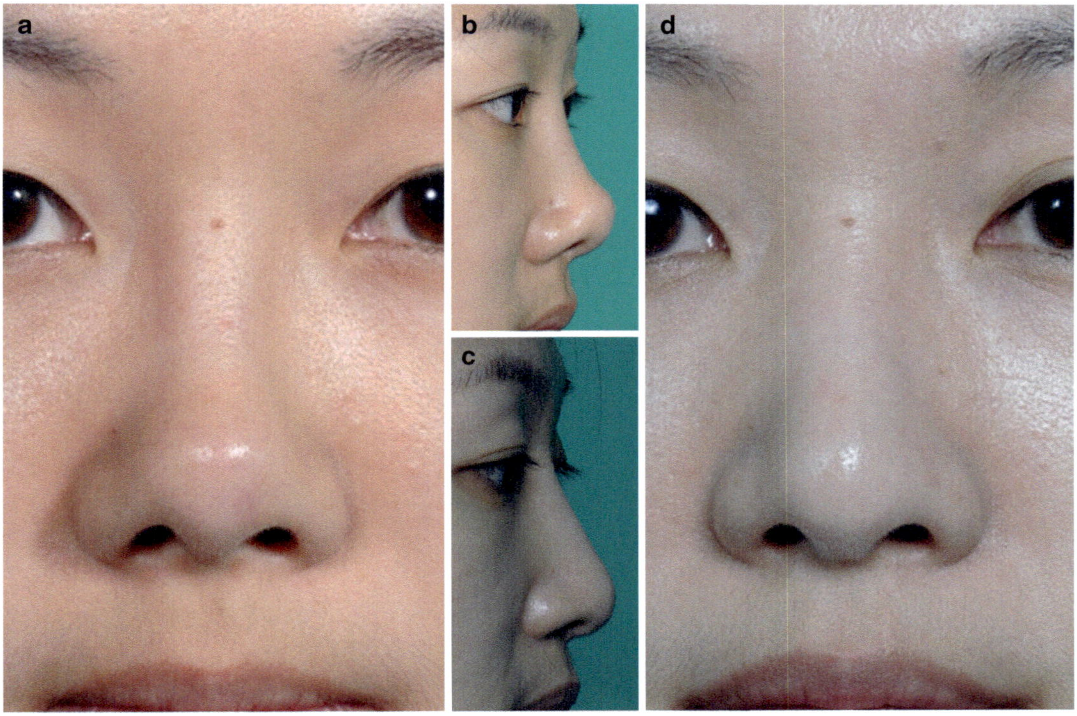

Fig. 1.15 Demarcated silicone implant with contracture (**a**, **b**) preoperative view, (**c**, **d**) postoperative view

References

1. Oliver JD, Eells AC, Saba ES, Boczar D, Restrepo DJ, Huayllani MT, et al. Alloplastic facial implants: a systematic review and meta-analysis on outcomes and uses in aesthetic and reconstructive plastic surgery. Aesthet Plast Surg. 2019;43(3):625–36.
2. Toriumi DM, Pero CD. Asian rhinoplasty. Clin Plast Surg. 2010;37(2):335–52.
3. Hong S-T, Kim D-W, Yoon E-S, Kim H-Y, Dhong E-S. Superficial mastoid fascia as an accessible donor for various augmentations in Asian rhinoplasty. J Plast Reconstr Aesthet Surg. 2012;65(8):1035–40.
4. Wee JH, Mun SJ, Na WS, Kim H, Park JH, Kim D-K, et al. Autologous vs irradiated homologous costal cartilage as graft material in rhinoplasty. JAMA Facial Plast Surg. 2017;19(3):183–8.
5. Suh M-K, Ahn E-S, Kim H-R, Dhong E-S. A 2-year follow-up of irradiated homologous costal cartilage used as a septal extension graft for the correction of contracted nose in Asians. Ann Plast Surg. 2013;71(1):45–9.
6. Toriumi DM. Choosing autologous vs irradiated homograft rib costal cartilage for grafting in rhinoplasty. JAMA Facial Plast Surg. 2017;19(3):188–9.
7. Kridel RWH, Ashoori F, Liu ES. Long-term use and follow-up of irradiated homologous costal cartilage grafts in the nose. Arch Facial Plast Surg [Internet]. 2009. https://jamanetwork.com/journals/jama/fullarticle/407629.
8. Gryskiewicz JM. Waste not, want not: the use of AlloDerm in secondary rhinoplasty. Plast Reconstr Surg [Internet]. 2005. https://journals.lww.com/plasreconsurg/Fulltext/2005/12000/Alloderm_Lip_Augmentation.24.aspx?casa_token=4n4K7vf5ObQAAAAA:PaVJJEk65rVrb351MEjlbHdUyg8slWclJhHq_hv9jxM94EK2oq4w11e167Ow_7F4CnZhxFa_149dXC2oxEpE5SOo.
9. Dhong E. 11 management of alloplast-related complications. Aesthetic Plastic Surgery of the East Asian Face [Internet]. 2016. https://pdfs.semanticscholar.org/fc9e/a8e751045e2e299c8649a38b57c80ded9b72.pdf#page=153.
10. Peled ZM, Warren AG, Johnston P, Yaremchuk MJ. The use of alloplastic materials in rhinoplasty surgery: a meta-analysis. Plast Reconstr Surg. 2008;121(3):85e–92e.

Surgical Site Infection (SSI) Vs. Late-Onset Inflammation (LOI)

2

Pearls

- A septorhinoplasty is a clean-contaminated surgery. In a sense, a septorhinoplasty using an alloplastic implant is contaminated surgery.
- Therefore, pre-, peri-, and postoperative antibiotics should be used.
- Asian septorhinoplasty is a complicated surgery combining submucosal resection (SMR), many cartilage grafts, and sometimes an alloplastic implant.
- Septal surgery is the most crucial factor in deciding the duration of antibiotic use.
- SSI that occurs in the acute postoperative phase and LOI that occurs after the long term should be treated separately.

SSI

- The treatment principle of SSI is rapid I&D and removal of implants and grafts.
- The SSI of open rhinoplasty begins with septum and the columella.
- Surgery can be salvaged with appropriate antibiotics, but all grafts and implants should be removed immediately when pus drains or the degree of cellulitis becomes severe.
- It is contraindicated to do the immediate secondary surgery during SSI.

LOI

- The first clinical manifestations are skin lesions such as cyst formations on the nasal dorsum, tip, and nasal cavity.
- Along with the above condition, a puncture is formed over time, or pus is drained.
- The criterion for deciding whether to perform only I&D or do the revision surgery is the degree of cellulitis of the skin envelope. The severity of cellulitis determines the timing of surgery.
- In the case of pus-draining patients, it is recommended to delay surgery after eradicating the pus with irrigation and antibiotics. However, if the severity of cellulitis is low, pus-drainage is not a contraindication of immediate reconstruction.
- The cyst is found in the operation field as a mucus-containing "mucocele" in a capsule.
- In the case of Gore-tex use, mucus-filled cyst patterns were also found.
- Damaged capsules and ingrowth of endothelium-like mucosa or de novo proliferation of granulation tissues and inflammatory cells play a crucial role in late-onset inflammation related to alloplastic implants.

2.1 The Differences by Definition

Surgical Site Infection (SSI)

Surgical site infection is an infection that occurs after any rhinoplasty. It is superficial infections involving a surgical pocket. It occurs during the wound-healing process and occurs within

E.-S. Dhong, M.-W. Na, *Asian Septorhinoplasty*, https://doi.org/10.1007/978-981-16-0542-0_2

2 weeks from 5 days postoperatively. In the acute phase, redness, swelling, and pain are accompanied, and eventually, pus drains. When septal surgery is performed simultaneously, the clinical picture may be completely different compared to the case without septal surgery.

SSI After a Septal Surgery

SSI from the septal surgical pocket can have serious consequences. The reason for this is the clinical risk of bacterial dissemination, rather than the vast extent of surgery.

The existing literature argues that antibiotics do not eradicate staphylococcus, which is the most problematic during septoplasty, disrupt intranasal physiology by changing the normal flora, concludes that septal surgery does not require any antibiotics [1, 2]. However, the author cannot fully agree with this. Asian septorhinoplasty (SRP) covered in this book is not a simple surgery mentioned in the papers, but a completely different surgical category. Although simple septoplasty shows a low infection rate, Asian SRP should be considered as a clean-contaminated surgery due to the surgery's nature [3]. Patients should receive prophylactic antibiotics appropriate for their specific procedures. In principle, antibiotics rather than the first generation of cephalosporin should be used prophylactically or perioperatively [4]. It is essential to keep in mind that the patient is in a temporary bacteremia state during surgery [5].

- Since the septum and external nose have two different surgical pockets, care must be taken to ensure that the two pus pockets communicate with each other or not.
- Septal mucosal flaps coapt sooner than the dorsal flap heals. However, the septal pocket lies in a dependent position, the pus often accumulates in the septum (Fig. 2.1).
- The pus pocket confined to the septum should be irrigated with external drainage.
- For septal abscess, systemic symptoms should be monitored. There have been reports of cases of severe sepsis, even death.

Septal mucosal flaps coapt sooner before the dorsal flap heals. When pus drains, if antibiotics had been treated just for one time, most cultures are found to be no bacteria, but susceptible antibiotics appropriate for the cultured strains should be prescribed.

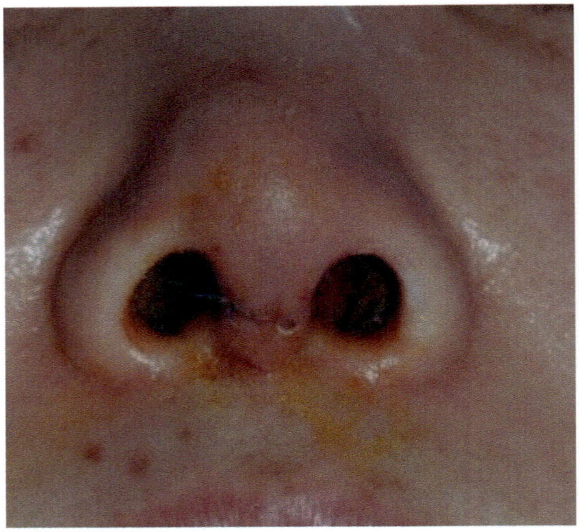

Fig. 2.1 SSI started from the septal abscess. The abscess pocket was connected from the septum to the dorsal pocket

- Monitoring the SSI begins with a flap color change of columella.
- Surgery can be salvaged with appropriate antibiotics, but all grafts and implants should be removed immediately when pus drains or the degree of cellulitis becomes severe.

SSI Without Septal Surgery

Since the surgical pocket is limited to the external nose, SSI is controlled by appropriate irrigation and systemic antibiotics. The essential principle is removing alloplastic implants and grafts quickly.

- As in the case of septal surgery above, immediate secondary surgery is avoided.
- The degree of dorsal cellulitis is the indicator of safe wound healing.

Late-Onset Inflammation (LOI)

Late-onset inflammation (LOI) is a rare complication that may occur several months to years

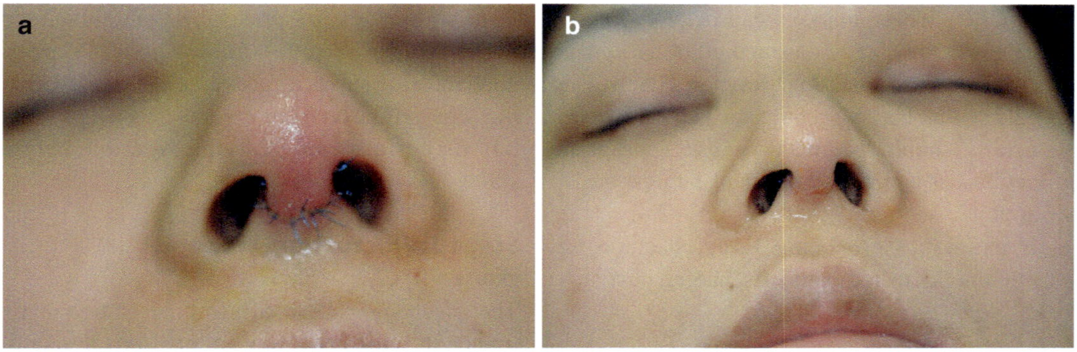

Fig. 2.2 Transient inflammation of the columella. (**a**) The redness was found 3 days postoperatively and changed the antibiotics from empirical cephalosporin to quinolone. (**b**) After 5 days, the redness improved without irrigation

after an uneventful rhinoplasty. It is an inflammatory stage utterly different from SSI, with or without pus-drainage seen in the acute stage of surgery. The inflammatory stage may progress to the last stage of infection that ends in pus-drainage. However, LOI is often accompanied by redness and mild repetitive swelling. Swelling subsides whenever empirical antibiotics are prescribed. LOI often occurs after pregnancy and when the patient's general condition is bad.

2.2 The Differences Between Clinical Features and Managements

Surgical Site Infection (SSI)

In case of simultaneous septal SMR, proper packing is critical. Nasal packing with appropriate antibiotics prevents hematoma, and at the same time it affects inhibiting colony [6]. The septal hematoma often results in a septal abscess. The causative agent of SSI, which occurs in the postoperative wound-healing process and occurs within 2 weeks from a few days after surgery, will be discussed in detail in Chap. 3.

In the early stages, redness usually begins from the columella. After removal of packing, endonasal inspection should be performed well. If the local fluctuation is found in the septum, actively do the puncture and drain. Besides, appropriate antibiotics should be started that match the culture. Whether columellar redness is temporary, cellulitis gets better, and the rhinoplasty will be salvaged in some cases (Fig. 2.2).

Adequate choice of antibiotics is the key, and the infected pocket usually improves within 1–2 days, so the wound should be observed daily. If an empirical antibiotic, first- to second-generation cephalosporin, was prescribed, it is necessary to switch to quinolones. If there is susceptibility, symptoms can improve after transient inflammation (Fig. 2.2b). However, when swelling gets worse or cellulitis progresses further, the breakage of the suture margin is observed. The pus starts to drain at an irreversible state, all graft materials and implants should be removed. Repeated irrigation is the only surgical maneuver.

Management of SSI

- Once the pus is drained, it is the principle to remove all implants and cartilages grafted from the nose.
- There are cases where an increase in CRP is found in the blood inflammation index (ESR

or CRP). These markers can help, especially CRP, but they are not a standard of treatment.
- As a general condition, fever, tiredness, and cold symptoms are accompanied by early onset.
- Efforts should be made to use appropriate antibiotics and willing to change unresponsive antibiotics.
- If antibiotics are being taken, bacteria are often not detected in the discharged pus.

Late-Onset Inflammation (LOI)

There has been debate on the status of "subclinical infection": A state in which swelling and improvement have fluctuated. A status of weak infection drains discharges but not the pus. However, this term should be redefined. Repeated swelling may be attributed to the biofilm formed around the implant. However, it can be observed that the clinical picture is more complicated than the inflammation caused by biofilm. It has been reported that coagulase-negative staphylococci found in the breast's capsular contracture are the leading cause of the biofilm [7]. The biofilm around the implant may be the cause of contracture, there are similarities, but the pathologic findings are slightly different. The LOI is characterized by intermittent nasal dorsal swelling and sometimes granuloma-like skin lesions. In severe cases, puncture with fluid drainage on the external or intranasal area may be present. There are many cases where pus is drained to the puncture site.

A "mucocele-like cyst"is a characteristic pathology that is not found in breast implants.

The stages of late-onset inflammation (LOI) can be divided into the following four stages:

1. The fluctuation of swelling, which is the mildest stage. The soft tissue starts to contract.
2. The granulation with skin lesions forms a thick scar around the pocket.
3. The stage of skin puncture, which is the opening of a "mucocele-like cyst."
4. Full infection with cellulitis.

If antibiotics are prescribed and sustained at the stage of one, the clinical pattern repeats deterioration and improvement, but finally, the stage of severity increases, so it is essential to perform surgical intervention before stage 3.

Stage 1: Fluctuation: Wax and Wane

The recurring pattern of swelling is frequently found in patients using alloplastic implants. Usually, empirical antibiotics are prescribed, and taking NSAIDs subsides swelling, and in some cases, this process lasts for years (Fig. 2.3). However, the swelling becomes more extensive in the end, and the capsule becomes irreversibly thick. Moreover, "the nose becomes shorter" (Fig. 2.4).

Regardless of the silicone or Gore-tex, the fluctuation is found, and no clear evidence of worsening and improving symptoms from the biofilm has not been found. Trauma history, drinking, pregnancy, and childbirth can be heard, but most of them are idiopathic. The appearance of gradually changing and thickening is the formation of scar tissue around the capsule, and when palpated, the fluid inside can be touched.

- It is recommended to perform a secondary operation before skin puncture, and the standard timing for this operation is when swelling is not severe and subsided.
- At this time, a CT scan can be helpful in planning the operation and in identifying the volume to be reconstructed.
- The soft tissue starts to contract.

It is advantageous to check the septal state to obtain full information about the type and method of alloplastic material used in the previous operation for the secondary operation.

It is essential to inspect the maximal swelling, and the height of the dorsum to be reconstructed can be predicted.

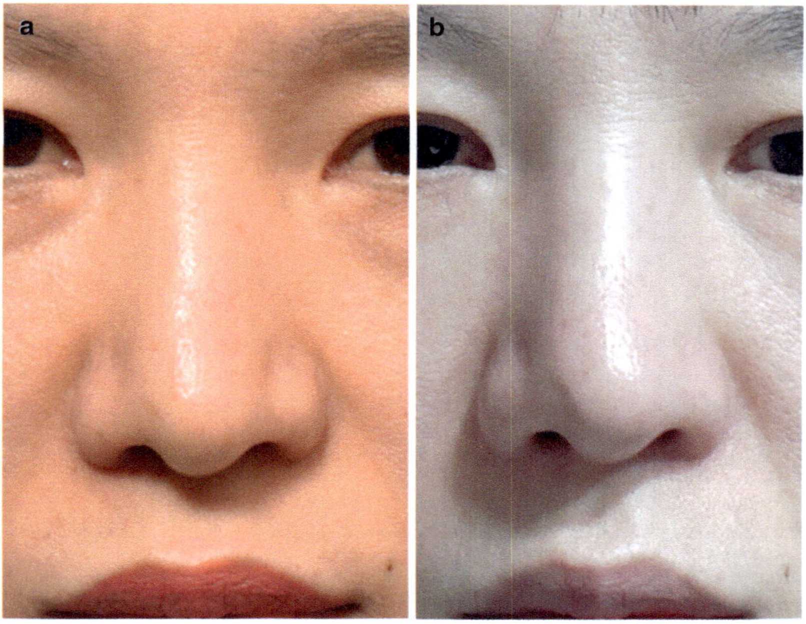

Fig. 2.3 The first stage of LOI: fluctuation. (**a**) Normal state after taking empirical oral antibiotics. (**b**) Swollen state

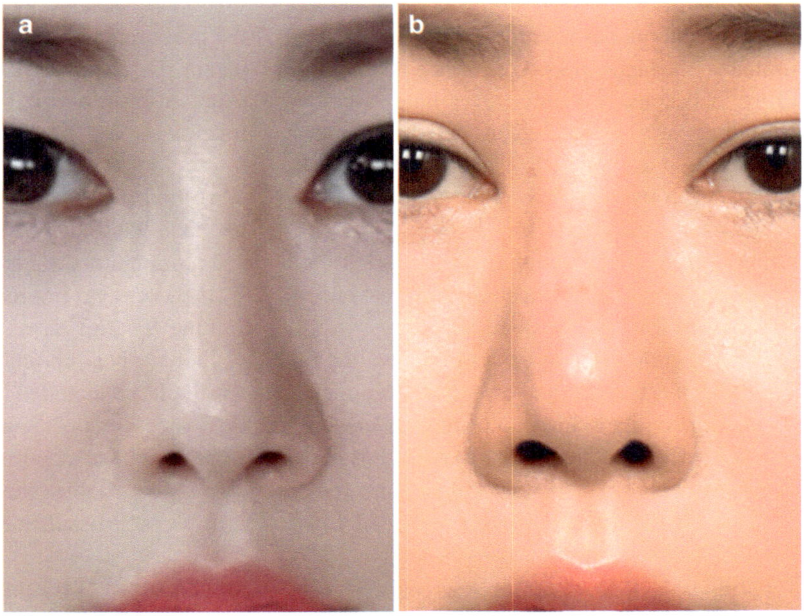

Fig. 2.4 The first stage of LOI: swelling does not subside. (**a**) The normal state, 1 year after the silicone implantation at another hospital. (**b**) Swollen state, which does not subside treated with quinolone. She was managed with secondary rhinoplasty using autologous materials

Stage 2: Skin Lesion: Out-Growth of the Granulation Tissue

The lesions found in the skin may show epidermal cyst patterns, but most are found as dark purple cysts with central thinning (Fig. 2.5a, b). It is found in various locations, even in the membranous septum (Fig. 2.5c).

Doctors who do not understand the LOI course perform skin biopsy or excision and encounter unpredicted sequels. This lesion's pathology is usu-

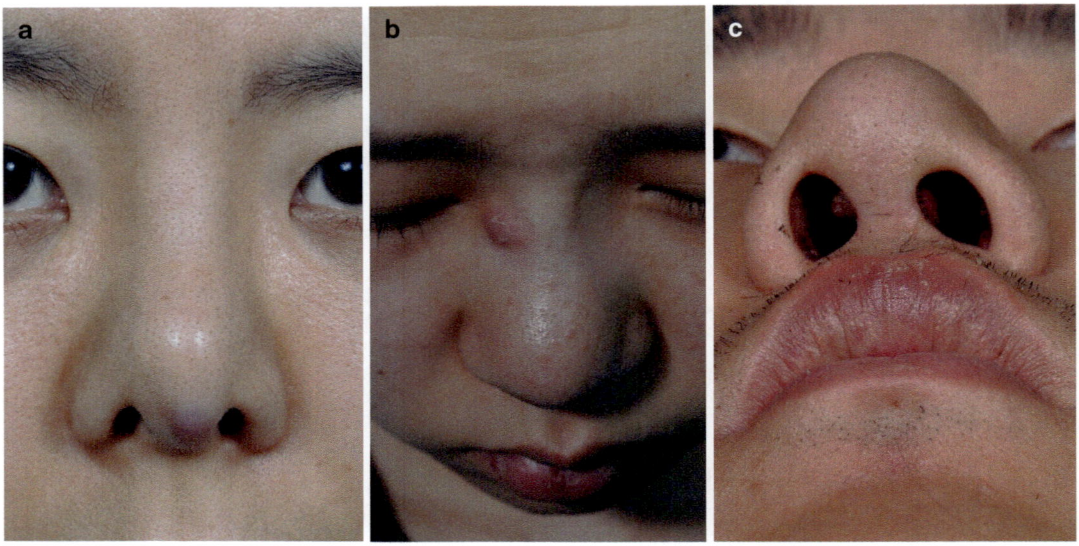

Fig. 2.5 The second stage of LOI: granuloma-like cysts. (**a**) Purple-colored thinning at the nasal tip. (**b**) Nasal root cyst misdiagnosed as an epidermal cyst by a dermatologist. (**c**) Granuloma-like cyst at the membranous septum

ally a granulomatous reaction with a mucous cyst, similar to the sinus mucoceles. Since this lesion is likely to become punctured over time, a definite septorhinoplasty should be considered at this stage.

- The mucous cyst should be eradicated from the whole lesion.
- Pockets made deep up to the anterior nasal spine or pockets connected to the nasion can be scraped with a small curette.
- The most challenging part is to dissect the thin dorsal skin surface. It is essential not to make a puncture on the skin as much as possible, but if it becomes punctured during surgery, it is necessary to apply appropriate soft tissue underneath. However, surprisingly it can be found that it heals well with the minimal scar left (Fig. 2.6).

Stage 3: Puncture with or Without Pus-Drainage

Discharge occurs at first and then develops into pus. The puncture heals by epithelization, but it requires a definitive excision. Only total resection is the solution (Fig. 2.7).

For pus, aggressive antibiotics should be treated, and for wounds with a puncture, the regimen should follow contaminated wounds. The first-generation cephalosporin cannot solve the problems overall. Ciprofloxacin (quinolone) meets the requirement of a single broad-spectrum antibiotic available in intravenous and oral form.

- If the primary choice of antibiotics should be made without the culture result, quinolone is recommended for stage 3 [8].
- If there is no improvement after using quinolone for 2–3 days, dual or triple antibiotics, including aminoglycoside or metronidazole, should be included.
- Besides many negative results in culture, selecting susceptible antibiotics as soon as possible enables secondary operation and prohibits soft tissue contracture.

This effort is for preparing secondary surgery and is not an end-point of treatment. If the underlying pathology containing mucocele is not resolved, improvement cannot be expected.

Level 4: Cellulitis with Pus-Drainage

Active irrigation and drainage are required. In principle, all grafts, along with alloplastic material in the nose, are removed. Check the cartilage condition, whether it is bleeding or not. It is essential to use appropriate antibiotics before

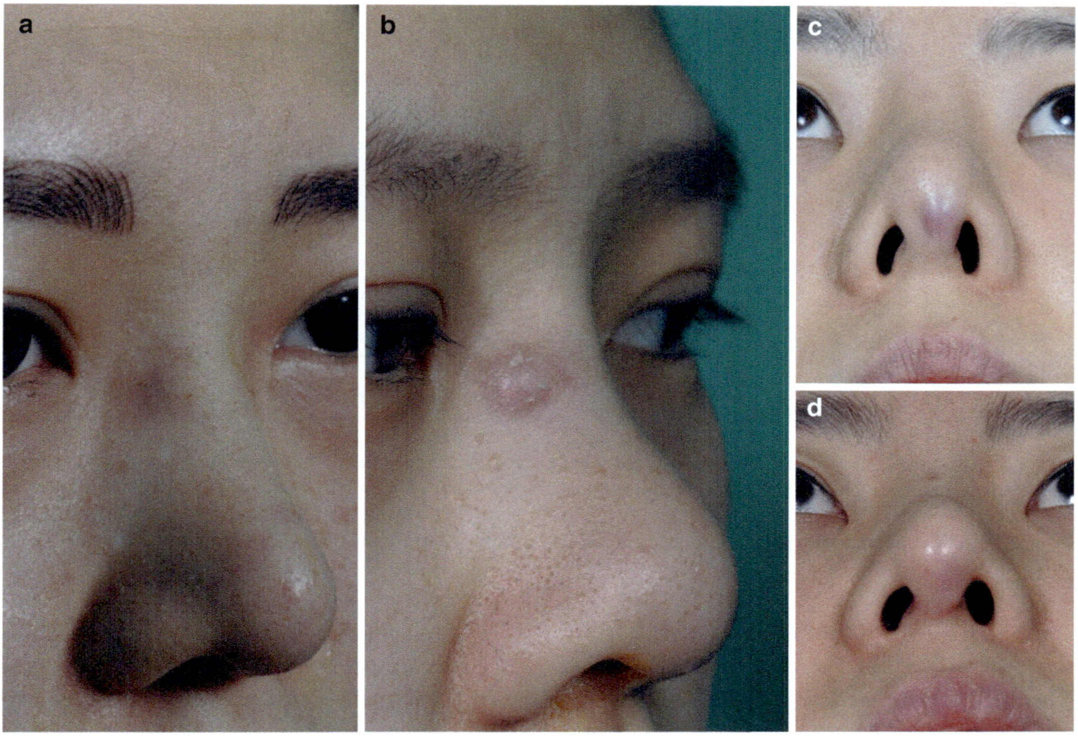

Fig. 2.6 Total excision of granuloma-like cysts that extends from root to tip inside the capsule. (**a**, **b**) Nasal root lesion, pre-, and postoperative state. (**c**, **d**) Columellar lesion, pre-, and postoperative state

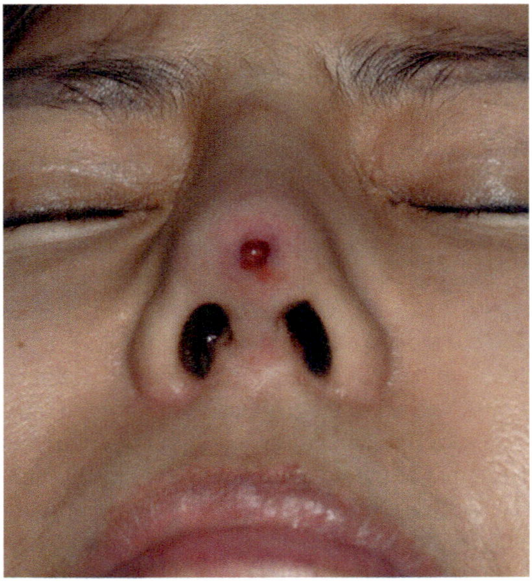

Fig. 2.7 The third stage of LOI: skin puncture, mucous cystic outbreak without pus-drainage

surgery, and it is crucial to reduce cellulitis as much as possible and undergo surgery.

- The degree of cellulitis is an index that determines whether a secondary operation is possible as in the SSI.
- Active reoperation is possible when cellulitis decreases, and the color of the skin flap returns to normal.
- However, if severe cellulitis is found, graft or septal surgery other than removing the pathogen is contraindicated (Fig. 2.8).
- It is good to plan step-by-step surgery, but note that if aggressive capsule removal is not performed, contracture occurs during the wound-healing period.
- The degree to which the nasal framework remains is a condition that determines the presence or absence of devastating deformation after surgery.

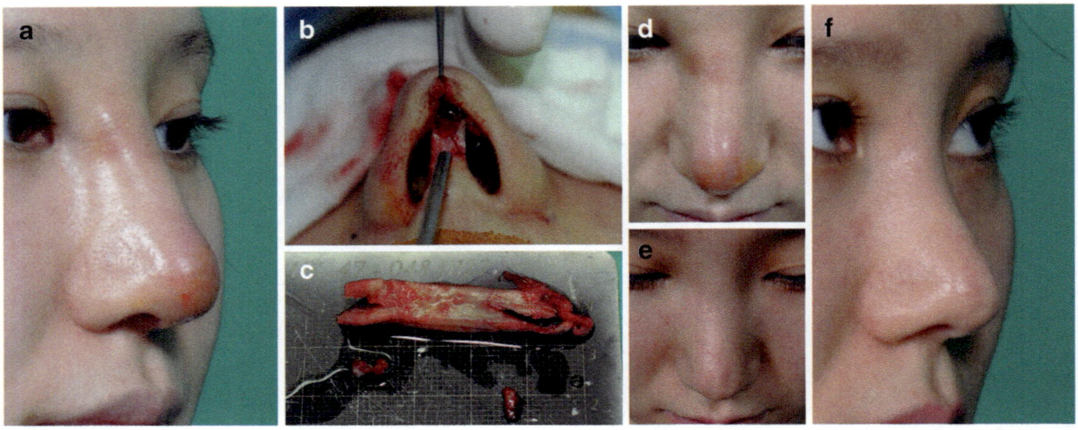

Fig. 2.8 The fourth stage of LOI: severe cellulitis with pus-drainage. (**a**, **d**) A 23-year-old female had been operated with a surgifoam. Her secondary operation was performed using dermofat graft replacing the surgifoam by the same doctor 1 year before visiting the author. Preoperative view. (**b**, **c**) Pus was drained after the incision. Old capsule with mucocele was excised above the scarred dermis. (**e**, **f**) Postoperative view

Pathophysiology of LOI

There have been no analytic reports of LOI in alloplastic implant patients. Most reports regarded the total infection rate. The complications that can occur due to silicone implants are reported to be 4–24% [9], but there is no detailed study on infection timing for all complications. One study reported a long-term infection of 1.3% in the primary operation in patients with Gore-tex and 4.3–5.4% in secondary operations [10].

Biofilm

Biofilm formation has been believed to be the most significant cause of subclinical infection. However, biofilm cannot be confirmed in the actual surgical field. A biofilm is defined as an assemblage of surface-associated microbial cells enclosed in a protective extracellular, primarily the polysaccharide matrix [11]. Abiotic surfaces surrounded by bacterially produced extracellular matrix established 3-D aggregates of polarized cells able to produce mucoglycoproteins and stimulate mucus production [12].

A large amount of mucus is formed in the biofilm, but it looks like a mucocele in the operation field.

- It is found as a cyst containing mucus in a silicone capsule.
- In the case of Gore-tex, mucus-filled cyst patterns were also found.
- In the case of patients who have undergone multiple operations, the clinical features are more complicated, so it is essential to listen to the detailed medical history and to estimate the cyst size and location of the mucocele by CT scan.
- By adjusting the CT contrast, the mucocele size and the soft tissue volume to be reconstructed can be estimated (Fig. 2.9).
- However, in multiple surgeries, more research is needed because there are many cases of putting Gore-tex back into the existing silicone capsule.

Mucocele-Like Pathology

Most of the mucus found in late-onset inflammation is formed in the capsule, so it shows an intricate pattern related to the biotic surface different from that of the mucus derived from the biofilm. Mucocele is mucus extravasation forming pseudocyst with epithelioid macrophages and a bunch of mucin actually without any epithelioid tissue. However, the mucocele-like cysts seen in LOI are different from typical ranula, and more similar to the pus containing mucocele of the nasal sinus.

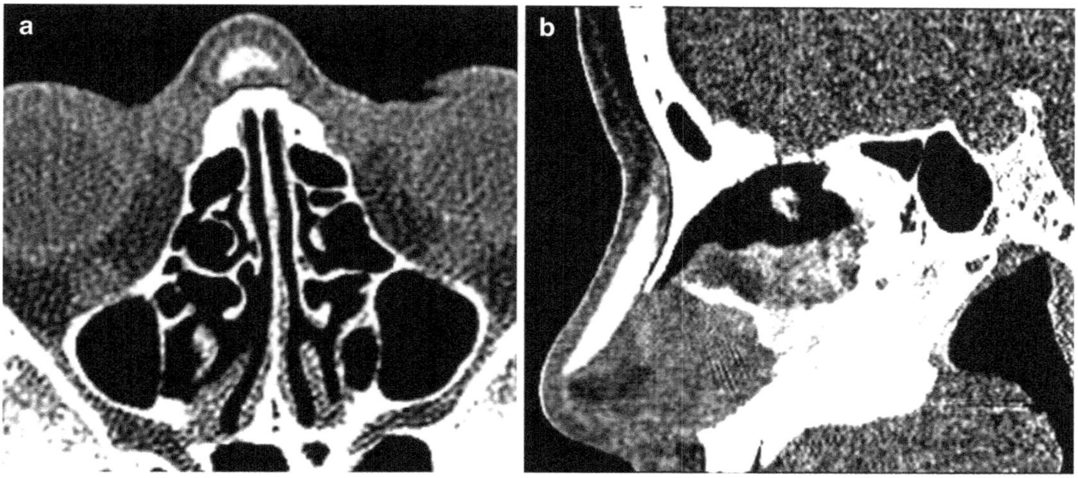

Fig. 2.9 Mucocele around the silicone implant, by adjusting the contrast, well-developed pericapsular space is identified. (**a**) Axial view. (**b**) Sagittal view

Histological Manifestations in Silicone Capsule

Healthy Capsule (HC)

The healthy capsule is in a stable state that does not show any aspect of LOI. Healthy silicone capsules with no inflammation signs are thin and can be separated as one layer during surgery. This capsule can be dissected well and used as a soft tissue graft. If necessary, the anterior capsule does not need to be removed when the anterior skin flap becomes too thin.

Thick capsules are not recommended to be used in situ because there is a risk of contracture. However, it is relatively safe to cut it out and use it on the tip or tissue depression.

Since the lateral capsulotomy alone can make a stable pocket, HC does not become a hurdle for secondary rhinoplasty.

Nonhealthy Capsule (NHC)

Nonhealthy capsules appear with LOI, and the capsules around the implants were thick and firmly adhered to the surrounding soft tissues of the nasal skin and cartilages. The thickness of the capsule depends on the patient's symptoms. Patients with contracture inflammation are found that the scar tissue around the capsule is thick (Fig. 2.10).

If this capsule and surrounding scar tissue are not removed, the nose will not be elongated comfortably. The capsule content has a fluctuation, and patients are divided into cases with or without surrounding cellulitis.

The Differences in the Histological Study [13]

Hematoxylin and Eosin Staining and Masson's Trichrome Staining

The HC group was organized into three tiers. The innermost layer adjacent to the implant is lined with a row of cells. Beyond this layer, synovial metaplasia was found. The outermost layer was a dense, regular layer of collagen (Masson's trichrome staining) with no signs of foreign body reaction or recruitment of inflammatory cells. All collagen layers were aligned relatively parallel to the implant compared to the NHC group (Fig. 2.11). In the NHC group, a synovial layer is found in the intermediate layer between the innermost silicone contacting layer, which is the contact surface with the implant, and the outermost granulation layer in a complex collagen arrangement. The outer layer looks similar to the granulation tissue. The content of inflammatory cells demon-

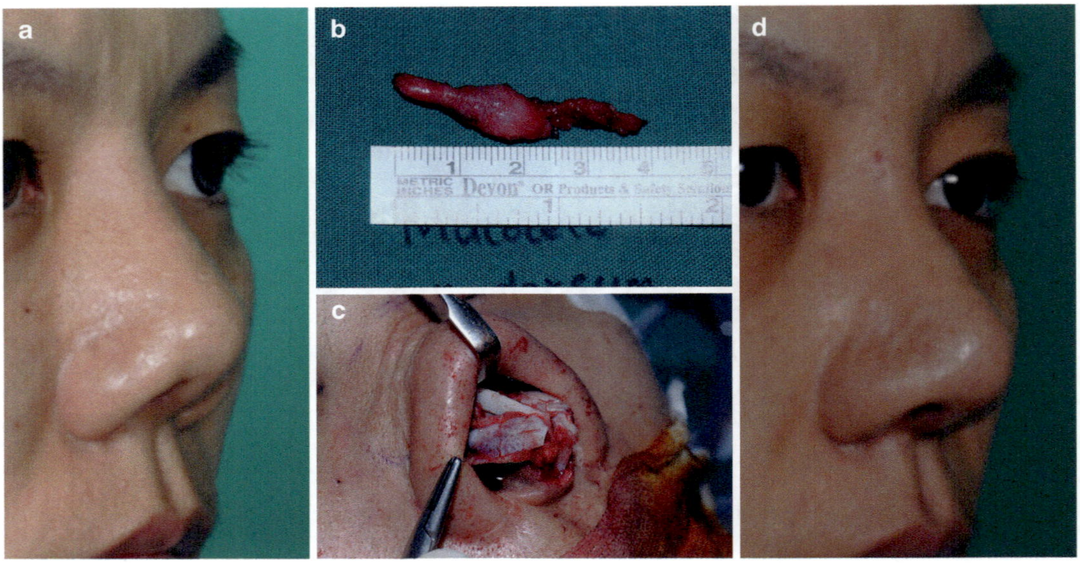

Fig. 2.10 Unhealthy capsule with contracture. (**a**) A 28-year-old female referred due to the severe contracture with dorsal fluctuation. (**b**) A thick pericapsular scar and a mucocele were removed. (**c**) Postoperative view. (**d**) Silicone was removed, and septal L-strut was extended using costal cartilage with anatomical crural batten graft

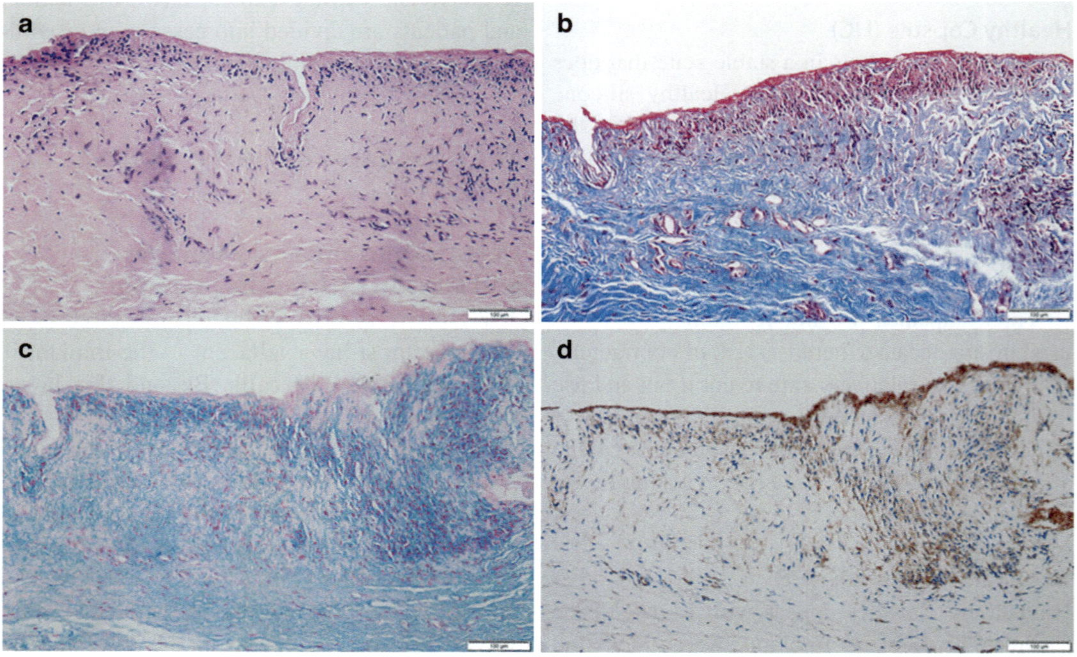

Fig. 2.11 Histology of a healthy capsule. (**a**) Hematoxylin and eosin staining, (**b**) Masson's trichrome staining, (**c**) Colloidal iron histochemical staining, (**d**) CD31 immunohistochemical staining of a healthy capsule at 200× magnification (Material from: Moon et al. Late-Onset Inflammation in Asian Rhinoplasty Using Alloplastic Implants, Aesthetic Plastic Surgery, 2020, Springer)

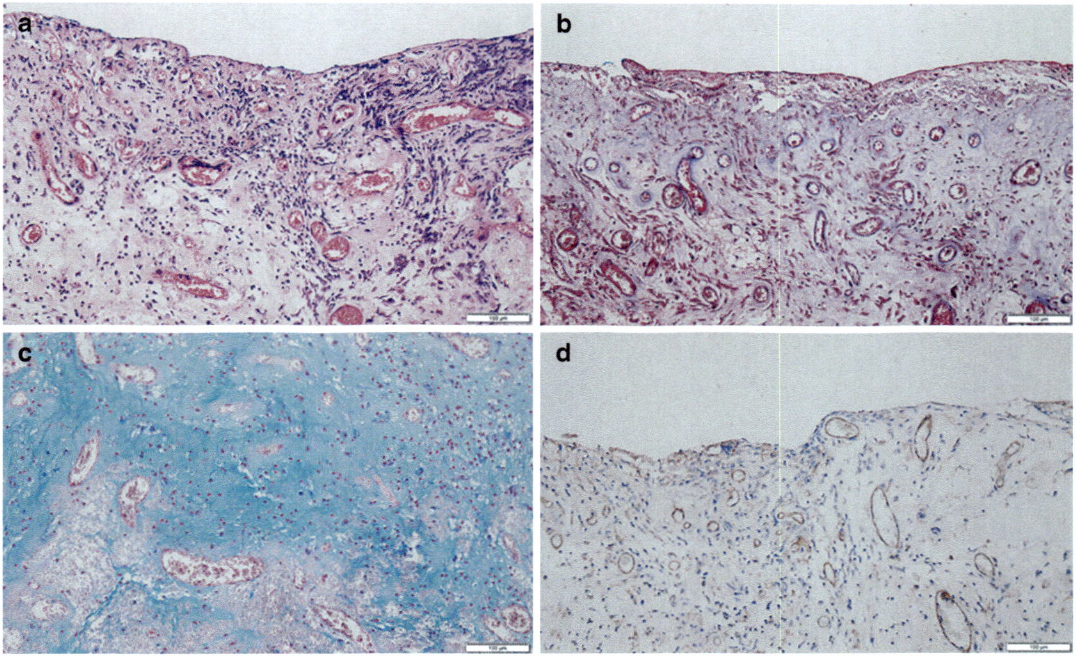

Fig. 2.12 Histology of a nonhealthy capsule. (**a**) Hematoxylin and eosin staining: irregular arrangement of collagen fibers. (**b**) Masson's trichrome staining: severe collagen degeneration. (**c**) Colloidal iron histochemical staining: intense blue staining shows mucin deposition. (**d**) CD31 immunohistochemical staining at 200× magnification. (Material from: Moon et al. Late-Onset Inflammation in Asian Rhinoplasty Using Alloplastic Implants, Aesthetic Plastic Surgery, 2020, Springer)

strated by the presence of macrophages and neutrophils also increased. However, no evidence of anaplastic large cell lymphoma or T cell proliferation was observed in the patients (Fig. 2.12).

Colloidal Iron Histochemical Staining

This staining determines the presence or absence of mucin. Mucin was found only in NHC; it was collected inside the capsule and lining. Although there was no evidence that the origin of mucin was from EPS of biofilm, the inner layer secreted it [14]. The endothelial component has grown in the capsule. Its vast amount and the multiple layers were found at the inner lining. The discovery of the endothelial layer found in the capsule's inner lining requires more research on whether it is endothelial metaplasia or mucosal metaplasia exposed during surgery (Fig. 2.12).

Immunohistochemical CD31 Staining

In the NHC group, the innermost layer, which was the surface in contact with the implant, consisted of the dense stratified lining of CD31-staining cells dispersed throughout the capsule. Breakage of endothelial or epithelial lining is also found, but it looks different depending on the site (Figs. 2.12 and 2.13).

The function of the inner layer and the synovial metaplasia around the implant can be seen as a good effect as a coating for sliding and lubrication between tissues and tissues to maintain synovial fluid around the implant. The late-onset inflammation response itself contributes to the development of tissue destruction through the continuous recruitment of pro-inflammatory cells such as macrophages and lymphocytes and the release of inflammatory mediators and proteases [15]. More research is needed to determine why complex inflammatory reaction

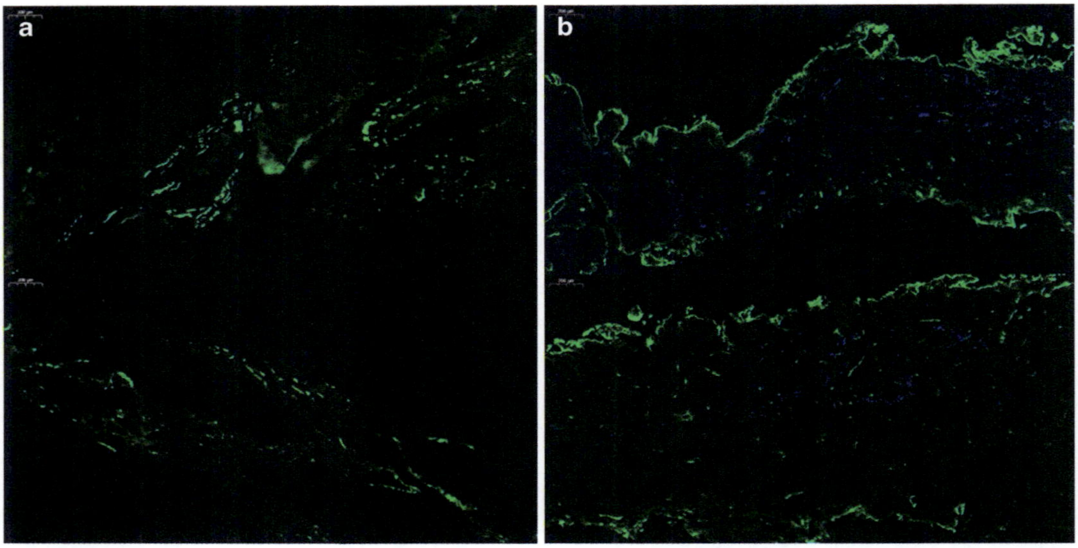

Fig. 2.13 Immunohistochemical staining of CD31 using a fluorescent dye at 200× magnification. (**a**) Healthy capsule: (**b**) Nonhealthy capsule: nonhealthy capsule shows continuous staining at the lumen with green color, which is endothelial hyperplasia of the inner layer

occurs in NHC, and mucus was accumulated inside while a thin single-layer capsule in HC does not. The author's conclusions to date are as follows.

- Damaged capsules and ingrowth of synovium-like mucosa or de novo proliferation of granulation tissues and inflammatory cells may play a crucial role in late-onset inflammation related to endothelial hyperplasia (or metaplasia).

Case Study 1: Granuloma-like Skin Lesion with Contracted Nose

A 28-year-old female underwent augmentation rhinoplasty using a silicone implant 8 years ago. During secondary septorhinoplasty, a silicone implant was found and removed. The lower lateral cartilages were mostly destroyed. The intracapsular space was filled with purulent fluids, and the capsule was totally excised. In the histological study, colloidal iron staining was markedly positive and Masson's trichrome staining showed collagen degeneration. She was managed with secondary septorhinoplasty using autogenous cartilage grafts after total release of contracted band (Fig. 2.14).

- A dense scar band forms the capsule in NHC. It attaches the upper lateral cartilage to the scroll area connecting the lower lateral cartilage.
- Resecting this contracture band is the surgical goal of the foreshortened nose correction.
- In some cases, until only the mucosal lining of the nasal cavity remains, LLC cannot be freely transferred to the caudal direction without tension. As more septal extension grafts are performed, the extent of release widens.

Case Study 2: LOI with the Loss of Mucosal Lining

A 22-year-old female patient was referred for intermittent swelling and a granuloma-like lesion on her right nasal mucosa that began 2 months ago. She underwent rhinoplasty using a silicone implant 2 years ago at another clinic. During secondary rhinoplasty, the capsule was filled with purulent fluid, and the capsule was totally

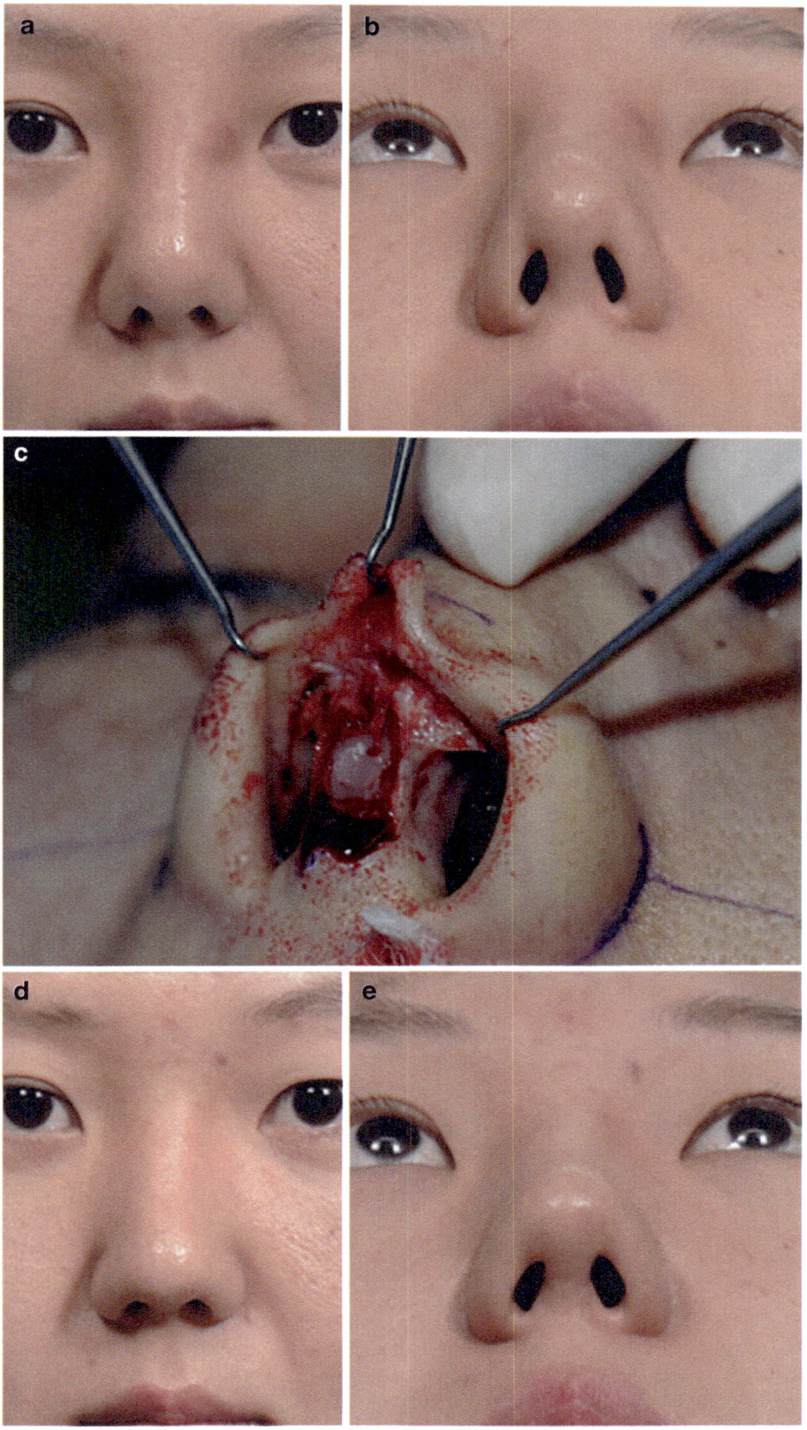

Fig. 2.14 Granuloma-like skin lesion with a contracted nose: A 28-year-old female underwent augmentation rhinoplasty using a silicone implant 8 years ago. (**a**, **b**) Preoperative views. (**c**) Intraoperative views. (**d**, Management of alloplast-related complications. Aesthetic Plastic Surgery of the East Asian Face) Six months after revisional septorhinoplasty. (Material from: Moon et al. Late-Onset Inflammation in Asian Rhinoplasty Using Alloplastic Implants, Aesthetic Plastic Surgery, 2020, Springer)

excised. For correction, two conchal cartilage were used. A sacral dermofat graft was grafted for nasal dorsal augmentation. The defect of the right membranous septum was sutured from inside and a small defect still remained after the repair. The wound was managed with wet dressing and prolonged antibiotics and healed after 5 days postoperatively.

- If the mucosal lining is damaged, the nasal cavity can be seen from the surgical pocket. It may not be possible to suture appropriately.
- Mucocele grows and ruptures into the nasal cavity, and the mucosal lining tends to be defective upon removal of a cyst.
- Care must be taken not to expose directly the graft cartilage and try to approximate the defect if the gap is located at the membranous septum.

Alloplastic materials should not be reused. Autograft should be adopted, and it is essential to use appropriate antibiotics for more days after the operation (Fig. 2.15).

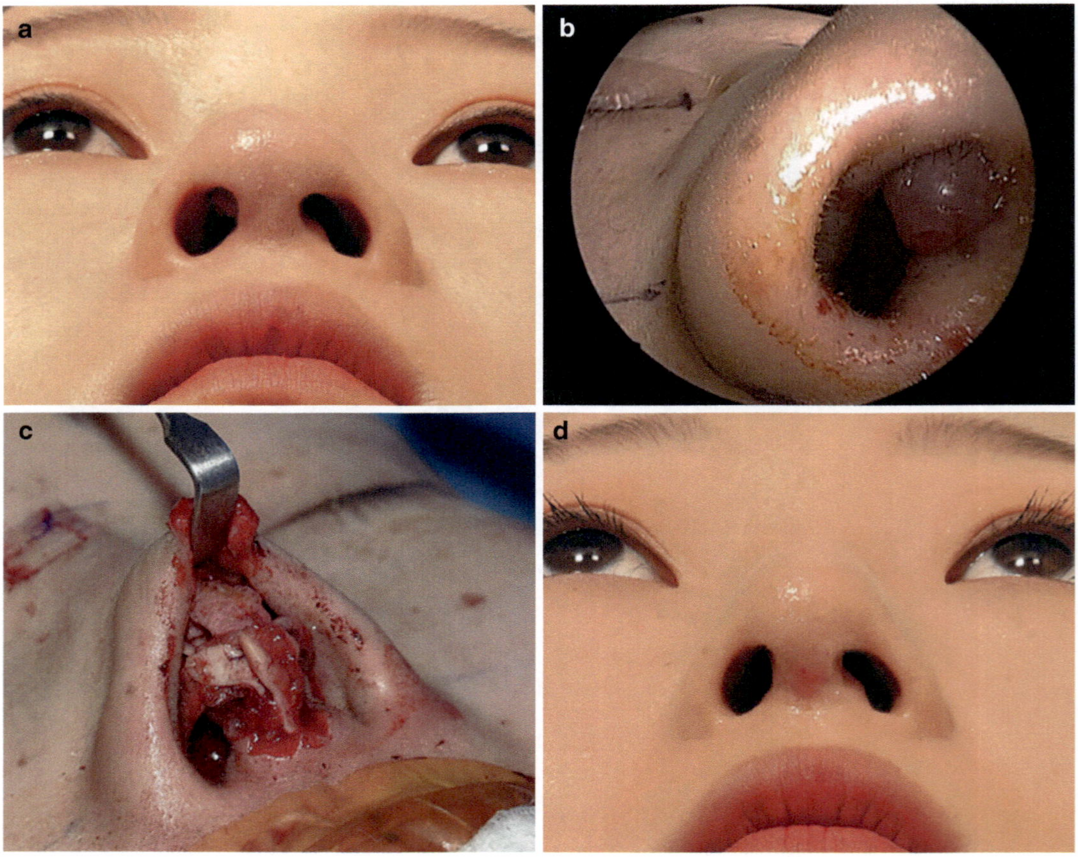

Fig. 2.15 LOI with the loss of mucosal lining: A 22-year-old female patient was referred for intermittent swelling and a granuloma-like lesion on her right nasal mucosa that began 2 months ago. Microbiological culture of the purulent fluid was identified as Staphylococcus aureus. She was successfully managed with purulent fluid drainage, silicone implant removal, capsulectomy, secondary septorhinoplasty using autogenous cartilage grafts, and intravenous antibiotics. (**a**) Preoperative views. (**b**, **c**) Intraoperative views. (**d**) Six months after revisional septorhinoplasty

References

1. Ottoline ACX, Tomita S, da Penha Costa Marques M, Felix F, Ferraiolo PN, Laurindo RSS. Antibiotic prophylaxis in otolaryngologic surgery. Int Arch Otorhinolaryngol. 2013;17(1):85–91.
2. Karaman E, Alimoglu Y, Aygun G, Kilic E, Yagiz C. Effect of septoplasty and preoperative antibiotic prophylaxis on nasal flora. B-ENT. 2012;8(1):13–9.
3. Mäkitie A. Postoperative infection following nasal septoplasty [Internet]. Acta Otolaryngolog. 2000;120:165–6. https://doi.org/10.1080/000164800454297.
4. Salkind AR, Rao KC. Antibiotic prophylaxis to prevent surgical site infections. Am Fam Phys. 2011;83(5):585–90.
5. Okur E, Yildirim I, Aral M, Ciragil P, Kiliç MA, Gul M. Bacteremia during open septorhinoplasty. Am J Rhinol. 2006;20(1):36–9.
6. Bandhauer F, Buhl D, Grossenbacher R. Antibiotic prophylaxis in rhinosurgery. Am J Rhinol. 2002;16(3):135–9.
7. Pajkos A, Deva AK, Vickery K, Cope C, Chang L, Cossart YE. Detection of subclinical infection in significant breast implant capsules. Plast Reconstr Surg. 2003;111(5):1605–11.
8. Patzakis MJ, Bains RS, Lee J, Shepherd L, Singer G, Ressler R, et al. Prospective, randomized, double-blind study comparing single-agent antibiotic therapy, ciprofloxacin, to combination antibiotic therapy in open fracture wounds. J Orthop Trauma. 2000;14(8):529–33.
9. Tham C, Lai Y-L, Weng C-J, Chen Y-R. Silicone augmentation rhinoplasty in an oriental population. Ann Plast Surg. 2005;54(1):1–5; discussion 6–7.
10. Jang YJ, Moon BJ. State of the art in augmentation rhinoplasty: implant or graft? Curr Opin Otolaryngol Head Neck Surg. 2012;20(4):280–6.
11. Donlan RM. Biofilms: microbial life on surfaces. Emerg Infect Dis. 2002;8(9):881–90.
12. Moreau-Marquis S, Stanton BA, O'Toole GA. Pseudomonas aeruginosa biofilm formation in the cystic fibrosis airway. Pulm Pharmacol Ther. 2008;21(4):595–9.
13. Moon K-C, Lee K-I, Lee J-S, Kim A-R, Dhong E-S, Kim D-W, et al. Late-onset inflammation in Asian rhinoplasty using alloplastic implants. Aesthetic Plast Surg [Internet]. 2020. https://doi.org/10.1007/s00266-020-01648-8.
14. Kasprzak A, Adamek A. Mucins: the old, the new and the promising factors in hepatobiliary carcinogenesis. Int J Mol Sci [Internet]. 2019;20(6). https://doi.org/10.3390/ijms20061288.
15. Galdiero M, Larocca F, Iovene MR, Martora F, Pieretti G, D'Oriano V, et al. Microbial evaluation in capsular contracture of breast implants. Plast Reconstr Surg. 2018;141(1):23–30.

3 Nasal Swab Culture: The Preparation for the Safe Surgery

Pearls

- Asian rhinoplasty can be categorized into two surgeries: septorhinoplasty and rhinoplasty that does not dissect the septum.
- Septorhinoplasty combining autografts is a clean-contaminated surgery that creates a complicated wound.
- Septorhinoplasty combining alloplastic implants is reasonably regarded as contaminated surgery.
- Reduction rhinoplasty is relatively safe from infection.
- A nasal swab is the simplest method and provides evidence of guidance for antibiotic therapy.
- SSI after the complicated septorhinoplasty results in a disastrous foreshortened nose.
- A nasal swab study showed that the prevalence rate of potentially infectious nasal flora (PINF) approximately 85%; MSSA and MSSE are most often identified.
- Using empirical antibiotics without a nasal swab study revealed the probability of resistance to these antibiotics up to 17%; In 3–17% of all patients, more than the first- and second-generation antibiotics are required for the undiagnosed PINF.
- According to the nasal swab results, applying mupirocin or quinolone ointment reduce PINF negative in 53% of positive patients.
- The nasal flora changes even after the surgery, so monitoring the bacterial change is necessary postoperatively, and if any inflammation is detected, efforts to change the primary antibiotics should be made.
- If the nasal swab is not available, quinolones will be appropriate for the complicated septorhinoplasty for the prevalent PINF.

Case Study 1

A 22-year-old female underwent primary septorhinoplasty with a dorsal silicone implant. SMR was performed for septal extension graft; since the nasion was low, a 3.5 mm-thick silicone implant was inserted into the dorsum. There were no other events during surgery, but the pocket bled more during septal surgery than others, but aPTT and BT were normal. Empirical first-generation cephalosporin was used from the day of surgery. The nasal packing was removed on the second day after surgery, and columellar stitches were removed on the fifth day. The septal hematoma was found at this time, and it was immediately drained, and the nose was repacked. However, she complained of generalized malaise and fever on the seventh postoperative day, and she was prescribed antipyretics. The packing was removed but swollen again. On the 11th postoperative day, pus was drained from the septum. Immediate revision underwent on that day, and all cartilages with the implant were removed. As a result of culture, pseudomonas aeruginosa was identified afterward. Antibiotics were changed to third-generation cephalosporin and aminoglycoside. After switching to susceptible antibiotics,

E.-S. Dhong, M.-W. Na, *Asian Septorhinoplasty*, https://doi.org/10.1007/978-981-16-0542-0_3

pus decreased, and cellulitis was also improved. However, cellulitis was improved entirely after switching to IV tobramycin and ceftazidime. For 3 months, pseudomonas was persistently cultured in the nasal swab (Fig. 3.1).

She later reconstructed using costal cartilage and is still awaiting more tip plasty (Fig. 3.2).

Case Study 2

A 46-year-old female visited the author with Lefort I and III fracture, and she underwent surgery. After 1 year, the L-shaped cantilever graft using costal cartilage was performed. An empirical second-generation cephalosporin was prescribed. On the fifth postoperative day, severe swelling and redness were noted. On the eighth day, cellulitis with the fluctuation deteriorated, so the pus was drained, and all rib cartilage was removed. As a result of culture, MRSA and MRSE were identified. After replacing the antibiotic with vancomycin, the amount of pus was reduced, and the cellulitis improved (Figs. 3.3 and 3.4). Subsequently, MRSA was intermittently identified in a nasal swab study until 1 year after the outpatient visit.

Fig. 3.1 Culture results of the pus drained; pseudomonas aeruginosa was positive by nasal swab study 3 months after the wound healed. (*R* resistant, *I* intermediate, *S* susceptible)

F/22 Primary: SRP: Septal extension + silicone
- Pseudomonas aeruginosa : for 3 months

Ticarc/K Clavulanate	S < = 16	**Gentamicin**	**I 8**
Amikacin	S 8	Imipenem	S < = 4
Aztreonam	S < = 8	Levofloxacin	R > 4
Ceftazidime	**S 4**	Meropenem	S < = 4
Ciprofloxacin	R > 2	**Tobramycin**	**S 2**
Ceftriaxone	I 32	Piperacillin/Tazobac	S < = 8
Cefotaxime	I 16		
Cefepime	S 4		

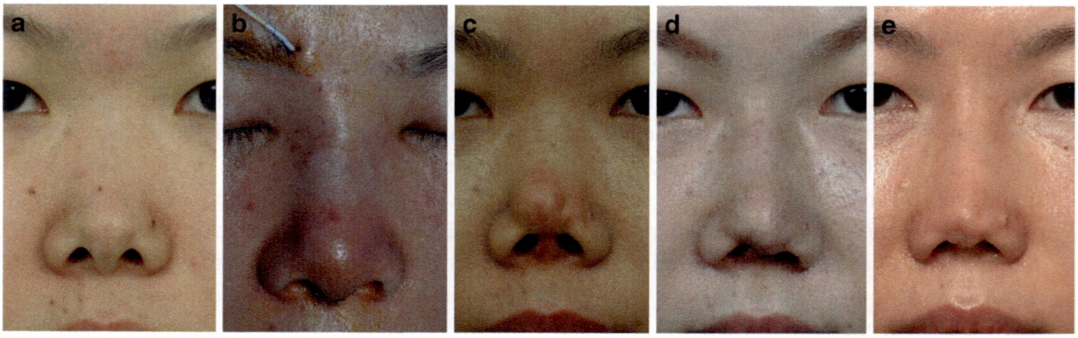

Fig. 3.2 Sequential AP photos. (**a**) Preoperative view. (**b**) After the pus was drained, all implants and grafts were removed, then a catheter was inserted for intermittent irrigation. (**c**) After the wound healed, severe foreshortening progressed. (**d**) After the nose was reconstructed using costal cartilages. (**e**) After the tip revision: The patient is awaiting a revision soon

F/46 Revision: Costal Cartilage SRP.
- POD 8th day - For 1 year MRSA

Fusidic Acid	R > 16	Imipenem	R > 8
Teicoplanin	S < = 4	Meropenem	R > 8
Ticarc/K Clavulanate	R > 8	Ofloxacin	R > 4
Ampicillin	R > 8	**Oxacillin**	**R > 2**
Amox/K Clav(c)	R > 4/2	Penicillin	R > 8
Chloramphenicol	I 16	**Rifampin**	**S < = 1**
Clindamycin	R > 2	Trimethoprim/Sulfa	S < = 2/38
Cephalothin	R > 16	Synercid	S < = 1
Ciprofloxacin	R > 2	Tetracycline	R > 8
Cefotaxime	R > 32	**Vancomycin**	**S < = 2**
Cefuroxime	R > 16		
Cefazolin	R > 16		
Erythromycin	R > 4		
Cefepime	R > 16		
Gentamicin	R > 8		

Fig. 3.3 Culture results of the pus drained on the eighth postoperative day; MRSA was cultured by scheduled nasal swab study for one more year. (*R* resistant, *I* intermediate, *S* susceptible)

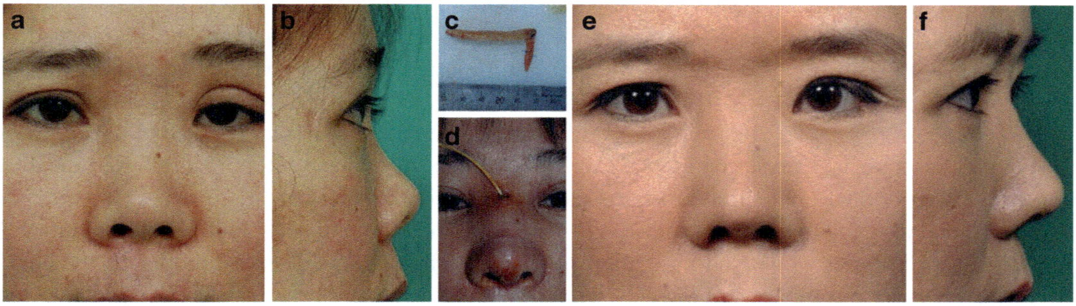

Fig. 3.4 Sequential photos. (**a**, **b**) Preoperative views: low nasion with foreshortening and Lt. eyelid ptosis. (**c**) Cantilever graft using costal cartilage before insertion. Ptosis correction was performed simultaneously. (**d**) After the pus was drained all grafts were removed, then a catheter was inserted for intermittent irrigation. (**e**, **f**) Three years later, she wanted a secondary rhinoplasty using silicone implants

3.1 What Did I Learn from these Patients?

The most painful moment in the author's Asian rhinoplasty-learning curve was the case of surgical site infection (SSI) involving septal pocket. These experiences are not well shared, but most doctors will have similar ones. Moreover, if a complex operation for several hours leads to bad results, the pain will be significant, and the patient's pain will be more profound.

- There are cases in which the surgical site infection cannot be prevented even with proper irrigation and antiseptic procedures.
- Empirical antibiotics are not enough.
- The complex wounds should be treated with susceptible antibiotics.
- A nasal swab study may be necessary for the procedure and preparation of the surgery.
- When pus-drainage occurs, it falls into an irreversible course, and there is no effect of continuous irrigation for cartilage salvage.

3.2 The Impact of SSI in Asian Septorhinoplasty

Framework Destruction

The technique of septal extension grafts in Asian rhinoplasty is increasing. Since submucosal resection (SMR) weakens the remaining septal strut, and even more frightening consequence is the septal framework's collapse after SSI (Fig. 3.1).

Once the framework collapses, continuous contraction or contracture occurs while waiting for a secondary operation, resulting in a foreshortened nose. The soft tissue results in irreversible contraction, which makes the secondary surgery difficult. Even when SSI is alleviated, inflammation of the soft tissues remains afterward.

Most secondary Asian rhinoplasty is an operation to lengthen the nose. Reconstruction of the framework is more difficult where the Medpor used.

- For patients who have undergone septal extension graft after SMR, the nasal dorsum is recommended to use autograft as possible.
- Conversely, patients who plan to use alloplastic materials for nasal dorsum are advised not to perform SMR concurrently.

3.3 The Potentially Infectious Normal Flora (PINF)

Among the potential bacterial pathogens (PBP), Staphylococcus aureus is the most problematic, and it has been reported that 33% and 41% were identified in the nasal vestibule and cavity, respectively. In other words, because Staphylococcus aureus was identified in the cavity where two-third of the total population was the vestibule, biofilms must also be taken into account in the nose. The inherent resistance to antimicrobial agents may be at the root of persistent and chronic bacterial infections [1].

However, many papers are claiming the uselessness of redundant antibiotic treatment in further studies. Assuming that the SSI rate after rhinoplasty is less than 1%, it is argued that antibiotic use is not supported [2, 3]. There is even a paper saying that topical antibiotics do not need to be used in rhinoplasty accompanied by septal surgery and do not need to be used pre- and postoperatively [4].

In a recent meta-analysis, similar conclusions have been drawn, and the use of antibiotics in nose surgery is discussed. Subsequently, the authors agree that there would have been no difference in SSI occurrence, whether used or not. Of course, when revision rhinoplasty and graft are required, there are cases where it is reported that the use of prophylactic antibiotics is meaningful [5]. However, as the author understands, the uselessness of antibiotic use has gained more sympathy until recently. There will be many refutations of the importance of the author's use of antibiotics in this chapter. The authors agree that redundant antibiotics lead to antibiotic resistance, while the patient's systemic condition deteriorates. However, reduction rhinoplasty should be distinguished from complex rhinoplasty. Reports are based on simple septoplasty-related surgeries, which quickly finish in a short time. If grafts and implants are not applied in Asian septorhinoplasty, the characteristics are entirely different. Asian septorhinoplasty is considered to be equivalent to or more complex than Western revision rhinoplasty.

PINF in Asian Septorhinoplasty

According to the author's study, Gram-positive microorganisms, such as Staphylococcus aureus (MSSA) and Staphylococcus epidermidis (MSSE), are frequently cultured. Among them, MRSA and MRSE strains cause problematic SSIs. Corynebacterium striatum is also cultured. Gram-negative microorganisms include Enterobacter aerogenes, Klebsiella pneumoniae, and Citrobacter spp. are frequently cultured [6] (Fig. 3.5). Among these, the problem would be the strain that resisted the first- and second-generation cephalosporin.

Preoperative Microbiology Profiles

	Cohort 2 (%)	Cohort 3 (%)	*p*
No. of patients	72	326	
Negative	10 (13.9)	50 (15.3)	0.756*
Positive	62 (86.1)	276 (84.7)	0.756*
Gram-positive microorganisms	42 (58.3)	194 (59.5)	0.854*
Staphylococcus aureus (MSSA)	29 (40.3)	77 (23.6)	0.004*
Staphylococcus epidermidis (MSSE)	6 (8.3)	48 (14.7)	0.152*
Staphylococcus aureus (MRSA)	2 (2.8)	13 (4.0)	1.000†
Staphylococcus epidermidis (MRSE)	3 (4.2)	42 (12.9)	0.035*
Corynebacterium striatum	2 (2.8)	14 (4.3)	0.747†
Gram-negative microorganisms	20 (27.8)	82 (25.2)	0.978*
Enterobacter aerogenes	14 (19.4)	56 (17.2)	0.648*
Klebsiella pneumoniae	3 (4.2)	8 (2.5)	0.427†
Citrobacter spp.	1 (1.4)	8 (2.5)	1.000†
Others	2 (2.8)	10 (3.1)	1.000†

MSSA, methicillin-sensitive S. *aureus;* MSSE, methicillin-sensitive S. *epidermidis;* MRSA, methicillin-resistant S. *aureus;* MRSE, methicillin-resistant S. *epidermidis.*
*Pearson χ^2 test.
†Fisher's exact test.

Fig. 3.5 Preoperative microbial profiles of nasal swab study; 72 patients in Cohort 2 and 326 patients in Cohort 3 were analyzed. (Material from: Moon et al. Preoperative Nasal Swab Culture: Is It Beneficial in Preventing Postoperative Infection in Complicated Septorhinoplasty?, Plastic and Reconstructive Surgery, 2020, Lippincott Williams & Wilkins)

Clean-Contaminated Wound

Septorhinoplasty should be considered a clean-contaminated surgery. Nose with late-onset inflammation (LOI) should be regarded as contaminated wounds if there is a puncture of the skin or drained discharge.

- For LOI with severe cellulitis, susceptible antibiotics should be used for at least 1 week before surgery. It is recommended to perform surgery after cellulitis decreases.

Complicated Septorhinoplasty for Asians

Among Asian septorhinoplasty, many surgeries correspond to septal surgery, cartilage graft, osteotomy, alloplastic material use, and secondary rhinoplasty. Most of them are considered complicated septorhinoplasty, and it is essential to take appropriate measures. The current description does not refer to a simple surgery that does not perform septal surgery with a simple rhinoplasty so that ULC and septum dissection are not performed.

Bacteremia During Operation

It is reasonable to assume that the patient is in a transient bacteremia during septal surgery. Of the septorhinoplasty, 13.5% of patients reported a bacteremia state, and the incidence was high in patients with severe postoperative bleeding. The bacteremia state worsened by nasal packing [7]. In most cases of head and neck surgery and maxillofacial surgery, it is essential to be aware that transient bacteremia may occur in patients from the moment of mucosal incision [8].

Nasal Packing: Intraoperative and Postoperative Management

Temporary nasal packing is essential during surgery. The author uses small-sized sponges soaked in a solution consisting of 50 CCs of 10% Povidone-iodine (Betadine), 1 g cefazolin, 80 mg gentamicin, and 500 CCs normal saline. Whenever transferring the instruments into the nasal vestibule, the instruments are cleansed with 70% alcohol. Cleansing is also applied when inserting and taking out an endoscope. While operating the external nose, the nasal cavity is packed with small sponges repeatedly. The author prefers much irrigation into the dissected pocket using the same solution 3–4 times (Fig. 3.6).

- While the external rhinoplasty is performed, the nasal cavity is packed with the soaked sponge. While the author performs septal surgery, packing is removed.
- All surgical instruments that have touched the nasal cavity should be cleaned with alcohol gauze during surgery.

For patients who underwent septal surgery, nasal packing is applied for 2–3 days postoperatively after surgery. The author uses a sufficient amount of susceptible ointment to the foam and pack. The authors prefer NasoPore® bioresorbable nasal dressing, which does not require packing out. On the second or third postoperative day, all packing is removed by suction.

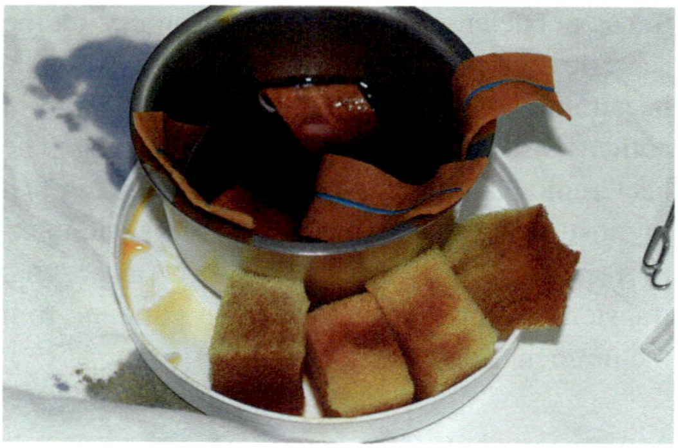

Fig. 3.6 Small sponges and nasal packing soaked in irrigation solution

3.4 Nasal Swab Study for PINF [6]

The efficacy of nasal swab study is high. One of the detection systems, VITEK2 (Biomérieux, Marcy-l'Étoile, France), reported excellent sensitivity/specificity of 99% and 96% for antibiotic susceptibility, according to MRSA, and the reporting time was quick within 6–18 h. Of course, there may be an error in the test method, and there is a possibility of a false-negative study. It is still the most convenient and rapid method of the nasal cavity in the existing and advantageous method for identifying vestibule strains. Although it costs, there is no reason not to do it for good results. Although extensive studies on septorhinoplasty have spoken about the ineffectiveness of antibiotics, the author cannot agree, at least in Asian septorhinoplasty [9].

Nasal Swab Negative

In our retrospective study, the number of patients with a culture-negative was 13.9–15.3% of the total when nasal swabs performed two weeks preoperatively. These patients do not experience SSI, even with empirical antibiotics. First- or second generation cephalosporin or amoxicillin-clavulanate may be prescribed.

Nasal Swab Positive

In the same study, the results of PINF were 84–86% of the total (Fig. 3.5). The prevalence of MSSA and MSSE was 23.6%–40.3% and 8.3%–14.7%, respectively. Then, MRSA and MRSE, which were not usually susceptible to empirical antibiotics, showed a frequency of 2.8%–4.0% and 4.2%–12.9%, respectively. Also, enterobacter aerogenes such as E-coli and Klebsiella pneumoniae showed 17.2%–19.4% and 2.5%–4.2% frequency, respectively. All these patients were identified to have resistant or intermediate sensitivity with empirical first or second-generation cephalosporin.

It is significant that MRSA, MRSE, and enterobacter, which are resistant to the empirical antibiotics of our hospital, were found at 4–17%. It was high, at least more than 4% of the total who undergo surgery, the empirical selection of antibiotics does not make any sense. At least it means that the antibiotic regimen of Quinolone or higher is correct.

Second Nasal Swab Positive

The results of the nasal swab performed immediately before surgery are shown in Fig. 3.7. MRSE was the most common at 9.8%, and the identification of MRSA was 1.8%, and the identification of Gram-negative microorganisms accounted for a large proportion of 8.9%. According to this result, antibiotics were changed and P.O. medication was also determined.

Changes in Microbiology

Positive to Negative Change

Two weeks before surgery, a susceptible ointment was applied to the found strain in the nasal cavity and swab again before the surgery to observe the change. As a result, the strain was no longer identified in 53.7% of the patients who showed positivity before surgery. There is no evidence that preoperative antibiotic ointment application to the nasal cavity prevents SIS. It is also risky that the application of lesional antibiotics with lesional irrigation may increase resistance to antibiotics. It has been reported that the effect of prophylactic antibiotic irrigation performed on intraoperative wounds is equivocal [10]. However, in terms of the effect of changing positive nasal swabs to negative, the authors judge that there is significant clinical significance (Fig. 3.8).

Negative to Positive Change

Instead, in the group of patients with negative cultures 2 weeks ago, 4.6% of patients showed positive nasal swab immediately before surgery. Here, there may be a new outbreak of PINF because ointment treatment was not performed before the surgery, or the first test may have been a false negative.

Positive to Positive

Even though the ointment was applied, 31% of patients showed identification of PINF. Most of them were identified with the same strain, and in a few, a change occurred as different strands. Because

Fig. 3.7 Microbiology profiles performed immediately before surgery; 326 patients in Cohort 3 were analyzed. (Material from: Moon et al. Preoperative Nasal Swab Culture: Is It Beneficial in Preventing Postoperative Infection in Complicated Septorhinoplasty?, Plastic and Reconstructive Surgery, 2020, Lippincott Williams & Wilkins)

Microbiology Profiles Performed Immediately before Surgery

	Cohort 3 (%)
No. of patients	326
Negative	210 (64.4)
Positive	116 (35.6)
Gram-positive microorganisms	88 (27.0)
Staphylococcus aureus (MSSA)	15 (4.6)
Staphylococcus epidermidis (MSSE)	23 (7.1)
Staphylococcus aureus (MRSA)	6 (1.8)
Staphylococcus epidermidis (MRSE)	32 (9.8)
Corynebacterium striatum	12 (3.7)
Gram-negative microorganisms	28 (8.9)
Enterobacter aerogenes	4 (1.2)
Klebsiella pneumoniae	5 (1.5)
Citrobacter spp.	0 (0.0)
Others	19 (5.8)

MSSA, methicillin-sensitive S. *aureus;* MSSE, methicillin-sensitive S. *epidermidis;* MRSA, methicillin-resistant S. *aureus;* MRSE, methicillin-resistant S. *epidermidis.*

Microbiology Profile changes in Cohort 3

	Cohort 3 (%)
No.	326
Negative → negative	35 (10.7)
Negative → positive	15 (4.6)
Positive → positive	101 (31.0)
Positive → negative	175 (53.7)

Fig. 3.8 Microbiology profile change in 326 patients of septorhinoplasty. (Material from: Moon et al. Preoperative Nasal Swab Culture: Is It Beneficial in Preventing Postoperative Infection in Complicated Septorhinoplasty?, Plastic and Reconstructive Surgery, 2020, Lippincott Williams & Wilkins)

the area where the ointment is applied is mainly the nostril, where the columella and marginal incision will be made, the bactericidal role may be insignificant. Applying ointment may not affect the nasal vestibule's bacteria, and there is a possibility that the bacteria will remain in the nasal cavity.

- In our study, 4.6% of the total were negative in the first nasal swab and then changed to positive in the second, so empirical antibiotics may be of no use in some of this patient group.

3.5 My Protocol for a *SAFE* Asian Septorhinoplasty

Nasal Swab Culture: Two Times

All patients underwent preoperative nasal swab cultures 2 weeks before surgery. After the internal nose was cleaned using a cotton swab wetted with saline solution, the nasal vestibule was swabbed using a culture swab. The nasal swab sample was immediately stored in an aseptic tube for subsequent culture. The nasal swab culture is repeated immediately before surgery in the operating room using the same method as the first preoperative nasal swab culture.

- The reason for doing two nasal swabs is that the strain of PINF may change in the timeline, or there may be false negatives in the initial nasal swab.
- If the second strain changes, an effort should be made to replace the primary antibiotics with a susceptible one.

Applying Antibiotic Ointment

Topical antibiotics were not applied in culture-negative patients. However, when microorganisms were isolated, the patients were taught to apply ointment at home for 5 days before the surgery at least three times a day. Two types of antibiotic ointments were used, mupirocin (Bactroban, GlaxoSmithKline, London, United Kingdom) and ofloxacin (Tarivid, Santen, Japan). In brief, mupirocin ointment was used for the decolonization of mupirocin-sensitive microorganisms. Ofloxacin ointment was used in sensitive microorganisms, including mostly such as MRSE, MRSA, and enterobacter.

- There are criticisms that the use of preoperative antibiotic ointment may lead to antibiotic resistance, but previous studies have reported that the identification of PINF decreased when antibiotic was applied to nasal packing during surgery.
- The author's study also confirmed that the strain found before surgery in 53.7% of patients disappeared, which is the basis [6].

The Choice of IV Antibiotics

The empirical antibiotics for the culture-negative patient and MSSA patients were the first-generation cephalosporin. In the case of patients whose strains were identified in the culture, susceptible antibiotics were administered pre- and postoperatively as a rule. Typically, many patients with MRSE and enterobacter were sensitive to ciprofloxacin. Simultaneously, MRSA mostly received vancomycin as the first-line prophylactic antibiotics. For patients with both methicillin- and ciprofloxacin-resistant S. aureus and S. epidermidis, intravenous teicoplanin, or vancomycin was administered.

However, when de novo bacteria were isolated in the second preoperative nasal swab cultures and were resistant to the previous prophylactic antibiotics, the intravenous prophylactic antibiotics were changed. The new antibiotic was administered intravenously for 3 days and then orally for the next 4 days (Fig. 3.9).

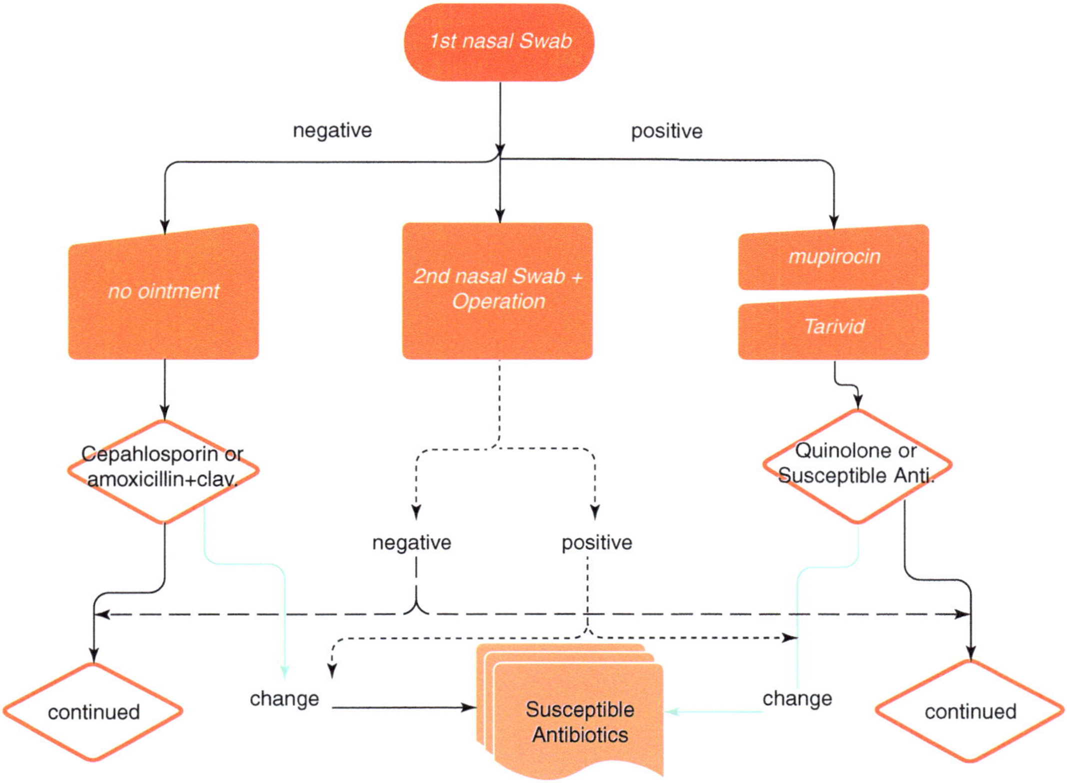

Fig. 3.9 Flow sheet of my protocol for a safe septorhinoplasty

References

1. Glück U, Gebbers JO. The nose as bacterial reservoir: important differences between the vestibule and cavity. Laryngoscope. 2000;110(3 Pt 1):426–8.
2. Nuyen B, Kandathil CK, Laimi K, Rudy SF, Most SP, Saltychev M. Evaluation of antibiotic prophylaxis in rhinoplasty: a systematic review and meta-analysis. JAMA Facial Plast Surg. 2019;21(1):12–7.
3. Georgiou I, Farber N, Mendes D, Winkler E. The role of antibiotics in rhinoplasty and septoplasty: a literature review. Rhinology. 2008;46(4):267–70.
4. Yoder MG, Weimert TA. Antibiotics and topical surgical preparation solution in septal surgery. Otolaryngol Head Neck Surg. 1992;106(3):243–4.
5. Schäfer J, Pirsig W. Preventive antibiotic administration in complicated rhinosurgical interventions—a double-blind study. Laryngol Rhinol Otol. 1988;67(4):150–5.
6. Moon K-C, Jung J-E, Dhong E-S, Jeong S-H, Han S-K. Preoperative nasal swab culture: is it beneficial in preventing postoperative infection in complicated septorhinoplasty? Plast Reconstr Surg. 2020;146(1):27e–34e.
7. Okur E, Yildirim I, Aral M, Ciragil P, Kiliç MA, Gul M. Bacteremia during open septorhinoplasty. Am J Rhinol. 2006;20(1):36–9.
8. Koc S, Uysal IO, Uysal EB, Yenişehirli G, Duygu F. The comparison of bacteremia and amount of bleeding during septoplasty. Eur Arch Otorhinolaryngol. 2012;269(4):1139–42.
9. Kullar R, Frisenda J, Nassif PS. The more the Merrier? Should antibiotics be used for rhinoplasty and septorhinoplasty?—a review. Plast Reconstr Surg Glob Open. 2018 Oct;6(10):e1972.
10. de Jonge SW, Boldingh QJJ, Solomkin JS, Allegranzi B, Egger M, Dellinger EP, et al. Systematic review and meta-analysis of randomized controlled trials evaluating prophylactic intra-operative wound irrigation for the prevention of surgical site infections. Surg Infect. 2017;18(4):508–19.

4 Medpor: The Hurdle of Secondary Rhinoplasty

Pearls

- Medpor has high tissue integration; the destruction of the surrounding tissue is devastating when the Medpor is removed.
- When Medpor was applied to the septum, the part that contacts the septal cartilage causes damage to the adjacent quadrangular cartilage, and the part that reaches the mucosa causes mucosal thinning and perforation.
- Extrusion or infection cannot be treated with antibiotics. Medpor should be removed.
- Micropore can be a breeding ground for bacterial growth, causing late-onset inflammation.
- Dorsal alloplastic implant and septal Medpor use are the worst combinations in late-onset inflammation communicating the septal pocket with dorsal implant capsule.

4.1 Physical Properties

The Medpor implant is made of a medical-grade, high-density polyethylene that is sintered to create a somewhat flexible framework of interconnecting pores [1]. The pore size ranges from 160 to 368 μm and more than half of these pores are larger than 150 μm in diameter. Since 1985, MEDPOR porous polyethylene implants have provided you with a range of off the shelf, biocompatible implant options for esthetic and reconstruction. Microthin, ultrathin, and sheet form is ready up to 0.25–3 mm. The vascular and fibrous ingrowth leads to excellent integration and stabilization of the implant and decreased rates of infection once the implant complex has formed [2]. Mainly, thin Medpor has been used for the nose in Asia. Thin Medpor is used for the septal application, and thick Medpor is used for nasal dorsum. Currently, it is mainly used for septal extension in Asian rhinoplasty.

4.2 Complication Reports

There are still many debates in the Asian rhinoplasty society. Medpor shortens surgery time, is easy to use for septal extension or extended septal extension, has an excellent functional outcome and reports that complication is not a problem in the long-term follow-up [3–6]. It is argued that only two of the 27 patients had a long-term extrusion, but due to their thin physical properties, the nasal cross-sectional area was wider than that of the septal cartilage after surgery. Here, two out of 27 are 7%. In one meta-analysis, the removal rate of silicone was 6.1%, and the removal rate of Medpor was 3.1%, and the safety of tissue integrating was reported [7]. However, the infection rate was reported as 4% for silicone and 6% for Medpor, and the extrusion of Medpor as 2%. The difference between these reports is that the

Supplementary Information The online version of this chapter (https://doi.org/10.1007/978-981-16-0542-0_4) contains supplementary material, which is available to authorized users.

E.-S. Dhong, M.-W. Na, *Asian Septorhinoplasty*, https://doi.org/10.1007/978-981-16-0542-0_4

Medpor use would be different. It remains unfortunate that this report comes only with complication rates. Each author might use Medpor at different sites such as the septum, membranous septum, columella, or dorsum.

The author has only bad memories of Medpor. Every single case was problematic due to the Medpor use. It is necessary to rethink the stability of this material based on science.

Due to the physical characteristics, Medpor provides stable support even with a thin thickness and maintains stability by the tissue's ingrowth. However, refutation on long-term stability without resorting to suture is below.

- The tissue ingrowth of Medpor, upon removal, destroys the surrounding tissue.
- When applied to the septum, the contact causes damage to the adjacent quadrangular cartilage and mucosal tear or perforation.
- Extrusion or infection cannot be treated with drugs. It must be removed.
- Silicone makes soft tissue called capsule or scar around, while Medpor is challenging to remove and cause soft tissue loss.
- The pore can be a breeding ground for bacterial growth.
- Secondary surgery is complicated due to adhesion.

The above reasons alone indicate that Medpor use is the leading cause of the most challenging complications in Asian septorhinoplasty. Any surgery cannot be convinced that it is the patient's last surgery.

Since the surgeon is not sure that he or she is the last surgeon, consideration should be given to reoperations that may occur next. Therefore, Medpor is not a good material for any septorhinoplasty.

As shown in Fig. 4.1, the vast high septal perforation is very difficult to reconstruct because of its location. Such complications would be a peculiar complication found only in Asia. Multiple septal perforations are also a typical complication due to Medpor. Septum reconstruction is impossible if these patients accompany framework collapse.

4.3 Why Is Medpor Such a Big Hurdle for Secondary Operation?

The physical characteristics of stiffness, micropores, and tissue integration are obstacles to the secondary operation.

The bilateral ingrowth of surrounding tissues should be removed and damaged while Medpor is removed.

- When Medpor is applied directly to the quadrangular cartilage, the septal cartilage and mucosa are simultaneously inflicted.
- If Medpor is applied to both sides of the quadrangular cartilage, the damage is more severe.

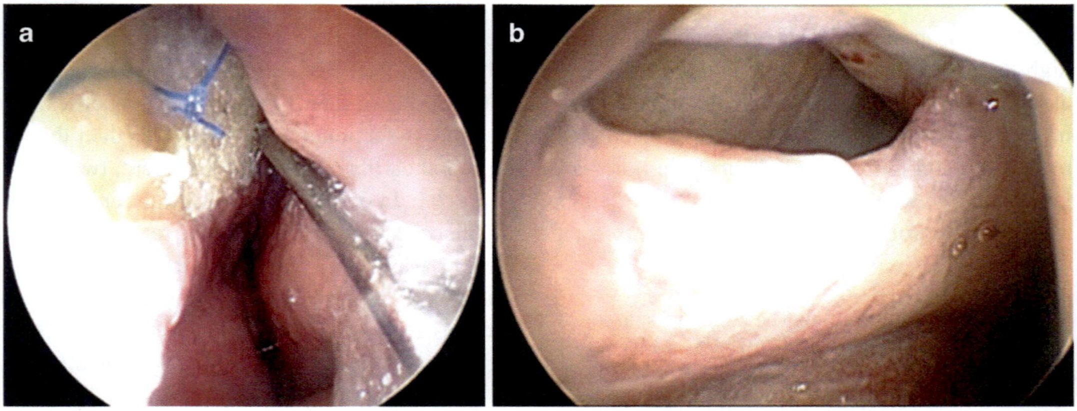

Fig. 4.1 Huge high septal perforation. (**a**) Before removing the Medpor and crust. (**b**) After removing the Medpor

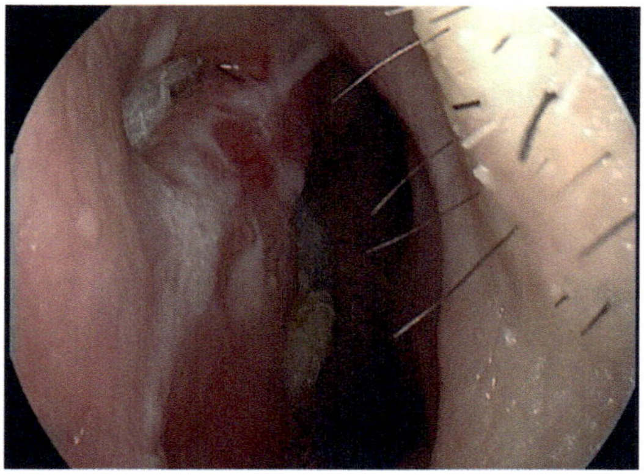

Fig. 4.2 Multiple perforations of the septum at the high septum and ethmoid-quadrangular cartilage junction

- In many cases, the reconstruction is impossible; multiple septal perforations would be the worst cases (Fig. 4.2).
- Microscopically, Medpor was covered with fibrous collagenous tissue, partially bridging through the pores. Inflammatory cells had infiltrated around the polyethylene [8].
- Micropores can cause late-onset inflammation.

In our study, 22% of the patients found Medpor in secondary septorhinoplasty. Of these patients, 28% had extrusion or puncture. In other words, in the author's experience, it is reasonable to say that Medpor can be found in one of five secondary surgeries in which the alloplastic materials are scheduled to be removed.

Patients are divided into cases with and without accurate previous operative information. 21% of them were draining pus or swollen with dorsal fluctuation. Most patients were inserted silicone or Gore-tex implants on the nasal dorsum and Medpor at their septum. Therefore, it is impossible to distinguish whether the cause of late-onset inflammation is Medpor or dorsal implant. However, based on the fact that the most pus pocket is connected to the Medpor, it is evident that the inflammation starts from Medpor.

- Since Medpor has high tissue integration, dorsal inflammation is not transferred to septal Medpor.
- Relatively, late-onset inflammation caused by Medpor is more likely to spread to the dorsal capsular pocket. This is why the LOI starts from septal Medpor.

The complication is characterized by intermittent nasal dorsal tenderness, swelling, and sometimes granuloma-like skin lesions. In severe cases, puncture with fluid drainage on the external or intranasal area may be present. Late-onset inflammation may result in significant esthetic and functional complications. In any case, the problem is fundamentally solved by removing the entire Medpor.

Dissectiblity

It is difficult to dissect the area where Medpor was applied. The greater the integration between tissues, the more difficult it is to dissect. If nasal framework damage occurs after excision, it may not be possible to remove the entire Medpor. It is advantageous for subsequent reconstruction leaving as much of the adjacent soft tissue as possible.

The preservation of mucosa is the most critical factor in the success or failure of the surgery.

4.4 What Do you Have to Prepare for the Reconstruction?

CT Scan: The Only Aid for Preoperative Diagnosis

It is impossible to obtain all surgical records or the history of accurate alloplastic use from patients with 3–6 previous surgeries. Of course, it is helpful for reoperation if there are detailed surgical records. However, if there is scanty information, computed tomography is the only diagnostic tool.

In the bone setting, there is no help other than checking the dorsum's alloplastic material. Changing the contrast to the abdomen (W 250 L50) or mediastinum (W450 L 45) and rotating the axial view would show "hypolucent Medpor shadow." Based on CT information, then the intranasal inspection should be accurately repeated by pressing the dorsum with a finger, and carefully observing the caudal septum through anterior rhinoscopy.

- A septal extension graft should be suspected if the caudal septal end cannot be observed with an anterior rhinoscope without the gap of the membranous septum.
- Pushing down with a finger touches the hardness or causes pain in the patients; suspects the Medpor use.

However, it is more important than anything else to control the contrast in CT scan and find a shadow with hypodensity (Video 4.1).

In the first case of each patient, the patient was not aware of Medpor use, and the actual operation for this image is shown (Fig. 4.3). Batten type septal extension graft can be seen in two layers under the silicone implant [9]. Since the pus pocket did not invade the septal Medpor, in this case, the pus was not drained from the septum, and the destruction was relatively small. Still, Medpor was in contact with the pus pocket, so the complete removal was necessary. In the second video, the operation was performed due to pain, and the anterior-caudal part of the septum was severely destroyed (Video 4.2, Fig. 4.4). In CT, Medpors with hypolucent density were found in a wide area.

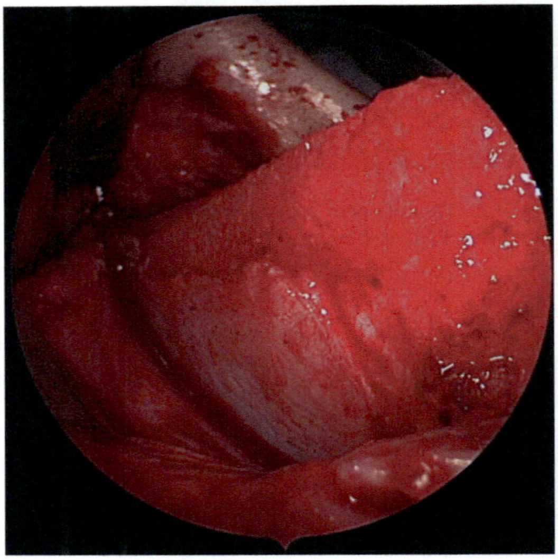

Fig. 4.4 A long and huge Medpor was found in one piece at the anterocaudal septum. The anterocaudal margin was destructed already before removing it

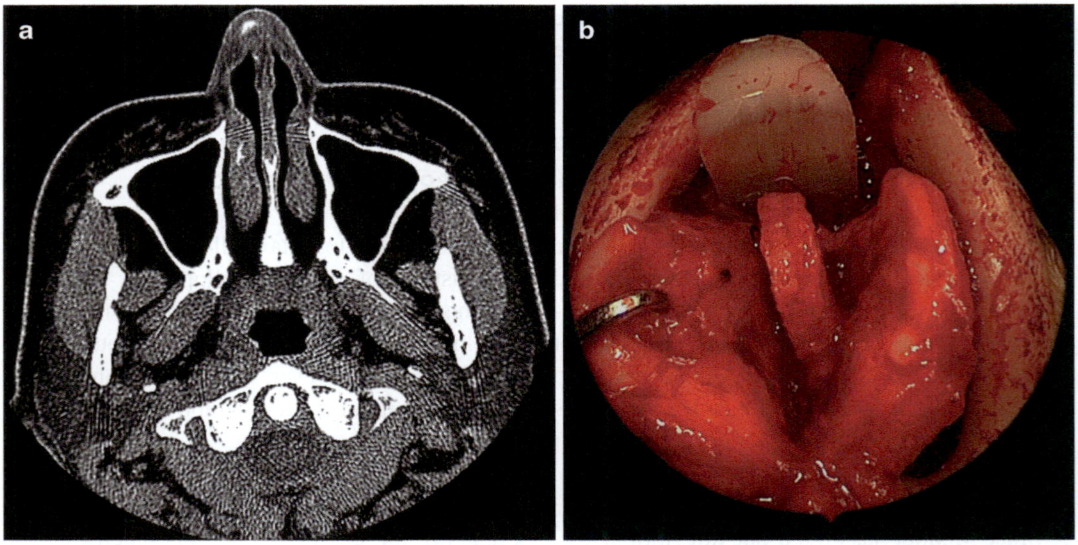

Fig. 4.3 Batten type septal extension by Medpor was found under the silicone implant. (**a**) Axial CT scan. (**b**) Intraoperative view

Autograft for the Septal Reinforcement

To rebulid the detroyed septum, the amount required should be larger than the actual size. Since the destruction of the rhinion weakens the fixation force, there is a high possibility of saddle nose deformity after surgery. Also, much effort is required to get the dorsal esthetic line smooth. There are many problems because the septal part is also fragile, and there is no supporting force. Significantly, the posterior septal angle is often required to obtain strong support. The extent to which the mucous membrane on the other side has been destroyed determines the operability.

4.5 Patterns of Medpor Application

Septal Application

Anterior Application

This is a method for applying Medpor in the same way as Dr. Byrd's spreader type septal extension. It leads to severe deficits, as shown in Fig. 4.1. Particularly crucial in part is that it involves the rhinion, which makes the reconstruction difficult. Ten years ago, this technique was popular in the form of a projection by emphasizing the boomerang type nasal tip. The high septal destruction is the most difficult of all complications.

Case Study 1: Deviation with Pain and Stiffness

A 24-year-old female underwent septorhinoplasty 2 years before the referral. The history described SMR, harvesting ear cartilage, and corrective osteotomies. One year later, 2 mm thick silicone was inserted for the esthetic dissatisfaction.

The patient complained of pain and stiffness in the nose and implant deviation in the nose.

The biggest problem was nasal congestion, and the NOSE score was 14/20 points. There were no records or information on Medpor use. A spreader type Medpor was found in the surgical pocket (Fig. 4.5).

The dorsal and tip projection did not change much, but all of the alloplastic materials were replaced with autografts. Pain has disappeared. That is a significant change (Figs. 4.6 and 4.7).

Caudal Application

Mainly Dr. Byrd's batten type, Medpor attaches to the caudal portion of the quadrangular cartilage, extends to the membranous septum, and projects the nasal tip. Injury to the cartilage in the caudal portion can be detected, and a severe reduction of the tip projection that loses support should be prepared after removal (Fig. 4.8).

Anterocaudal Application

Anterocaudal application yields the most severe case. The Medpor applied to the entire anterocaudal septum can be found along the patient's L-strut. Most patients complain of pain. The patient's nose is moving left to right but has restrictions in the anterocaudal direction. Therefore, even subtle nose movements can cause pain and discomfort. In particular, patients feel discomfort in mimetic movement, especially in making the "o" pronunciation. The tip of the nose is stiff. If Medpor is found in late-onset inflammation, salvaging the nose length would be difficult.

Case Study 2: Late-Onset Inflammation

A 31-year-old man, a patient with a nasal bone fracture 14 years ago was transferred to the author after four surgeries. Septoplasty was performed after a nasal bone fracture, but the exact history was not remembered. Two years ago, augmentation rhinoplasty underwent using silicone implants. One year later, the tip plasty and silicone were replaced twice. In history, the information of Medpor use was unclear, and for several months before the visit, the swelling and subside was repeated after taking empirical antibiotics. Just before the visit, the scar band and hard foreign body descending to the columella were palpable, and the skin thinning was found to the extent that impending puncture was suspicious

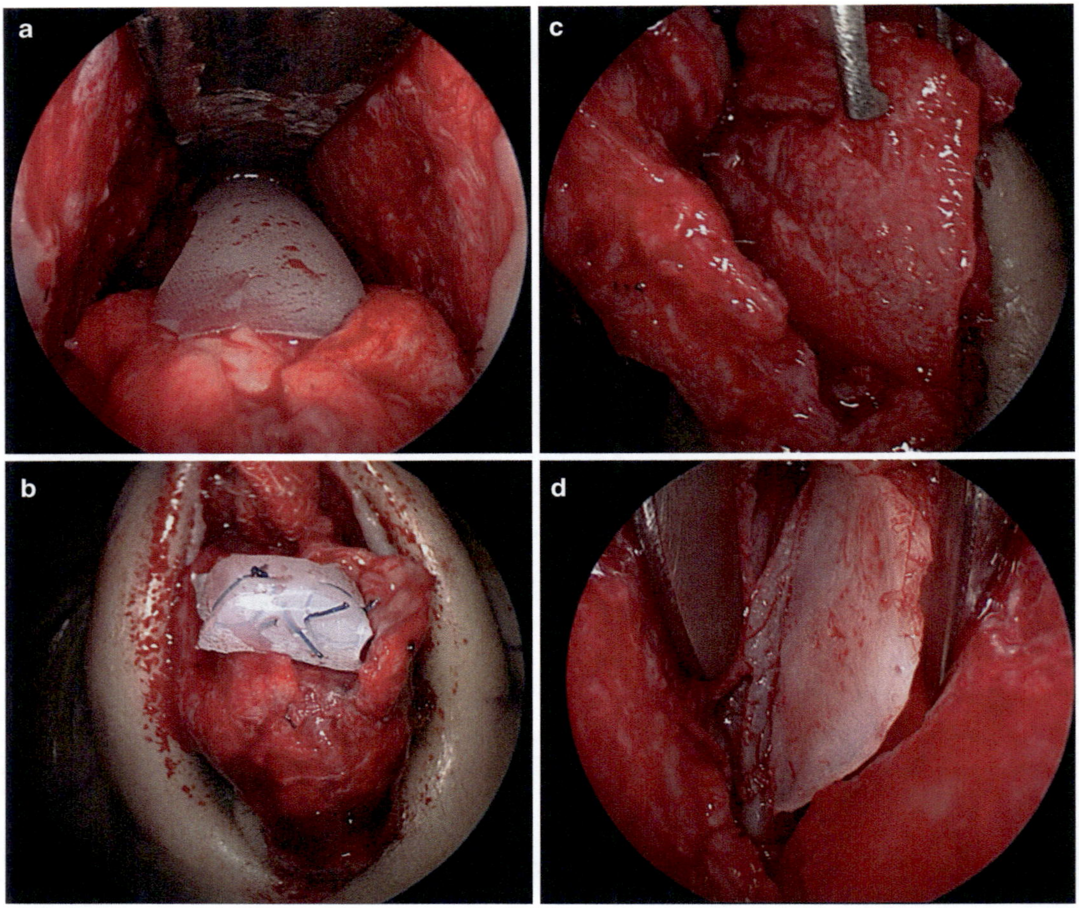

Fig. 4.5 Dorsal silicone implant with septal Medpor use. (**a**) Dorsal silicone. (**b**) Tip silicone was found first before approaching the dorsum. (**c**) Batten type one-piece Medpor at the right caudal margin. (**d**) After removing the Medpor, the caudal septal margin was attenuated and fractured

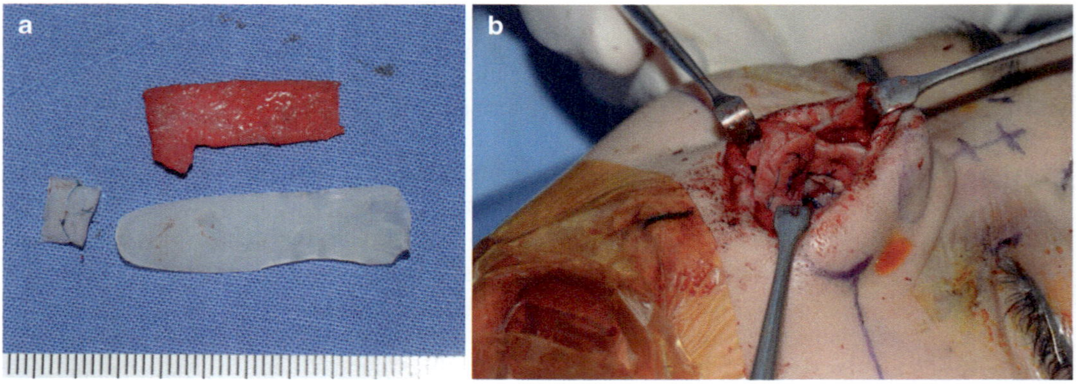

Fig. 4.6 Substitutes of the surgery. (**a**) Removing the alloplastic materials: dorsal silicone, tip silicone, and septal Medpor. (**b**) Reconstructing the L-strut using two conchas

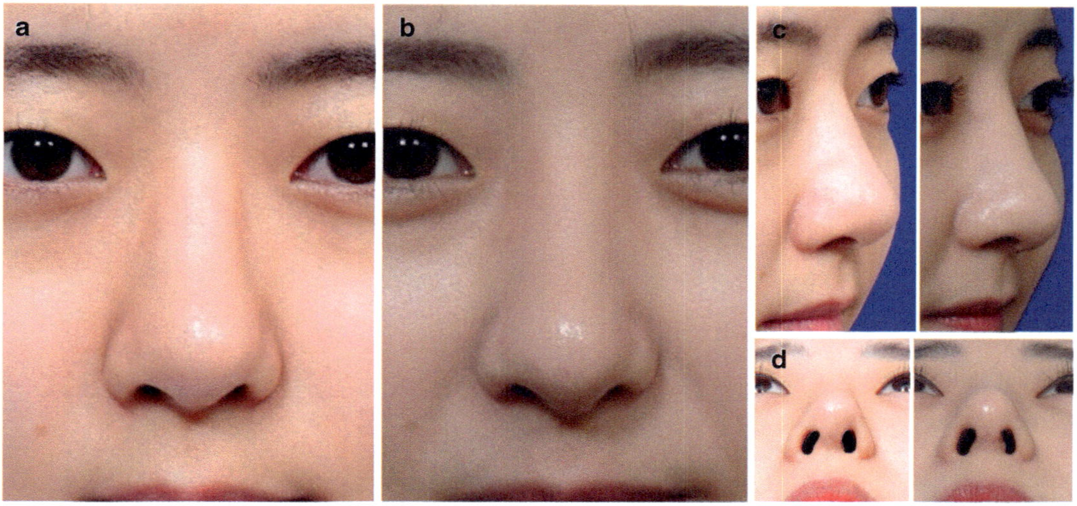

Fig. 4.7 Pre- and postoperative views. (**a**) Preoperative view: dorsal implant deviation to Lt. side. (**b**) Postoperative 1 year view. (**c**) Quarter view: Lt. preoperative, Rt. postoperative view. (**d**) Basal view: Lt. preoperative, Rt. postoperative view

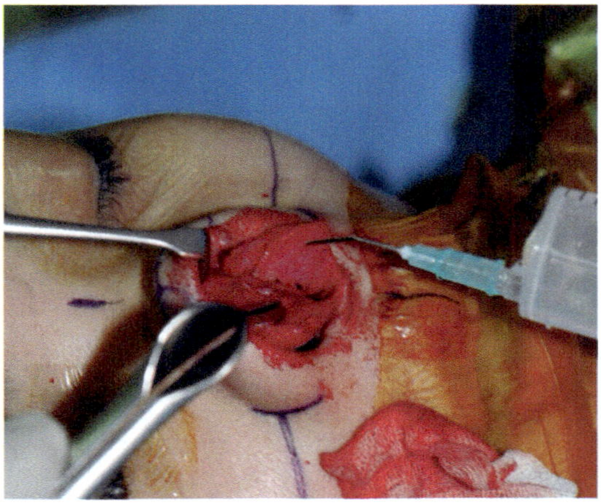

Fig. 4.8 Caudal unilateral batten type application of Medpor

(Fig. 4.9). Several silicone pieces were found in the surgical field, and Medpors applied in two layers to the anterior septum, and two layers to the caudal septum were found, and the capsule existing in the surrounding scar had to be removed (Fig. 4.10). Also, as shown in the following method, the septal L-strut was rebuilt using two ear cartilage. The superficial mastoid fascia was grafted to minimize dorsal irregularity (Fig. 4.11).

Case Study 3: Pain with Saddle Nose Deformity

A 21-year-old female patient came to the hospital with persistent discomfort after surgery. Recently, she felt a pulling down sensation and pain when speaking and laughing. A saddle nose and drooping nose deformity were found. In the surgical field, four pieces of Medpor were found at the anterocaudal portions of the L-strut. She underwent L-strut reconstruction using two conchal cartilage using the same technique (Figs. 4.12 and 4.13).

Columella Application

A relatively small amount of Medpor can be found in the columella, and if the LLC surrounds, it is relatively less in the case of extrusion. Even the smallest amount of Medpor cannot be said to be without problems.

Nasal Pain

A characteristic symptom of patients who are applied Medpor is unknown pain; pain is believed

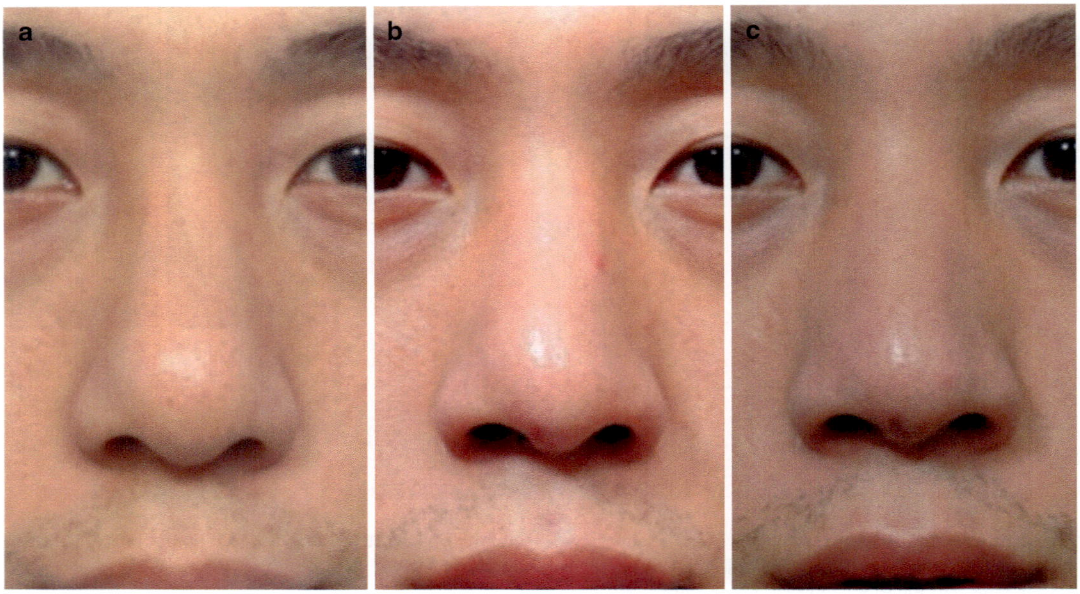

Fig. 4.9 Repetition of swelling and skin puncture due to Medpor. (**a**) He visited the author with a swollen nose. (**b**) He visited 2 months later for the secondary surgery. The swelling has subsided after the columellar discharge and antibiotics. (**c**) Postoperative view

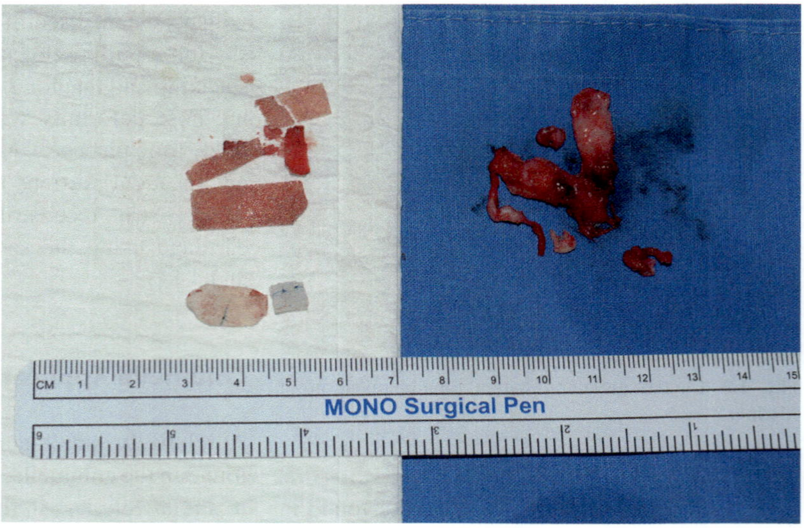

Fig. 4.10 Excised alloplastic materials: Medpors, two silicone pieces at the dorsum, and old nonhealthy capsules

to be due to the physical properties. The plate is more rigid than the autogenous tissue, so constant physical pressure is applied to the surrounding tissue. The good thing about tissue incorporation is that it is closely attached after the suture loses integrity. There must be constant movement in the normal scroll area or hinge area. However, the central component with Medpor is not as movable as the lateral component. Mucoperichondrium, Pitanguy ligaments, and mucosa trilogy connect the ULC and LLC to the septum enabling the micromovement central component of Medpor to make this impossible. Pain is proportional to the degree of stiffness at

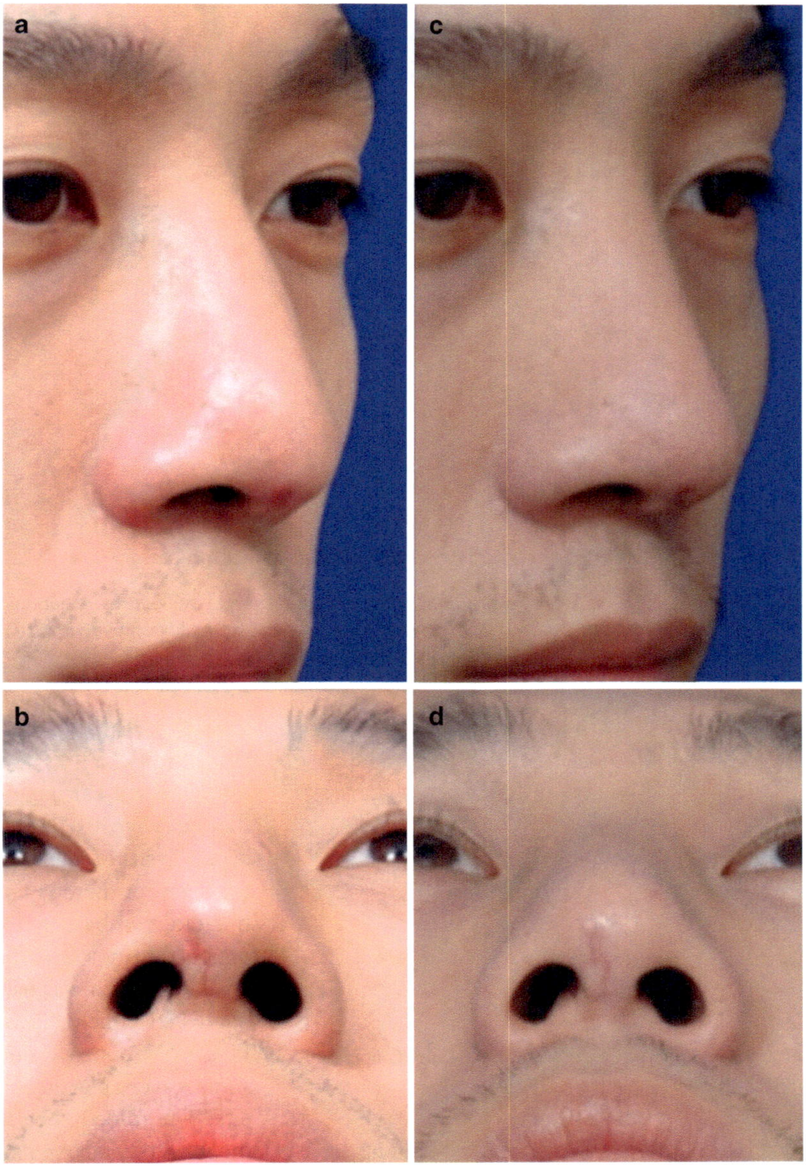

Fig. 4.11 Pre- and postoperative 1 year. (**a**, **b**) Preoperative views. (**c**, **d**) Postoperaive views

the tip and dorsum. The pain when breathing should be compared with the pain from its stiffness. Breading pain is related to nasal dryness and obstruction.

4.6 Operative Technique of Reconstruct the Collapsed Septum

There are two ways to restore nasal length: septal L-strut reconstruction and cantilever graft. It is impossible to reconstruct without cartilage transplantation at the site of destruction. Since Medpors is attached in various forms, it varies depending on the situation. However, when a thin Medpor is applied, the destruction of the tissue is relatively vast.

Septum Reconstruction

The cartilage that can be replaced is ear cartilage and costal cartilage.

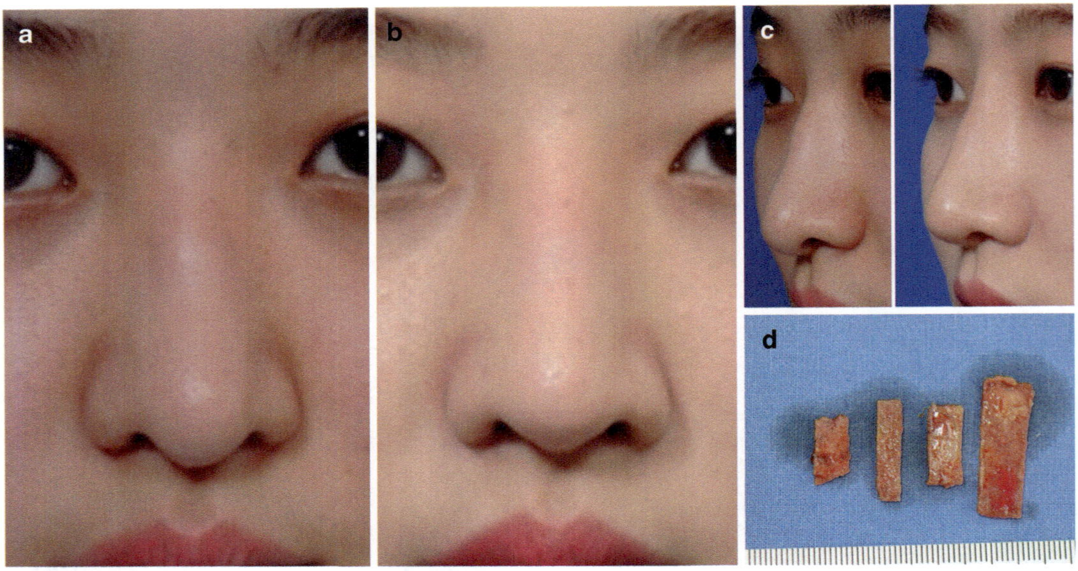

Fig. 4.12 Saddle nose with tip drooping: anterocaudal septal extension by Medpor. (**a**) Preoperative AP view, (**b**) Postoperative 1 year, (**c**) Quarter view, Lt. preoperative view, Rt. postoperative view. (**d**) Four pieces of Medpor

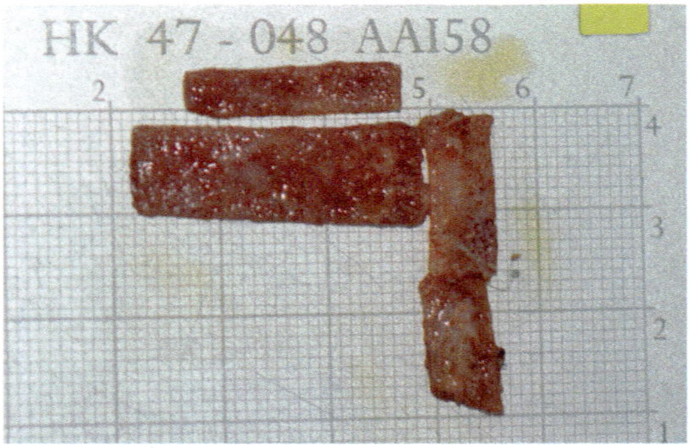

Fig. 4.13 Four pieces of Medpor: bilateral application anteriorly, and caudally

In the author's case, since most patients have a stiff nose, they want to change to a softer nose. Therefore, the first choice is ear cartilage, and the costal cartilage is chosen as the last choice. In many cases, since the ear cartilage has been used on one side, all cartilages are collected from the ear. Cymba concha is used where long cartilage is needed, and cavum concha is used where the relatively short cartilage is needed. Moreover, tragal cartilage can also be harvested.

Septal L-strut Reconstruction Using Two Conchal Cartilages [10]

Two conchal cartilage (cymba and cavum) from the ear were used as the primary selection for septal L-strut reconstruction. If the patient's ears are small or there is no cavum conchal cartilage, bilateral cymba conchal cartilage is used. If the patient did not have bilateral conchal cartilage, costal cartilage was used for reconstruction. This harvested conchal cartilage was folded face to face on the concave side. Two horizontal mattress sutures were placed using 5-0 or 6-0 polypropylene. The folded conchal cartilage was placed in the ANS (septal extension graft type) in a tongue-in-groove manner.

The folded cartilage was attached to the ANS's periosteum and surrounding soft tissue using 4-0 polydioxanone (PDS) without drill holes. Other conchal cartilage was also folded in the same manner and used in a tongue-in-groove method for the anterior septum (spreader type). The graft was sutured to the remaining anterior square cartilage using multiple fixation sutures with 4-0

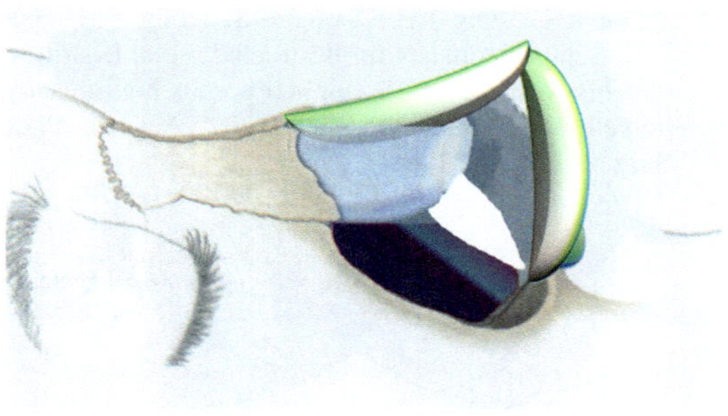

Fig. 4.14 Septal L-strut extension graft using two conchal cartilages

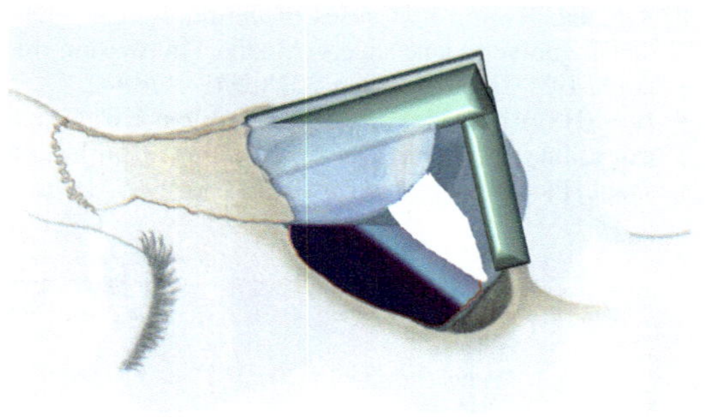

Fig. 4.15 Septal L-strut extension graft using sliced costal cartilages

Vicryl and 5-0 PDS. When severe destruction of the keystone was observed, cartilage was attached to the nasal bone through both drilled holes. After that, the two-folded conchal cartilage was sutured together to create a de novo anterior septal angle and suture to the middle crura using 4-0 PDS (Video 4.3). Small cartilage pieces, sculpted from previously harvested conchal cartilage, can be applied as reinforcing rafters between two folded conchal cartilage. After the reconstruction of the septal L-strut, tip plasty and dorsal autograft was performed (Fig. 4.14).

Septal L-strut Reconstruction Using Sliced Costal Cartilages

For reconstructing the septal L-strut, the seventh costal cartilage was usually used with an incised costal cartilage. Harvested rib cartilage was carved lengthwise. Divide into several pieces approximately 1–2 mm thick. The sculpted cartilage was immersed in a saline-filled container for at least an hour to reveal a tendency to warp. Two costal cartilages were applied facing the concave side of the anterior septum. The caudal septum was created and sutured to the anterior septum using the other two rib cartilage slices. The rectus abdominis fascia was taken and wrapped with a cut rib cartilage. They were applied onlay graft to project and smooth the nose dorsal profile (Fig. 4.15).

Cantilever Graft

If no septal reconstruction is possible, only the reconstruction of the external nose should be focused. This method without septal dissection may be more difficult as it is difficult to loosen enough constricted soft tissue. Considering that most Medpor is applied to the nasal septum, this is not a fundamental solution. The author does not use this method because the septal dissection has to be done to remove Medpor.

References

1. Frodel JL, Lee S. The use of high-density polyethylene implants in facial deformities. Arch Otolaryngol Head Neck Surg. 1998;124(11):1219–23.
2. Sclafani AP, Thomas JR, Cox AJ, Cooper MH. Clinical and histologic response of subcutaneous expanded polytetrafluoroethylene (Gore-Tex) and porous high-density polyethylene (Medpor) implants to acute and early infection. Arch Otolaryngol Head Neck Surg. 1997;123(3):328–36.
3. Kim YH, Kim BJ, Jang TY. Use of porous high-density polyethylene (Medpor) for spreader or extended septal graft in rhinoplasty: aesthetics, functional outcomes, and long-term complications. Ann Plast Surg. 2011;67(5):464–8.
4. Skouras A, Skouras G, Karypidis D, Asimakopoulou F-A. The use of Medpor© alloplastic material in rhinoplasty: experience and outcomes. J Plast Reconstr Aesthet Surg. 2012;65(1):35–42.
5. Sykes JM, Patel KG. Use of Medpor implants in rhinoplasty surgery. Oper Tech Otolaryngol Head Neck Surg. 2008;19(4):273–7.
6. Niechajev I. Facial reconstruction using porous high-density polyethylene (Medpor): long-term results. Aesthet Plast Surg. 2012;36(4):917–27.
7. Peled ZM, Warren AG, Johnston P, Yaremchuk MJ. The use of alloplastic materials in rhinoplasty surgery: a meta-analysis. Plast Reconstr Surg. 2008;121(3):85e–92e.

8. Kim JH, Hwang K. Causes of the removal of high-density polyethylene sheets (Medpor) in revision rhinoplasty. J Craniofac Surg. 2018;29(7):1730–2.
9. Byrd HS, Andochick S, Copit S, Walton KG. Septal extension grafts: a method of controlling tip projection shape. Plast Reconstr Surg. 1997;100(4):999–1010.
10. Moon K-C, Jung J-E, Dhong E-S, Jeong S-H, Han S-K. Septorhinoplasty for destructed septal L-strut in patients with previously applied porous high-density polyethylene implants (Medpor®). Aesthet Plast Surg. 2019;43(5):1286–94.

5 Nasal Obstruction in Asian Rhinoplasty

Pearls

- Patients with sudden worsening of symptoms or the presence of new symptoms with purulence on physical examination imply an acute exacerbation of CRS (chronic rhinosinusitis), and the operation should be postponed at least 4 weeks.
- Symptoms of nasal obstruction do not always coincide with those examined with nasal or nasal endoscopy and CT scans.
- The most important defense is to take a history of nasal congestion before surgery.
- Patients in the post-SMR state have weak L-strut. At this time, the pressure applied to the lower part of the implant in the tight soft tissue pocket worsens the septum's deviation.
- Atypical causes of nasal obstruction that can be seen after the Asian septorhinoplasty are mainly related to the exaggerated tip projection with dorsal augmentation.
- The most significant cause of functional deterioration is found at the minimal cross-sectional area (MCA) of the internal nasal valve (INV).
- "Exaggerated tip extension anchoring (sutures)" pushes down the INV.
- If the nasal framework is weak, dorsal alloplastic implants or thick dermis graft may destroy the healthy angle of the INV.
- Excessive tip projection causes a step ladder deformity from internal nares to MCA of INV area.
- To improve the function of INV, projection of the caudal portion of the ULC corresponding to the tip projection is necessary.

5.1 Diagnosis

History and Inspection

In nasal obstruction, the most important thing is taking the patient's history. The symptoms of nasal obstruction are not related as it looks. From the past, nasal obstruction is said to be located in the anterior part, visible by a nasoscope. However, the patient's subjective symptoms do not necessarily coincide with these findings. In other words, it is not what the patient feels as seen on the nasoscope or as seen on the CT scan. Always the patient's subjective symptom is more critical to the diagnosis. No objective measurement perfectly represents the subjective symptom [1, 2].

However, the use of minimal objective measurements to obtain surgical help or compare patients' surgical outcomes is necessary to protect the doctor's practice.

Supplementary Information The online version of this chapter (https://doi.org/10.1007/978-981-16-0542-0_5) contains supplementary material, which is available to authorized users.

E.-S. Dhong, M.-W. Na, *Asian Septorhinoplasty*, https://doi.org/10.1007/978-981-16-0542-0_5

Relying 100% on the subjective symptoms of the patient is because objectivity is poor.

Comparing the nasal airflow entirely to the intranasal cross-sectional area is not 100% physiologically correct, but too much worry is often detrimental to the surgery's decision. Based on the patient's symptoms, it is necessary to obtain appropriate auxiliary means for surgery. Even nasal inspiratory peak flow is not related to subjective symptoms, so it is challenging to implement accurate flow objectively [3]. Also, the limitations of acoustic rhinometry have been reported. It has been reported that there is a limit to the association of rhinomanometry with clinical symptoms [4].

There are various measurements for the patient's subjective symptoms, but the author mainly uses the NOSE scale (Nasal Obstruction Symptom Evaluation Scale© AAO-HNS Foundation 2002) and is used as the basis for clinical follow-up [5] (Fig. 5.1).

It is the simplest and most effective instrument for observing the patient's condition before and after surgery. It should be borne in mind that this single sheet can be a great resource to protect doctors from patients complaining of unexpected nasal obstruction after surgery.

Nasal Cycle

Naturally, everyone has a nasal cycle. It is an autonomous cycle and is affected by the patient's posture and emotion and shows a complex and subtle relationship such that the resting state and exercise, night and day, and left and right dominance exist [6]. It is necessary to listen to the patient's nasal cycle closely. Decongest to change the turbinate and closely observe the patient's nasal obstruction. It is recommended to visit the doctor when the patient's symptoms are the most severe and examine and compare even when there are no symptoms. It is also essential to accurately record the antihistamine formulation and nasal spray the patients are taking.

In the end, keep in mind that nasal obstruction, which can be improved with drugs, is contraindicated in surgery because the part that the doctor can help with is limited to the visible part.

Nasal Obstruction and Septoplasty Effectiveness Scale

Physician AAO-HNS#: ________ **Patient ID:** ____________ **Today's date:** __/__/____

➔ **To the Patient:** Please help us to better understand the impact of nasal obstruction on your quality of life by **completing following survey.** Thank You!

Over the past *ONE* month, how much of a problem were the following conditions for you?

Please circle the most correct response

	Not a Problem	*Very Mild Problem*	*Moderate problem*	*Fairly Bad Problem*	*Severe problem*
1. Nasal congestion or stuffiness	0	1	2	3	4
2. Nasal blockage or obstruction	0	1	2	3	4
3. Trouble breathing through my nose	0	1	2	3	4
4. Trouble sleeping	0	1	2	3	4
5. TUnable to get enough air through my nose during exercise or exertion	0	1	2	3	4

Fig. 5.1 Nasal Obstruction Symptom Evaluation Scale © AAO-HNS Foundation 2002

Rhinitis and Sinusitis

The worse the atmospheric environment gets, the more patients' nasal function deteriorates. It is necessary to remove the vibrissae to observe the intranasal structure from external nares to deep turbinate at the first outpatient clinic.

Based on the patient's medical history, rhinitis and sinusitis should be treated separately. Depending on the type of rhinitis, the surgery needs to be postponed. For mucosal whitish discoloration and secretions, which are signs of typical allergic rhinitis, medical treatment prioritizes first. Symptoms should be released first, then structural problems are considered for the surgery.

Also, acute and chronic sinusitis should be diagnosed differentially. CT scans at this time are helpful. It is possible to diagnose space-occupying lesions of the sinus or polyps of the meatus. Of course, it is necessary to observe the nasal septal deviation that causes obstruction.

Bacterial and viral rhinosinusitis are difficult to distinguish on a clinical basis. The clinical diagnosis of acute bacterial rhinosinusitis should be reserved for patients with nasal sinusitis symptoms lasting more than 7 days with maxillary pain or tenderness in the face or teeth and purulent nasal secretion. Patients with body temperature less than 38.3 °C and mild pain can be prescribed by amoxicillin or trimethoprim/sulfamethoxazole.

However, if these symptoms come and go for more than 8–12 weeks, it is better to postpone the operation and perform the operation after sufficient antibiotic treatment for at least 3 weeks. In addition to chronic rhinosinusitis, it is recommended to use irrigation and topical therapy along with priority to regular treatment by an ENT doctor. If there is a schedule for surgery, one of the antibiotics such as amoxicillin-clavulanate, clindamycin, sulfamethoxazole/trimethoprim, and levofloxacin or ciprofloxacin should be selected and treated. If the symptoms do not improve during treatment, you should try changing it [7]. There are many thesis and disagreements regarding antibiotics, but the patients awaiting septorhinoplasty should be rhinosinus-symptoms-free. The problem is that sudden worsening of symptoms or the presence of new symptoms with purulence on physical examination implies an acute exacerbation of CRS, which should be treated. These patients are managed by microbiological culture, determination of antibiotic sensitivities, and appropriate antibiotic therapy [8].

CT Scan

In nasal obstruction, the most important thing is taking the patient's history. However, the doctor has no choice but to operate as seen by the intranasal inspection. It should be remembered again that nasal obstruction is not correlated 100% as it looks. CT is beneficial to see the relationship between the shape of the nasal septum and the surrounding inferior turbinate. It is also essential to observe the shape of the internal nasal valve (INV) and judge the possibility of reconstructing it. According to one report, the INV of Asians is broader than that of Caucasians. The INV angle in Asians is 21.6° ± 4.5°, and it is significantly larger than that of Caucasians. The reconstructed CT method has better reproducibility than the endoscopic method in measuring the INV angle. Caucasians, which has been reported to be 11.4° ± 2.6° ($p < 0.001$) [9]. This study is useful for observing the shape of INV and determining the spreader graft. It is particularly beneficial for observing the position and type of alloplastic implants in determining secondary rhinoplasty and seeing how it has a relationship with INV.

Inferior Turbinate

In the inferior turbinate, it is necessary to determine whether the bone occupies the actual volume or the venous sinusoid is enlarged along with the lamina propria to determine the surgical method. If the lamina propria is thicker than the turbinate bone, simple coblation can be applied (Fig. 5.2).

Concha Bullosa

Anomalous pneumatization of the turbinate is occasionally found. Inferior turbinate can be treated easily, but middle turbinate is following a symptomatic treatment. The author prefers a simple method for collapsing if concha bullosa found on the concave side can cause nasal obstruction after septoplasty. The medial lamina and lateral lamina can easily collapse, but in the middle turbinate, concha bullosa can be resolved with lateral laminectomy, partial turbinectomy, or concha-pexy. However, since septum and middle turbinate contact can cause rhinogenic headache, a close diagnosis is required, and accompanying sinusitis should be observed (Fig. 5.3).

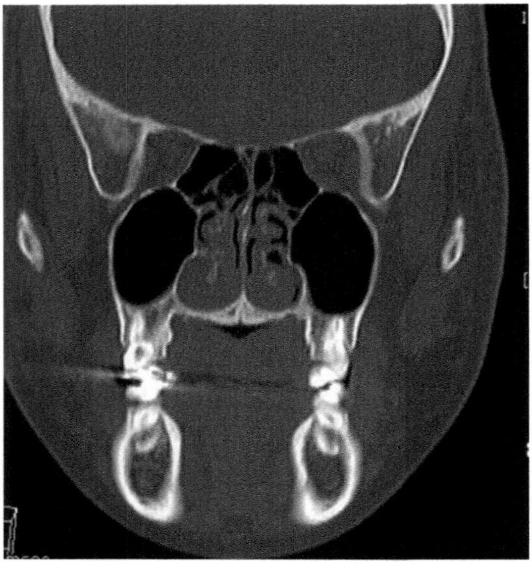

Fig. 5.2 Bilateral inferior turbinate hypertrophy: The lamina propria hypertrophied. The patient complained of severe nasal obstruction. Choanal patency is not observed

Acoustic Rhinometry

Among the objective measures, the author prefers acoustic rhinometry (AR) as an auxiliary. It is a method for viewing the cross-sectional area in the nasal cavity using acoustic reflection, and it is of sufficient value as a diagnostic aid, despite many criticisms [10].

Acoustic rhinometry is worthwhile to use as a means of getting help rather than relying on it. It is beneficial for comparing the left and right of the minimal cross-sectional area or for comparative evaluation before and after surgery. It is unreasonable to judge whether or not to perform surgery based on this. The graph is different according to the type of machine, and there may be an error in the part where the machine is inserted into the external nares, but the cross-sectional area from the inferior turbinate part forming the INV to 7 cm rear can be measured (Fig. 5.4) [11].

Even for rhinoplasty using alloplastic materials, a report recommends an examination before and after surgery using AR [12].

Many studies report on the changes before and after surgery using AR in reduction rhinoplasty, but there are few studies using AR of Asian septorhinoplasty, mainly augmentation rhinoplasty.

Case Study: A Case of CT Findings Do Not Correlate with AR

The patient with Video 5.1 complained more about nasal obstruction on the left. It is differ-

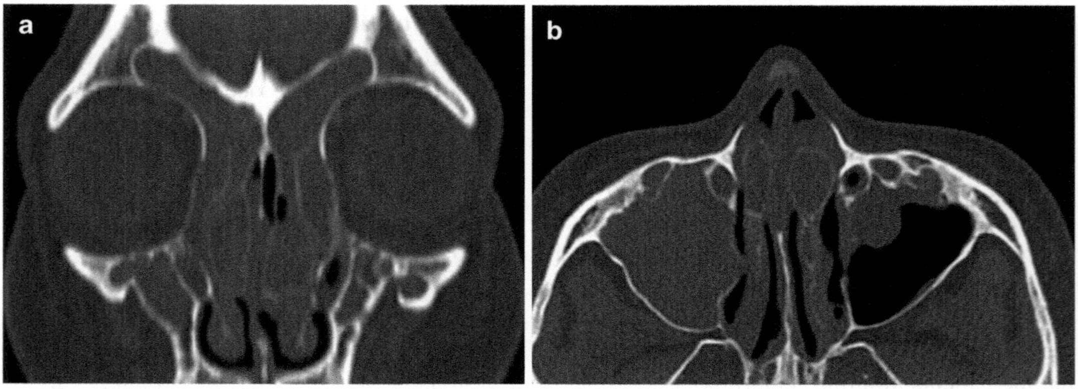

Fig. 5.3 Severe concha bullosa of the bilateral middle turbinate. (**a**) The frontal sinusitis is accompanied. (**b**) Middle turbinate concha bullosa with Rt. maxillary sinusitis and Lt. maxillary polyp

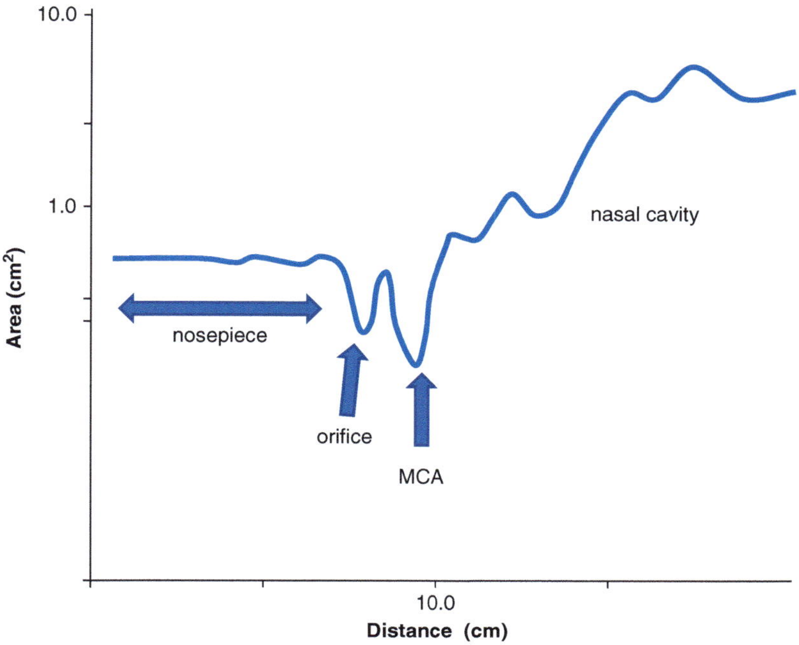

Fig. 5.4 AR: acoustic rhinometry: From the external nares, MCA exists (minimal cross-sectional area). Usually, the point is the most narrow internal valve. The picture on the left and right may change, but in general, it is interpreted as the width versus depth, the left vs. right sides, and before vs. after decongestion

ent from the findings of intranasal adhesion of the right nasal cavity. In the patient's AR, it can be found that the MCA on the left is located more anteriorly (Fig. 5.5). Since the slope of the peak is also steep in the left, it is judged that there will be more turbulence. What looks like and what the patient feels is often quite different.

Causes of Nasal Obstruction after Surgery

Intranasal Adhesion

Intranasal adhesion occurs when there is a slight wound after packing inside the nose and sticks to each other. This is the reason why gauze is not preferred as a material for nasal packing. If possible, using a more smooth surface or the recently preferred dissolving nasal packing material is a way to prevent this unwanted intranasal adhesion [13]. The author prefers Nasopore (Stryker Corporation, Kalamazoo, MI) because it has less bleeding, can be removed by suction after surgery, and results in relatively less mucosa bleeding. Severe intranasal adhesion found before surgery can be easily separated using a sharp freer elevator. At this time, the surgeon only needs to be careful with septal mucosal perforation (Fig. 5.6).

Neglected Preoperative Septal Deviation

Patients who had a septal deviation before surgery increase their concavity when heavy implants are placed at the dorsum. The cause may be due to gravity or the pressure of the tight pocket. Therefore, if the surgeon does not want the unexpected complaint of postoperative nasal obstruction, it is necessary to actively pay attention to the septum's concavity and convexity before surgery. If harvesting cartilage is required, submucosal resection inevitably leads to the weakening of the caudal septum. Therefore, it can be more easily transformed.

Aggravated Caudal Septal Deviation

Patients in the post-SMR state have a weak L-strut. At this time, the pressure applied from the implant in the tight soft tissue pocket worsens the septum's deviation. Above is a typical cause of nasal obstruction that can be seen after the Asian septorhinoplasty using implants. This situ-

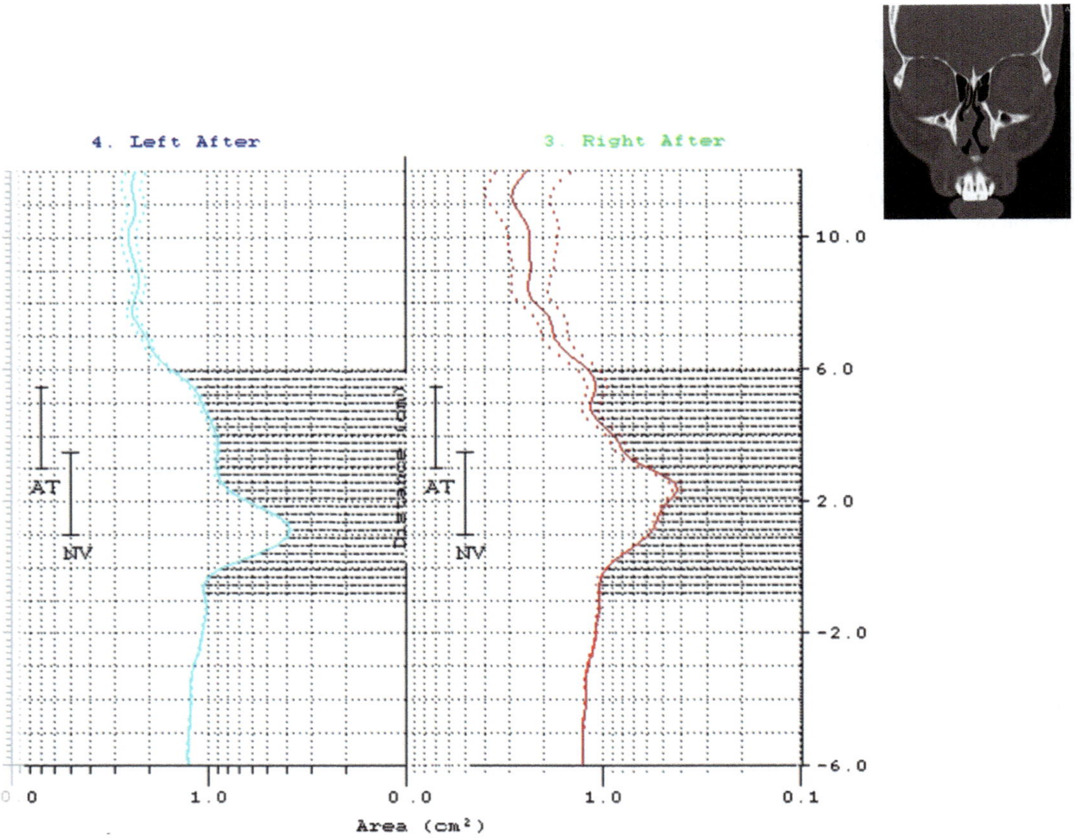

Fig. 5.5 The AR shows more anterior MCA of the left side. This is different from the findings seen on CT

ation is the most significant cause of functional deterioration and narrowing the internal nasal valve (INV).

Case Study

A 30-year-old male underwent septorhinoplasty with corrective osteotomy with the dorsal Gore-tex at another hospital 5 years before. The nasal obstruction was not severe before the operation, but after the operation, the left side became severely obstructed, and a headache occurred. A septum's convexity to the left was found in the nasoscope. The convexity of the left nasal septum was found even after decongestion. When the caudal septum was pushed with nasoscope, it recoiled again. Since the membranous septum exists, it was found that the septal extension graft was not performed (Video 5.2).

It is most important to find the caudal septum between the LLC in the middle of the surgical field, and it can be found that the convexity of the left side increases as the pocket overriding the caudal septum becomes tighter. The surgery was to securely place the caudal septum on ANS in the mid-center. Using a folded cymba concha, tongue in groove type reinforcement was performed to obtain the caudal septum's straightness (Video 5.3).

After the operation, the nasal obstruction was resolved, and the patient's headache also improved. These are the findings of the endo-

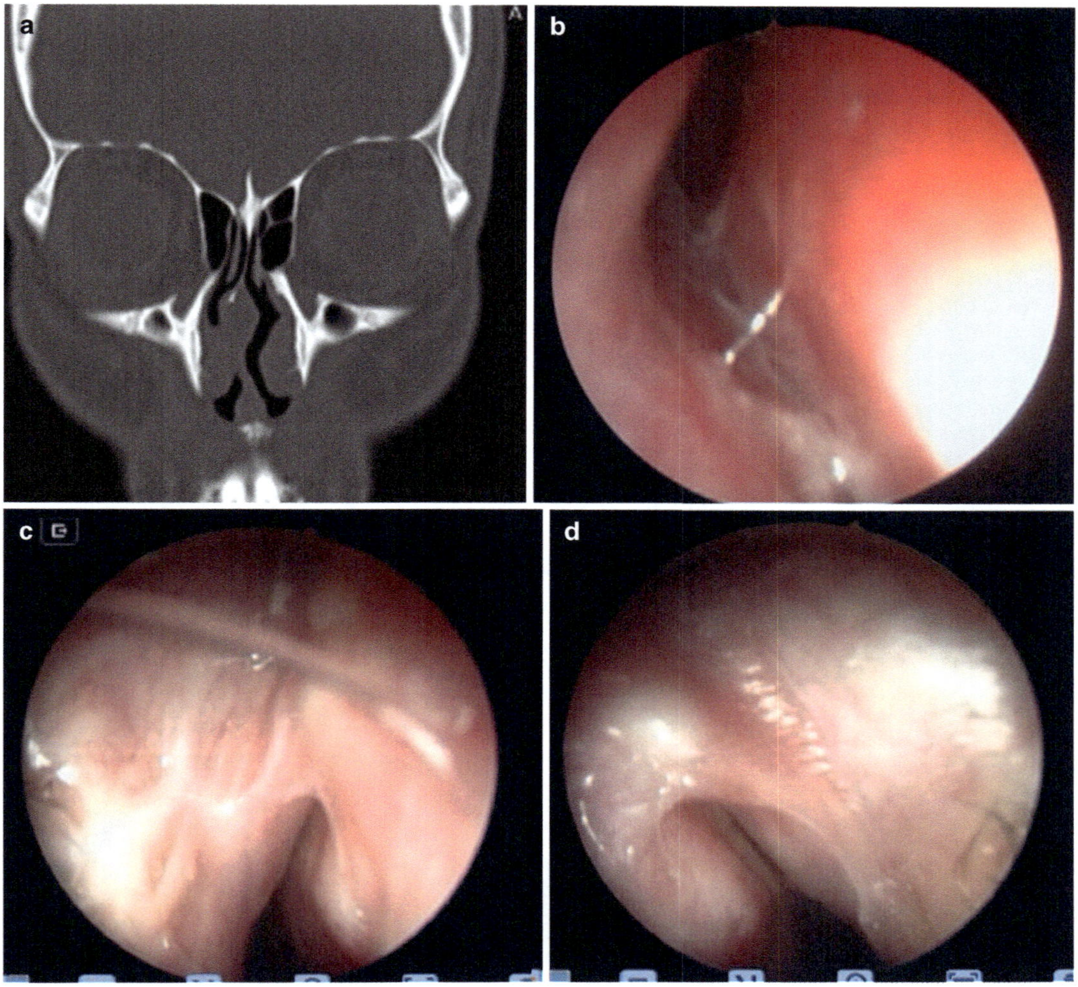

Fig. 5.6 Intranasal adhesion (**a**) CT shows Rt. side inferior turbinate attached to the septum. (**b**) The endoscopic view of the attached site was contacting and healing with each other. (**c**) The shape of Rt. the internal valve was acute, and there was synechia. (**d**) The attachment was found in the Lt. side internal nasal valve

scope after 2 years. NOSE scale also improved from 15/20 to 5/20 (Fig. 5.7).

Implant Instability over Weak Nasal Framework

Inserting the alloplastic implant into the nasal dorsum after corrective osteotomy, including the lateral osteotomy, delivers pressure to the nasal framework below, and the sinking implant can press INV.

Dorsal implanting requires the presence of a supportive cartilaginous framework. If the anterocaudal septal support is weak, the implant is easy to deviate to one side (Figs. 5.8 and 5.9). When the dorsal implant presses the INV, the INV on the pressed side or the opposite side nar-

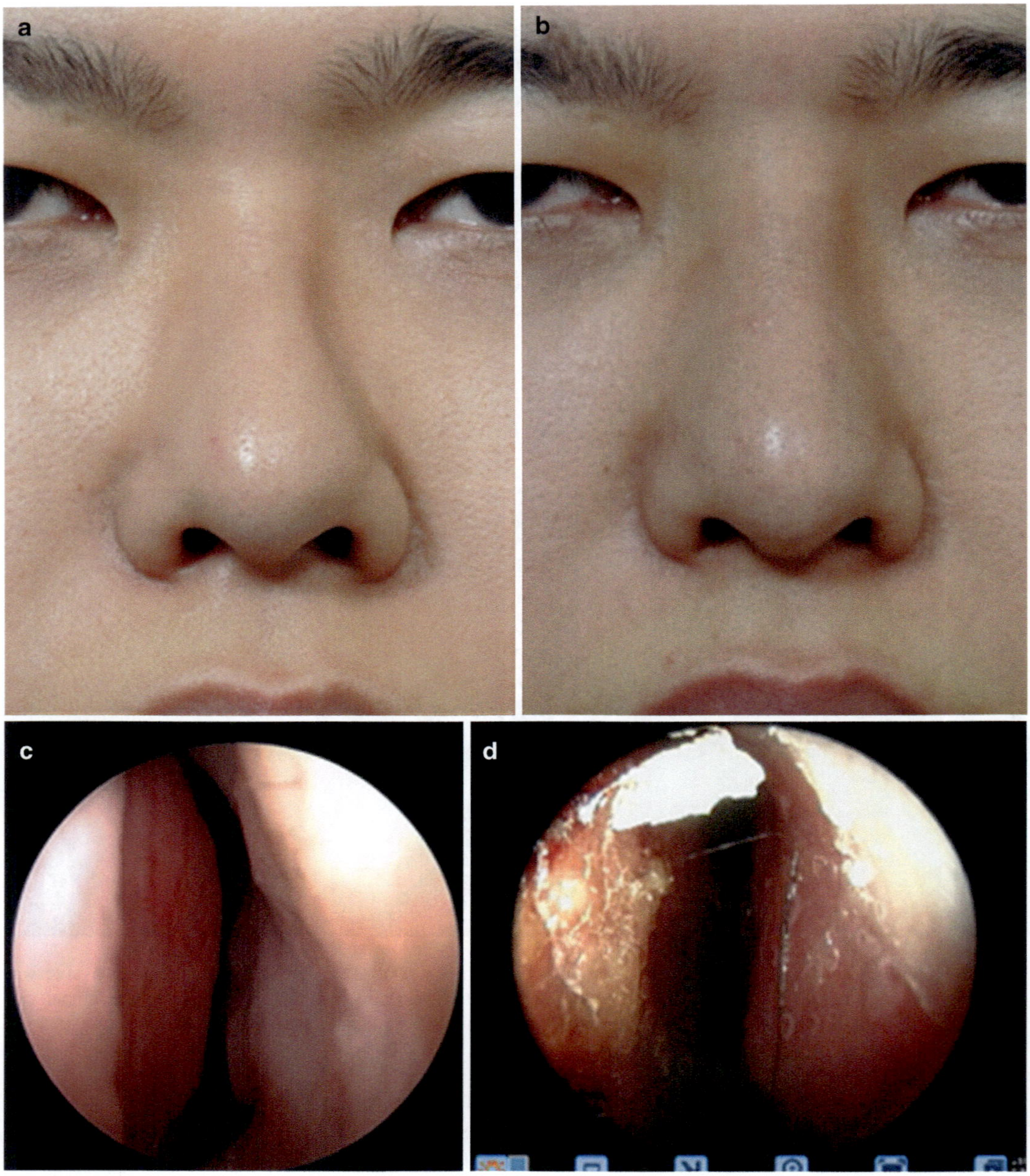

Fig. 5.7 Pre- and postoperative changes. (**a**) Preoperative AP view. (**b**) Postoperative AP view. (**c**) Preoperative Lt. nasal cavity. (**d**) Postoperative Lt. nasal cavity

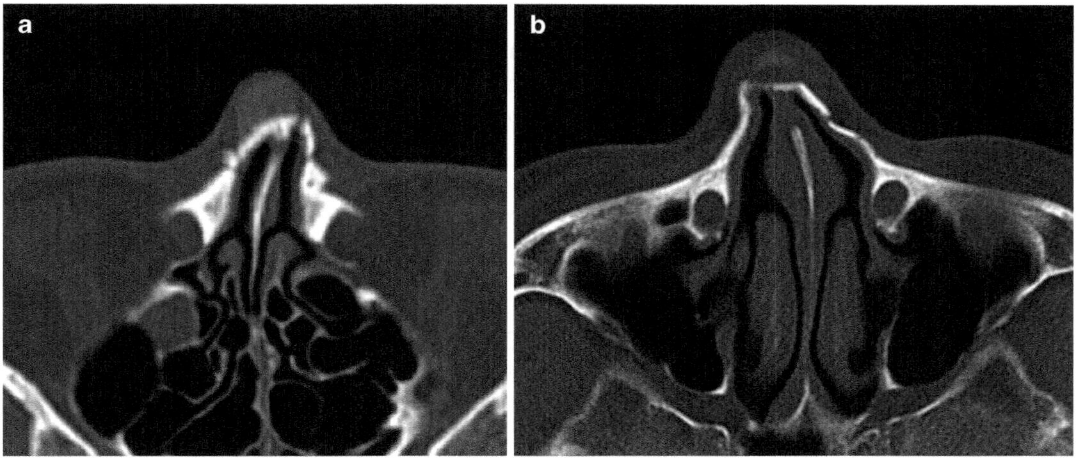

Fig. 5.8 Implant sinking on the unstable lateral wall was found. (**a**) Rt. lateral wall sinking. (**b**) Lt. lateral wall sinking

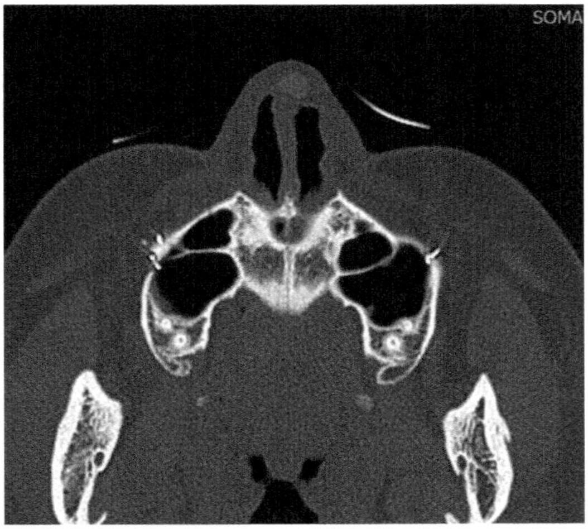

Fig. 5.9 Implant sinking on the Lt. side of ULC and INV was found. But this patient complained Rt. side nasal obstruction

rows, so it is necessary to observe what symptoms occurred in each situation.

Internal Valve Problem

Asian INV is characterized by pinching or a step ladder deformity after excessive tip projection or dorsal augmentation surgery. Most of them are not aware of an obstructive nose before surgery but the symptom aggravates after the surgery.

Patients tend to become hypersensitive to deteriorated nasal airways.

It is difficult to prove the association of nasal obstruction after surgery because meta-analysis for nasal obstruction after esthetic rhinoplasty is still insufficient.

Not all surgery will improve the symptoms, and it is essential to decide on the strategy after several interviews and long follow-ups. Surgery suitable for each cause should be chosen, and a careful surgical method should be determined after the diagnostic modalities mentioned above.

5.2 "The Tip Extension Anchoring (Suture)" Pushes down the INV

The method for stiffly anchoring lateral crus to get the tip projection excessively can have a harmful effect, which pushes down the INV when repairing above the high septum (Fig. 5.10).

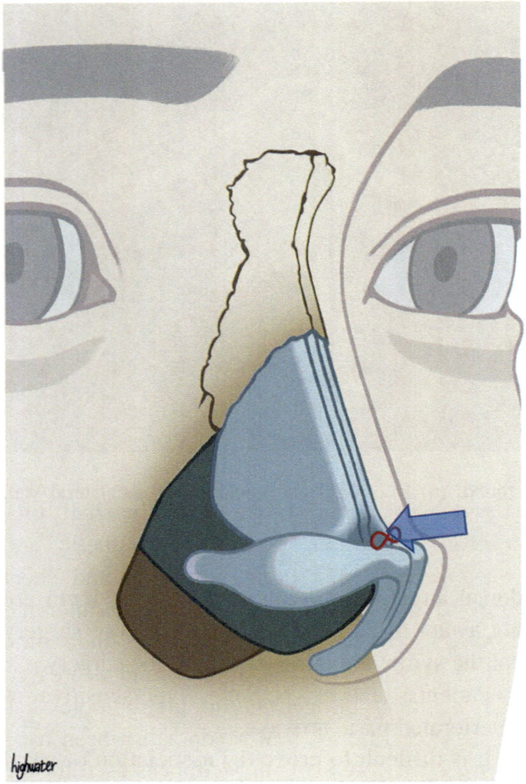

Fig. 5.10 Tip extension anchoring (suture) pushes down the INV and results in step ladder deformity

– "exaggerated tip extension anchoring (suture)" pushes down the INV.

It should be borne in mind that surgery for only the tip's projection can be a factor that degrades the entire nasal function. Most Asian rhinoplasty only pays attention to the tip's projection, and the dorsum is, of course, considered to be solved with a simple graft or alloplastic implant. Some surgeons do excessive medialization of the lateral crus for the tip projection without maintaining the angle between the long axis of the lateral crus. It has also been discovered that the long axis is located almost parallel.

For treatment, a method for increasing the height of the high septum itself should be performed by turning down the lateral crus's long axis by doing the entire tip plasty again and inserting a lateral crural spanning graft. This will be discussed again in Chap. 8.

If the anterior septum does not support the LLC, a strong force is applied to the scroll area. Moreover, the depression of INV occurs. Even if a dorsal implant is put in here, the depression will be overwhelmed.

Case Study: Exaggerated Tip by "The Tip Extension Anchoring (Suture)"

A 28-year-old female patient complained of a bulbous tip, alar flaring, and low nasal tip primarily underwent septorhinoplasty 2 months before at another clinic. SMR and right cavum concha and 3 mm silicone were used. The tip extension suture, dorsal augmentation, and alar reduction were done for the shaping. The patient complained of severe nasal obstruction and pain every time she breathed. In particular, she felt the right side tightening every time. In the surgical records, tip extension suture and derotation graft were performed for the tip projection, and the height of the tip was slightly lowered at the hospital immediately after the operation. However, she complained that nasal obstruction became more severe. She brought the pre- and postoperative CT scans. The nasal cavity was found narrowed a lot after the surgery. The INV angle is also much smaller. However, the biggest change was that the INV entrance from the external nares was abruptly lowered with a step ladder deformity (Fig. 5.11). The MCA was correlated with this deformity (Video 5.4). Although it is said that 3-mm silicone is inserted into the patient's dorsum, the cause of the sudden narrowing of the INV can be predicted that excessive tip extension anchoring occurred by pressing the upper lateral cartilage, considering the decrease in the INV angle and the increase in the tip projection.

Endoscopy: It can be seen as a typical acute angle at INV, but what stands out is that its relative position is low. However, the external dorsal

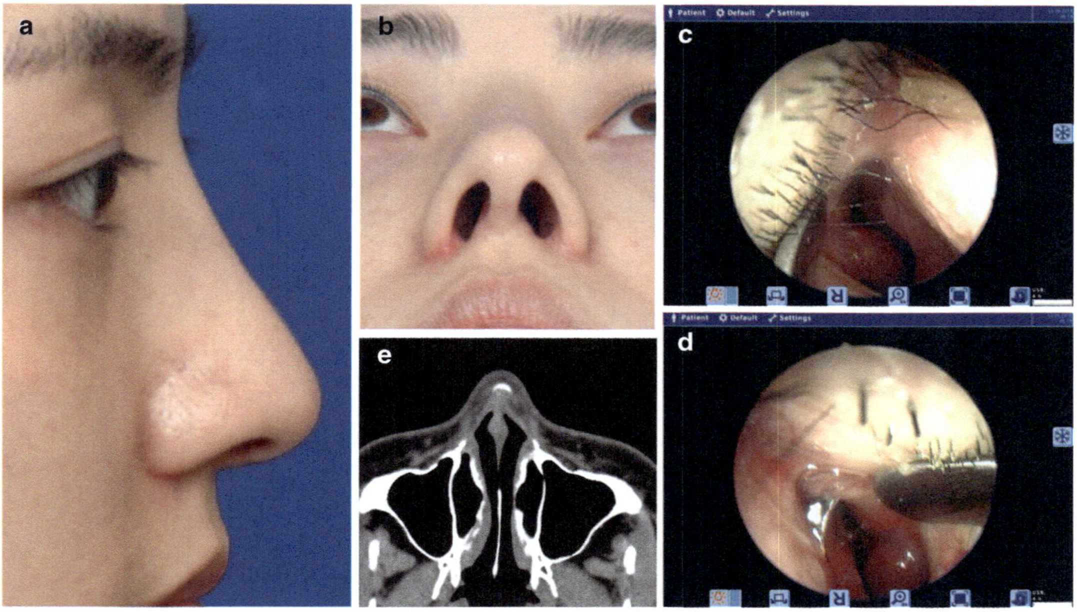

Fig. 5.11 Patient with severe nasal obstruction after septorhinoplasty: tip extension suture, derotation graft using ear cartilage, and dorsal 3 mm silicone and SMR were performed. (**a**) Postoperative lateral view. (**b**) Postoperative basal view. (**c**) Right INV angle was unfolded using a freer elevator for the inspection. (**d**) Left INV angle was unfolded for the inspection. (**e**) The nasal cavity was wide and patent without any turbinate problems

profile is smooth and high, so it can be assumed that LLC excessively projected the tip then the dorsum was augmented accordingly. Since it is only 2 months after surgery, surgery to increase the MCA in the INV area is necessary for sufficient observations.

AR: The MCA at the INV site decreased in the same way on the left and right, and the MCA on the right and left was the same. The patient complained more of obstruction on the right side (Fig. 5.12).

5.3 Aggravated Tip-Middle Vault Airway Discrepancy

As it happens in connection with the above concept, it cannot be distinguished. To respond to the tip's projection, too much a dorsal graft or thick alloplastic implant is inserted, which also affects pressing INV. This is a phenomenon that occurs during dorsal augmentation. However, in some cases, there is a phenomenon that the INV angle becomes more obtuse, thereby solving nasal obstruction. The case by case of the patient needs to be followed, and the method of resolution will differently depend on the cause.

– If the nasal framework is weak, the dorsal alloplastic implants or thick dermis graft may destroy the INV's healthy angle (Fig. 5.13).

Case Study: Too Heavy Dorsal Graft

A 45-year-old female underwent rhinoplasty 25 years ago, and 20 years ago, after failing two silicone surgeries, she underwent rhinoplasty with Gore-tex and Medpor 17 years ago. After that, nasal discharge started to appear recently, and all were removed. In addition, a dermofat graft was performed at another hospital.

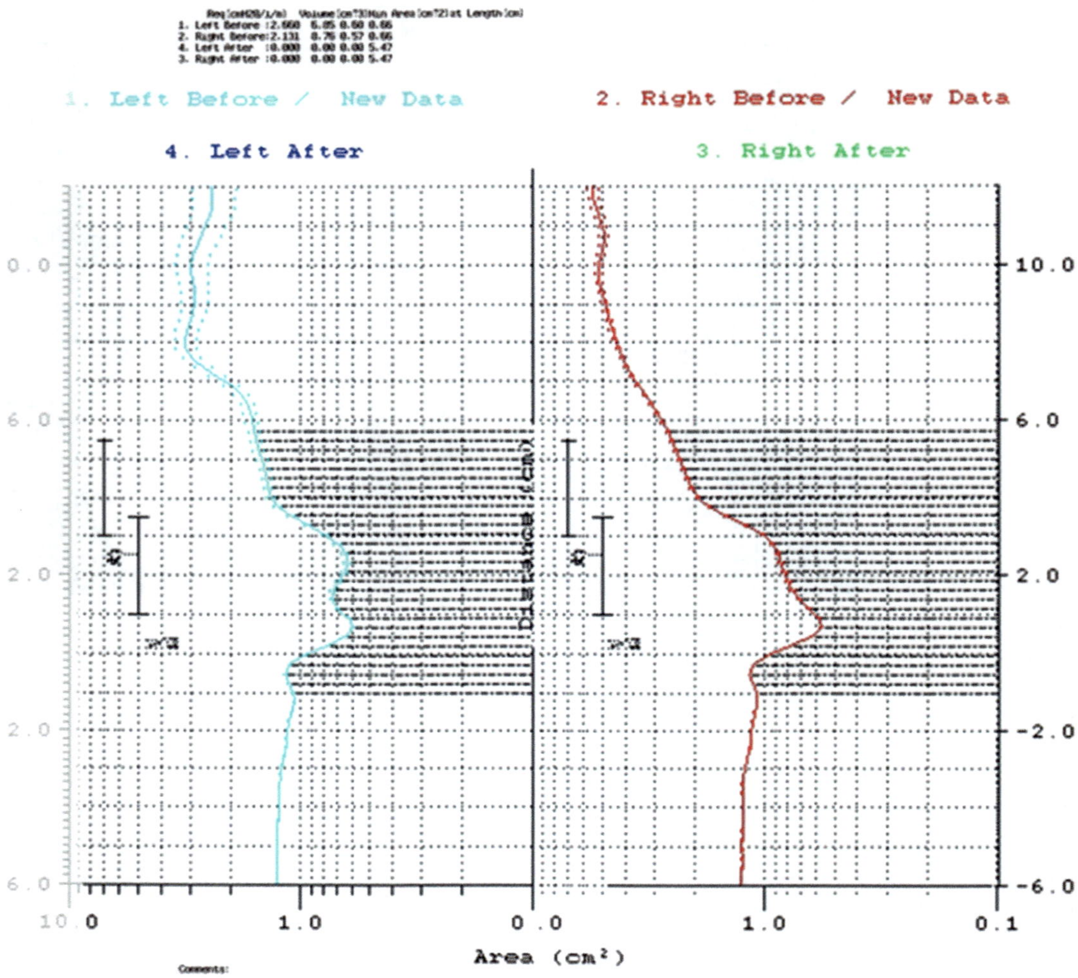

Fig. 5.12 AR showed MCA in the bilateral INV areas. Right side INV showed a stiffer notch

However, after the recent surgery, the nasal tip's asymmetry was revised 2 weeks later, and the ear cartilage batten graft inserted in the nasal tip was adjusted. At the time of referral, she was appealing for severe nasal obstruction. An excessive amount of dorsal graft was found in the pre- and postoperative axial views of CT. Since the recent surgery is dermofat, it is predicted that it will be absorbed for more than a year in the future, so the continuous observation is necessary, and if no improvement in symptoms, surgical intervention will be required. It cannot be said that the amount of the dermis is too much. The author believes that this would have been done because a large amount of absorption was expected.

Endoscopy: Severe bulging was found in the INV site ceiling, which was a dermofat graft inserted into the nasal dorsum (Fig. 5.14).

CT: When comparing the pre- and postoperative conditions, the Medpor was removed, and

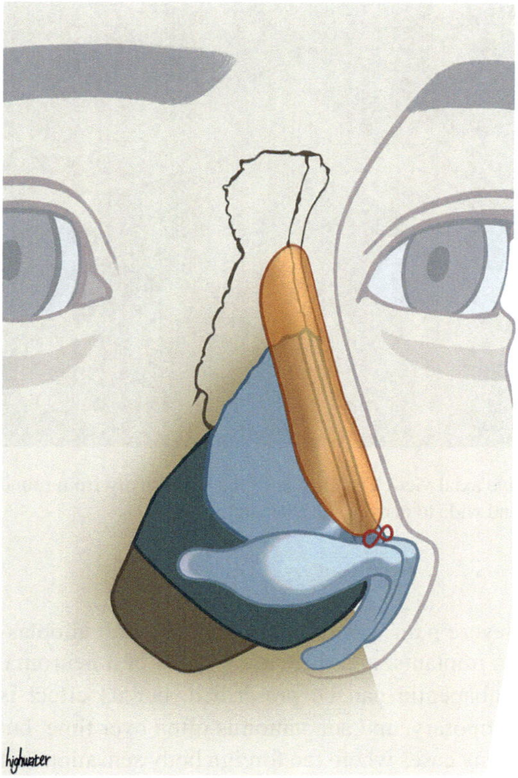

Fig. 5.13 Tip extension anchoring with dorsal onlay implant pushes down the INV and results in step ladder deformity

the ear cartilage was applied. The thickness of the dorsal graft in the INV area was increased (Video 5.5).

The dorsal contour's shape has improved with a dermofat graft, and this operation cannot be said to be wrong. I believe this would have been done because a large amount of absorption was expected.

5.4 Too Narrow INV Angle

The INV angle is too narrow, it is also related to excessive tip projection, and it can be assumed that it occurred as a result of excessive tip extension anchoring for tip projection and applying a strong strut to the tip. INV angle is less than 15°. This is the case of a typical spring graft indicated (Fig. 5.15).

Thickened Caudal Septum

When the graft applied to the columella is thick, MCA occurs from external nares before reaching INV. Therefore, care must be taken when applying rib cartilage or ear cartilage.

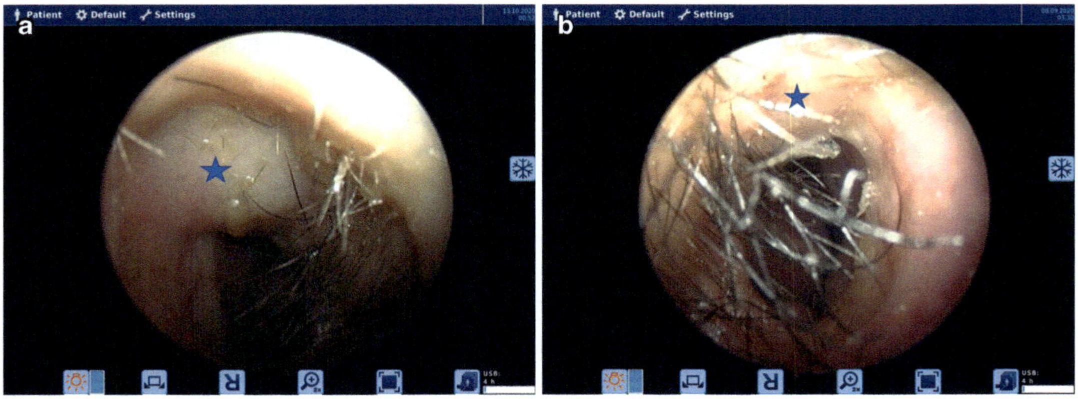

Fig. 5.14 The roof of the INV area was bulged down (the star mark), and the MCA notch was found here bilaterally. (**a**) Left side INV. (**b**) Right side INV

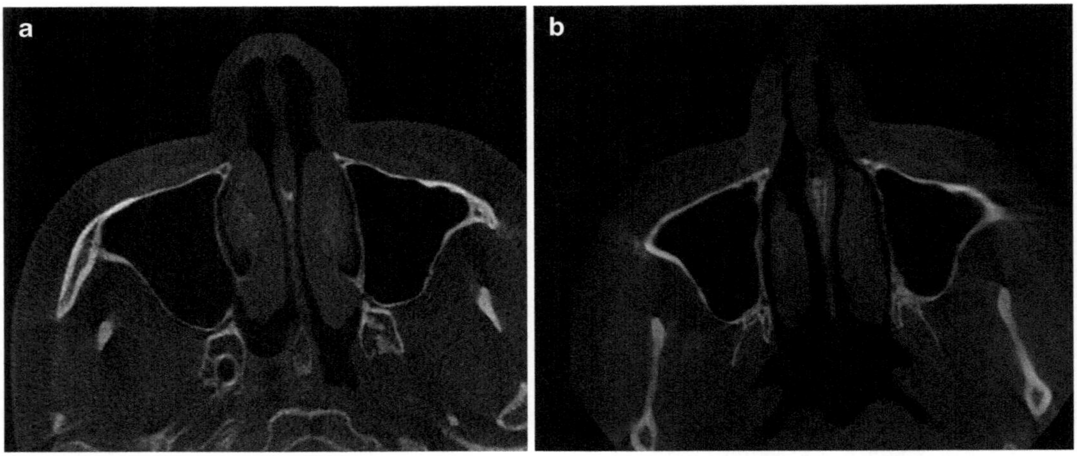

Fig. 5.15 Severe nasal obstruction after septorhinoplasty with tip extension suture and derotation graft without the dorsal implant. (**a**) Preoperative axial view. (**b**) Postoperative axial view. The change of the nasal cavity from round and wide to narrow and stiff angle

Unlike Westerners, Asians have alar flaring so that they can be relatively free from this problem. Even with severely thick columellar grafts, we can find cases where the nasal obstruction has not complained.

In the author's case, a folded cymba concha was applied to the caudal septum, and nasal obstruction complaints were found in patients with graft tilting, but there was no problem due to the thickening.

Other Combined Symptoms with Nasal Obstruction

Nasal Pain

Many Medpor users complain of nasal pain. It is proportional to the degree of stiffness at the tip of the nose, and pain when breathing should be compared with the resting pain. Sometimes it is associated with chronic nasal pain and rhinogenic headache, sometimes without.

In the case of patients who have undergone multiple surgeries, it is unknown when the pain begins. Of course, it is reported that 100% of the sensory of the skin flap returns over time [14], but in patients with more than four surgeries, the recovery is slow, and there are many cases of complaining of abnormal sensations. Severe pain was found in patients with alloplastic implants, and there were cases of a neuroma. Gabapentin can be prescribed, but its effect is temporary, and adaptation is often over time, but many cases where the foreign body sensation that has occurred once does not disappear. CT scans should be used to differentiate from pain such as rhinogenic headache, and reoperation should be selected depending on whether pain around the eyes, nasal dorsum, or tip pain.

In severe pain, the authors found that most of the cases in which Medpor was used, which is sensitive to micromovement due to strong tissue integration, and it is judged that the harness causes pain. It can be found that the pain decreases when switching to autograft.

Foul Odor

Many patients complain of a strange odor from the inside of the nose. It can be detected in patients with exaggerated transdermal suture for tip projection or acute middle to lateral crural angle. This can be found when nasal secretions or crusts are trapped between vestibules and produce foul odors or in cases where non-absorbable sutures are sometimes protruded from the tip to show local chronic inflammation. It is not the peculiar smell of chronic nasal obstruction or chronic sinusitis. It is recommended to clean the nasal tip frequently with water. If pinching is severe, securing the space under the middle crural medial crus or soft triangle of LLC reduces crust and sometimes improves symptoms.

References

1. Andre RF, Vuyk HD, Ahmed A, Graamans K, Nolst Trenité GJ. Correlation between subjective and objective evaluation of the nasal airway. A systematic review of the highest level of evidence. Clin Otolaryngol. 2009;34(6):518–25.
2. Kim CS, Moon BK, Jung DH, Min YG. Correlation between nasal obstruction symptoms and objective parameters of acoustic rhinometry and rhinomanometry. Auris Nasus Larynx. 1998;25(1):45–8.
3. Andrews PJ, Choudhury N, Takhar A, Poirrier AL, Jacques T, Randhawa PS. The need for an objective measure in septorhinoplasty surgery: are we any closer to finding an answer? Clin Otolaryngol. 2015;40(6):698–703.
4. Dadgarnia MH, Baradaranfar MH, Mazidi M, Azimi Meibodi SMR. Assessment of septoplasty effectiveness using acoustic rhinometry and rhinomanometry. Iran J Otorhinolaryngol. 2013;25(71):71–8.
5. Stewart MG, Witsell DL, Smith TL, Weaver EM, Yueh B, Hannley MT. Development and validation of the nasal obstruction symptom evaluation (NOSE) scale. Otolaryngol Head Neck Surg. 2004;130(2):157–63.
6. Kahana-Zweig R, Geva-Sagiv M, Weissbrod A, Secundo L, Soroker N, Sobel N. Measuring and characterizing the human nasal cycle. PLoS One. 2016;11(10):e0162918.
7. Suh JD, Kennedy DW. Treatment options for chronic rhinosinusitis. Proc Am Thorac Soc. 2011;8(1):132–40.
8. Lanza DC, Kennedy DW. Adult rhinosinusitis defined. Otolaryngol Head Neck Surg. 1997;117(3 Pt 2):S1–7.
9. Suh M-W, Jin H-R, Kim J-H. Computed tomography versus nasal endoscopy for the measurement of the internal nasal valve angle in Asians. Acta Otolaryngol. 2008;128(6):675–9.
10. Roithmann R, Cole P, Chapnik J, Shpirer I, Hoffstein V, Zamel N. Acoustic rhinometry in the evaluation of nasal obstruction. Laryngoscope. 1995;105(3 Pt 1):275–81.
11. Krouse J, Lund V, Fokkens W, Meltzer EO. Diagnostic strategies in nasal congestion. Int J Gen Med. 2010;3:59–67.
12. Daele JJ, Leruth E, Goffart Y. Consensus in rhinoplasty. B-ENT. 2010;6(Suppl 15):109–13.
13. Wang J, Cai C, Wang S. Merocel versus Nasopore for nasal packing: a meta-analysis of randomized controlled trials. PLoS One. 2014;9(4):e93959.
14. Bafaqeeh SA, al-Qattan MM. Alterations in nasal sensibility following open rhinoplasty. Br J Plast Surg. 1998;51(7):508–10.

6 The Various Preparations of Autologous Materials

Pearls
- Ear cartilage is the best donor cartilage that can be used with alloplastic dorsal implants.
- If enough cymba concha and cavum concha are collected from one ear, then L-Strut covering the anterior septum and caudal septum can be made.
- Deformity of the ear can be prevented by leaving a cartilage of 5 mm gap between cymba and cavum.
- Before collecting ear cartilage, a dental impression putty is used to make an embossed molding of the ear and prepare it.
- Conchal cartilage without perichondrium is brittle and fragile.
- The perichondrium on one side of the ear cartilage must be attached to the cartilage.
- The perichondrium on one side of the ear cartilage must be preserved in the skin flap.
- The superficial mastoid fascia (SMF) is not thick, but it comes out in a sufficient amount for use with a nasal tip, and it can be folded for dorsal augmentation.
- The consensus of doctors who do much dermal graft is that the dermis is absorbed until postoperative 12–18 months.
- When the absorption is considered, the dermal part is used as a double or triple layer, and the fat part is rarely used.
- If dorsal skin is too thin, a little fatty layer should be attached to the dermis. The fatty side is placed directly under the thin skin. It is suitable for shaping.
- When using sacral dermis-fat (SDF), if the fat layer is located outside the pocket, the graft appears less demarcated due to the tissue's characteristics.
- The thick SDF may appear demarcated under thin dorsal skin.

6.1 Auricular Cartilage

When cartilage graft is required in patients who do not require septal surgery, ear cartilage is the most preferred donor site in Asian rhinoplasty due to its elasticity and sufficient amount.

- In patients who do not require septoplasty, there are cases of SMR performed because of the need. In Asian rhinoplasty, this is not the best option with the dorsal alloplastic implants.
- Ear cartilage is the best donor site that can be harvested with dorsal implants.
- Surgeons who feel burdened with septal surgery should be familiar with the wise use of ear cartilage.

Supplementary Information The online version of this chapter (https://doi.org/10.1007/978-981-16-0542-0_6) contains supplementary material, which is available to authorized users.

E.-S. Dhong, M.-W. Na, *Asian Septorhinoplasty*, https://doi.org/10.1007/978-981-16-0542-0_6

Ear cartilage is the most used material in Asian rhinoplasty. It is because the septum is smaller and pliable than the Western or because more cartilage is needed after the septal cartilage is harvested. If a cartilage graft is needed in patients who do not require septal surgery, ear cartilage is the preferred donor site due to its elasticity and sufficient amount. It can be easily prepared in the same surgical field of view, so it is easy to collect, and it can be used as needed before and during surgery, and there is a donor part on the left and right. The width of the ear covering the cymba conchal cartilage was found to be 30.5 mm in African women, 32.5 mm for African men in a morphological study of 100 volunteers [1]. A study using facial computed tomography images (mid-sagittal view) of 200 Koreans reported that the mean boundary of the cartilaginous septum was 818 mm^2 [2]. Therefore, if the conchal cartilage can be harvested as much as possible without deformation of the donor site, the physical dimensions of conchal cartilage are theoretically large enough and similar to the septal cartilage. To harvest the maximum amount, Han et al. introduced a surgical technique with minimal donor site morbidity, the average size of cymba and cavum is 155.7 mm^2 and 210.2 mm^2, respectively. They could harvest the maximal amount without contour collapse leaving a helical crus of at least 5 mm [3].

However, clinically, some surgeons harvest all cymba and cavum without leaving the intermediate bridge cartilage, and depending on the situation, it can be found that patients do not complain (Fig. 6.1). Even though 5 mm bridge is left, hypertrophic and ugly scars can be created and depending on the patient's character, deformity of the ear may have complained (Fig. 6.2). The cause for the ugly scar will be covered in detail in the dissection, but the author thinks it depends on whether the perichondrium of cartilage is left or sacrificed. The author thinks that deformity can be reduced by leaving either of the perichondrium attached to one side's skin flap.

- When collecting ear cartilage, it is recommended to preserve the perichondrium on the anterior side by attaching it to the skin.
- The cartilage is harvested with the perichondrium attached on the posterior side.

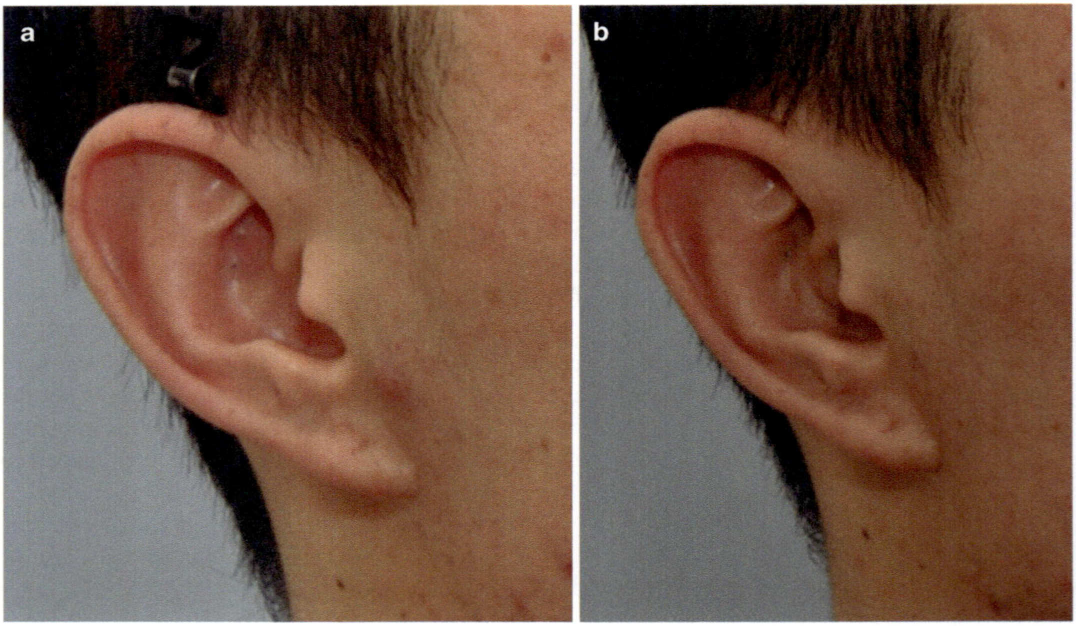

Fig. 6.1 The postoperative appearance of all patients, without the bridge between the cymba and the cavum concha, but this is not recommended. (**a**) Preoperative view. (**b**) Postoperative view

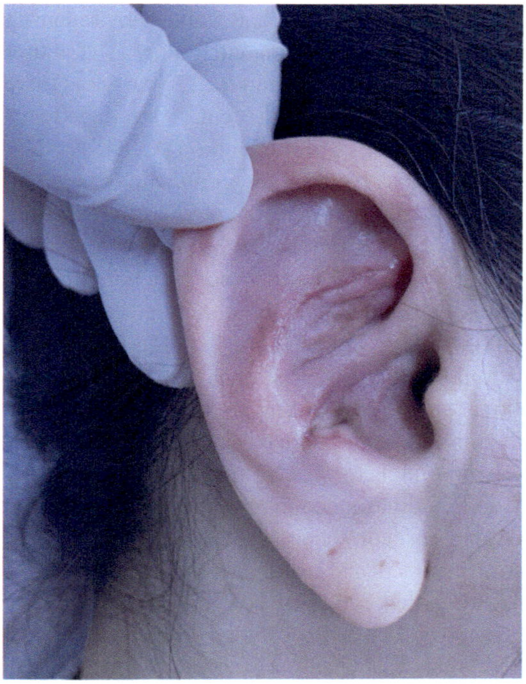

Fig. 6.2 Ugly scars; The middle bridge between the cymba concha and the cavum concha was left 5 mm, but the ugly scar remained; Both side perichondrium was harvested attached to the cartilage; the skin flap contractured after surgery

- This contributes to the stability of the skin flap on one side and the ear cartilage's stability on the other.
- If enough cymba concha and cavum concha are collected from one ear, then L-Strut covering the anterior and caudal septum can be made.

Dissection

There are two approaches for cartilage harvesting anterior incision and posterior incision. Few studies have reported on the occurrence of complications according to incision sites. Studies revealed only about the keloid or infection rate of the donor site after ear cartilage collection [4].

The author prefers the anterior approach from a direct view. According to the surgeon's skill, a posteriorly approach method leaves less scars. However, it is easy to collect the maximal width and length to separate the concavity side of the ear cartilage.

A solution containing 0.5% bupivacaine, epinephrine (1: 100,000), and hyaluronidase (50 units/100 mL) was injected at the anterior harvest site for vasoconstriction and hydrodissection. To obtain the maximum length, incisions were made as long as possible along the lower boundary of the antihelix without crossing the scaphoid. While uncovering the skin envelope, subperichondrial detachment was continued between the anterior circumcised skin and cartilage to the desired size. The antihelix and 5 mm bridge between cymba and cavum concha were preserved. The posterior skin was similarly dissected, and the posterior perichondrium was harvested and attached to the cymba concha. Then, the cavum concha was dissected in the same manner. The incision was made anteriorly at the lower border of the cavum concha. Like cymba concha, perichondrium was preserved and attached to the anterior skin.

6.2 Must Do and Must Not Do

Deformity of the ear can be prevented by leaving a cartilage of 5 mm gap between cymba and cavum concha. Collecting the entire cymba and cavum without an intermediate cartilage bridge can deform the ear width later. However, if the perichondrium is adequately preserved, there are cases where there is no significant deformity left, so choose according to the surgeon's confidence. Initially, the author preserved the anterior perichondrium attached to the skin, and then the cartilage was harvested. However, all perichondrium was attached to the cartilage for about 3 years after attending a fellow doctor's presentation. As a result, many patients complained of severe scars during follow-up. The author hopes that readers do not commit the mistake of listening to others and changing your own beliefs. It is impossible to trust 100% of the content that others are presenting, and the presentation without a published thesis is just an empty story.

- After cartilage harvesting, the patient needs to wear an auxiliary molding for an extended time to maintain the cymba and cavum's concavity.
- Before harvesting, a dental impression putty is used to make an embossed ear model and prepare it.
- The ear embossing model is worn for more than a month after surgery.
- The perichondrium on one side of the ear cartilage must be attached to the cartilage.
- Conchal cartilage without perichondrium is brittle and fragile.
- The perichondrium on one side of the ear cartilage must be attached to the cartilage.
- The perichondrium on one side of the ear cartilage must be preserved in the skin flap.
- If perichondrium is collected from both sides, contracture of skin flap may occur.

The author uses 3M™ Express™ VPS Bite Registration Material Putty (3M, Korea) to prepare an embossed model by putting it in the ear before surgery, preparing it in sterilization in advance then applying it immediately after sealing the skin for simple dressing. Instead of this method, concavity can be maintained by tie-over dressing for 4–5 days using a bolster suture, but since it is necessary to maintain steady concavity for more than 1 month after surgery, the author uses a putty orthosis. Be careful as excessive pressure can cause pressure-sore of the skin flap.

6.3 Folded Concha: Is it Large and Stable Enough?

Folded Cymba and Cavum Concha Technique: Straightening and Stability

The biggest drawback of the conchal cartilage is its convolution and instability. The way to overcome these two points is to repair and use concavity or convexity sites [5]. Alternatively, there is a way to make the shape of the nose by using the curvature well. The author's preferred method is to obtain straightness and stability by repairing concavity sides by facing each other. The author has been using this method for 15 years, and there have been reports that recently introduced this method and the opposite method (face to face vs. back to back) [6]. For surgeons who have experienced folding directly, the method for repairing concave sides is more straightforward, and in the author's method, there is no perichondrium of this concave side, and the perichondrium is preserved on the opposite convex side. For this, it would be advantageous for the perichondrium to exist outside. For folding, 4–5 mm of cartilage in the middle can be folded without applying a longitudinal incision to obtain a more potent force. A longitudinal incision is applied to the top and bottom, except the center to obtain maximum straightness. The incision should be made in the direction that can obtain the straightest shape by observing the cartilage's shape (Fig. 6.3). Using a non-absorbable suture such as Prolene 5.0, the straightness can be obtained from 1–2 point repair at the folding point (Fig. 6.4 and Video 6.1).

Average Length and Width of Folded Cymba

The analysis of 311 intraoperative photographs of the harvested auricular cartilage revealed that

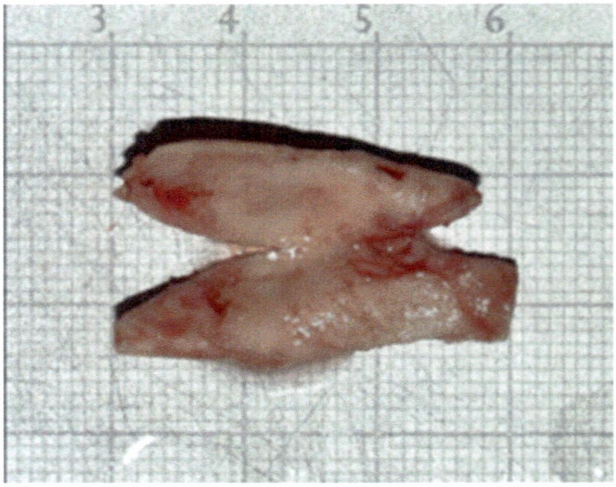

Fig. 6.3 Two longitudinal incisions were made to the mid-portion of cymba concha. More strength by folding can be achieved by leaving the middle portion

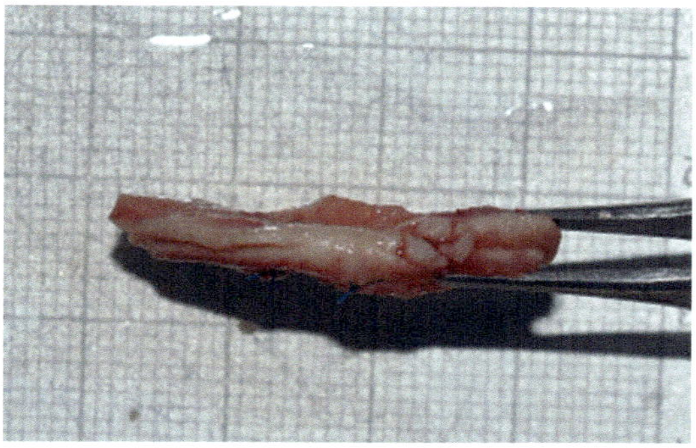

Fig. 6.4 Folded cymba concha

the mean (± SD) length of the folded cymba conchal cartilage was 24.2 ± 3.9 mm in men and 22.4 ± 3.7 mm in women. The mean width was 7.8 ± 1.9 mm in men and 7.2 ± 1.9 mm in women. This length and width are sufficient as the commonly used columella strut or spreader's length and width, making it a useful material. (data in publishing, Aesthetic surgery journal).

For Caudal Septal Extension Graft (CSEG)

Folded cymba concha or cavum concha has the advantage of being easy to apply to tongue-in-groove to anterior nasal spine (ANS) as its structural advantage.

Floating Type Columella Strut Graft

As a columellar strut, it can be used with a smaller width. That is, the maximal width mentioned above is not necessary. The authors do not prefer this method, only it is used as an auxiliary technique. The main reason is that the septal dissection is mandatory to support the caudal septum, so direct manipulation of the caudal septum is preferred. Strong coaptation between the posterior septum and ANS needs the tongue-in-groove technique. Columella strut is used as an auxiliary method.

Tongue-in-Groove Technique for CSEG

First, subperiosteal pockets were created on either side of the anterior nasal spine (ANS), leaving minimal soft tissue in the anterior pocket. While dividing both medial crura, the caudal septum was approached from ANS to the anterior septal angle, and at least 4–5 mm of the caudal edge was dissected in the subperichondrial plane. Any resection or correction of the caudal septum was performed before placing the folded concha. If necessary, a swing door procedure was performed to correct the septal tilt, and a figure of eight shaped suture was also applied between the posterior septal angle and the soft tissue part of ANS. Both columns of the folded conchal cartilage were inserted into the subperiosteal pocket with two or more transfixing sutures, and the folded cartilage was placed in the caudal septum as shown in the tongue-in-groove method [7] (Fig. 6.5). The horizontally contacted part of the conchal cartilage was sutured to the caudal septum.

Eventually, two points are under tongue-in-groove, one is ANS, and the other is the caudal septum. Various modifications are possible

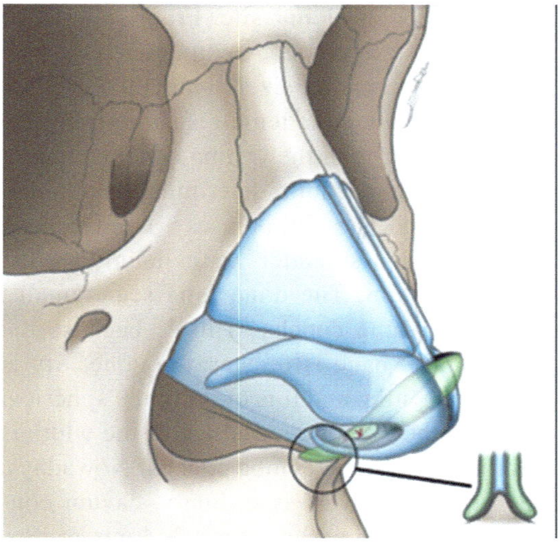

Fig. 6.5 Caudal septal extension graft: Inserting folded cymba concha by tongue-in-groove technique

depending on which part of the LLC and the CSEG tip to be repaired. When CSEG meets the anterior extended spreader graft (AESG), a de novo anterior septal angle can be created.

The Stability: Columellar Strut Vs. CSEG

To obtain the stability of the tip, the septal extension graft is more advantageous than the columella strut [8].

As mentioned earlier, the key factors determining the surgical method in Asian rhinoplasty are whether septoplasty is needed and whether alloplastic materials are used for the dorsum. Therefore, the degree of stability of the tip and the presence or absence of septal surgery are factors that determine whether to use the columella strut or CSEG. CSEG is preferred when strong tip support is required.

Cavum Concha

Along with cymba concha, cavum concha is also an excellent donor site. From experience in the anterior approach, cavum concha is harvested with a smaller size than cymba concha. If folding is done, the length is shorter, but the width is wider than the cymba concha. Taking this shape into account, determine the application location. The author uses cavum concha as an extended spreader graft, mainly on the anterior septum. The donor site scar remains less than cymba concha. This is because the tissue on the back is thicker, the concavity is relatively gentle, and it is close to the spherical shape, so the risk of contracture of the width is less than that of the cymba concha. Nowadays, when earphone wear is ordinary, cavum concha collection should preserve 3–4 mm to protect the orifice's margin that makes up external auditory meatus.

Tragal Cartilage

The third donor of the ear is tragal cartilage. This area can be accessed by retrotragal incision or incision using lateral margins. It has been reported that the size of 15 × 20 mm can be collected from here. Tragal cartilage has been used as flat cartilage [9].

However, it has no advantage over cymba or cavum concha because of the disadvantage that the amount of harvesting is less than the effort required for the incision. When the cartilage from all other places is used, it can be collected in a size of 10 × 15 mm [10]. There is no disagreement on the usefulness, a size of less than 10 mm is collected, and it also has a disadvantage in that the size is small because the marginal cartilage must be left in consideration of the inconvenience of ear phone users or projection of tragus.

The Superficial Mastoid Fascia (SMF)

The donors that can be collected for soft tissue transplantation are divided according to the dermis thickness. The thickest place is the sacral dermis, followed by the groin, but there is a disadvantage in that there is a hair-bearing. The author has also tried medial plantar but also prefers the thickest sacrum. However, there is a discomfort of having to prepare again, if necessary, during the operation. It will not be easy if the soft tissue is suddenly needed unless the operation is planned. The easiest way to access this is the superficial mastoid fascia, which is located behind the auricle [11].

Dissection

After injecting local anesthetics (0.5% marcaine, 1: 100,000 epinephrine, hyaluronidase 30 IU/mL), the area behind the ear is intended to raise a thin skin flap and leave most of the subcutaneous layer as the fascia layer. A 3–4 cm long incision made in the posterior

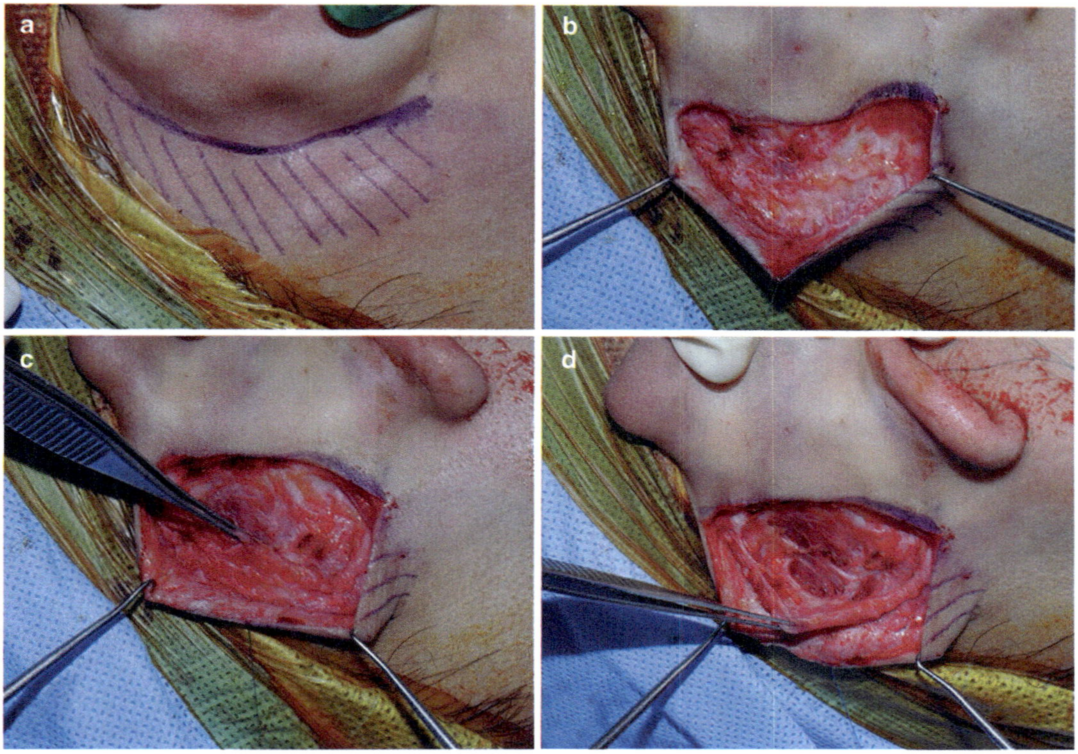

Fig. 6.6 Harvesting the superficial mastoid fascia; Clinical harvesting of the SMF from the right posterior auricular area. (**a**) Hydrodissection of the retroauricular area was done at the dashed area. (**b**) Thin skin flap measuring more than 1.0 cm wide was elevated. (**c**) Deeper dissection was performed into the incised site to find the retroauricular muscle. (**d**) The maximal SMF flap was elevated above the postauricular muscle. (Material from: Hong et al. Superficial mastoid fascia as an accessible donor for various augmentations in Asian rhinoplasty, Journal of Plastic Reconstructive & Aesthetic Surgery, 2012, Elsevier)

auricular circus placed a thin skin flap measuring a width of at least 1.0 cm. After raising the skin flap, a deeper incision is made in the incision site to locate the posterior auricular sulcus (Fig. 6.6). One or two bundles of posterior ear muscle fibers were easily found at the midpoint of the posterior incision (Fig. 6.7), and a full SMF flap was harvested over the posterior ear muscle (Fig. 6.8). The author considered this superficial subcutaneous layer of muscle as SMF. After the SMF was harvested, the skin flap was repositioned, Prolene 5.0 was used to close the incision, and a quilted suture and a light compression dressing were used to prevent hematoma (Video 6.2).

For Dorsal Augmentation

- The SMF is not thick, but it is a good material, and it comes out in a sufficient amount for use with a nasal tip, and it can be folded for dorsal augmentation (Fig. 6.9).

It is good to keep the volume by filling the diced cartilage inside the rolled SMF for more volume. Use a 1 cc syringe to seal the SMF around the periphery, and then remove the syringe and apply the space. It is a useful method of filling (Fig. 6.10). The cartilage should be minced finely. If transferring the cartilage is not easy, cut the syringe's front part to get the cartilage out.

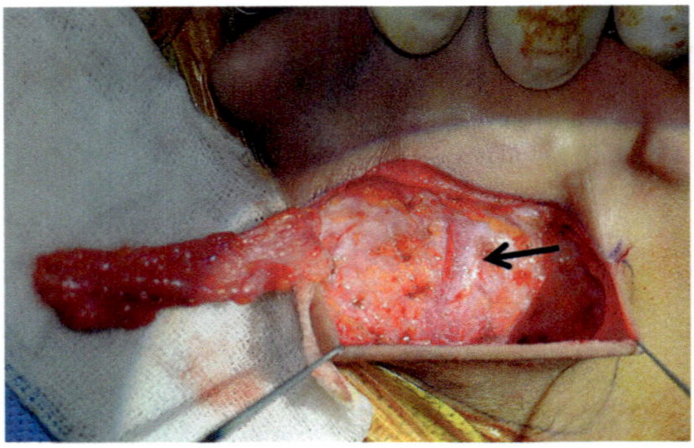

Fig. 6.7 Dissection plane and underlying posterior auricular muscle. At the midpoint of the posterior auriculocephalic sulcus, one bundle of posterior auricular muscle fibers was found (arrow). SMF flap was elevated so as not to dissect deeper than the plane of the posterior auricular muscle. (Material from: Hong et al. Superficial mastoid fascia as an accessible donor for various augmentations in Asian rhinoplasty, Journal of Plastic Reconstructive & Aesthetic Surgery, 2012, Elsevier)

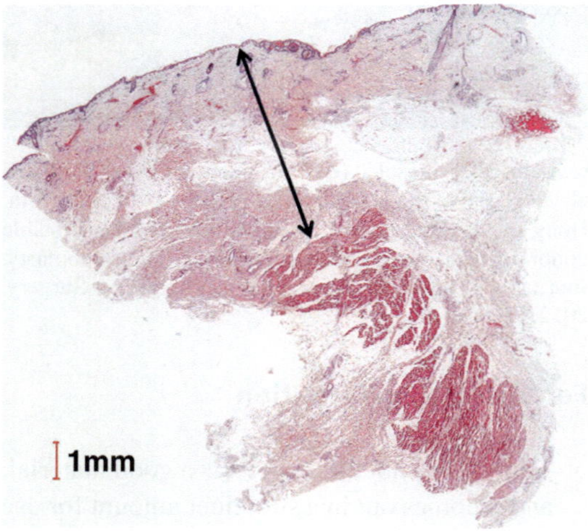

Fig. 6.8 H&E staining of transverse biopsy (×50). The histologic thickness of SMF was estimated between the skin and posterior auricular muscle plane (arrow). (Material from: Hong et al. Superficial mastoid fascia as an accessible donor for various augmentations in Asian rhinoplasty, Journal of Plastic Reconstructive & Aesthetic Surgery, 2012, Elsevier)

The Sacral Dermis-Fat (SDF)

From the early 1980s, the sacrum has been reported as the best donor site as a thick dermal graft in Korea [12]. Dr. Kim has performed more than 3000 primary and secondary nose augmentations with dermal fat grafts. He collected a

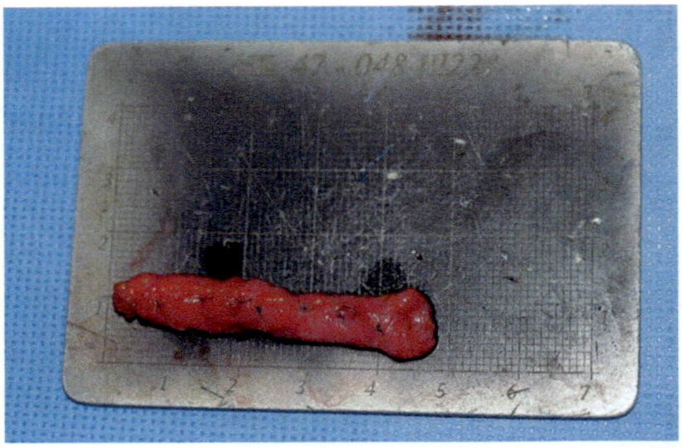

Fig. 6.9 The rolled superficial mastoid fascia

1.5 × 6.5 cm dermal fat graft between the anus and coccyx. He reported this donor tissue was denser and thicker than other areas such as the abdomen, groin area, or gluteal folds. Another study showed that the sacrum's dermis was significantly thicker ($p < 0.008$) than the other sites, and the panniculus adiposus was well developed. Moreover, they assume that dermal fat grafts harvested from the sacral region have greater viability and durability when transplanted. The sacrum is a suitable donation site for augmentation. This area boasts a thick dermis, a large number of fibroblasts and fibrocytes, dense subcutaneous tissue, and hidden scars [13]. There is no disagreement here, and the author prefers this as the first donor site when the highest dorsal projection is desired. Many doctors use the compact fold of multiple layers of the dermis.

- The consensus of doctors who do much dermal graft is that the dermis is absorbed until postoperative 12–18 months.
- When the absorption is considered, the dermal part is used as a double or triple layer, and the fat part is rarely used.
- If dorsal skin is too thin, a little fatty layer should be attached to the dermis. The fatty side is placed directly under the thin skin. It is suitable for shaping.
- When using SDF, if the fat layer is located outside the pocket (dermis-in rolling, in Chap. 7), the graft appears less demarcated due to the tissue's characteristics.
- The thick SDF dermis may appear demarcated under thin dorsal skin.

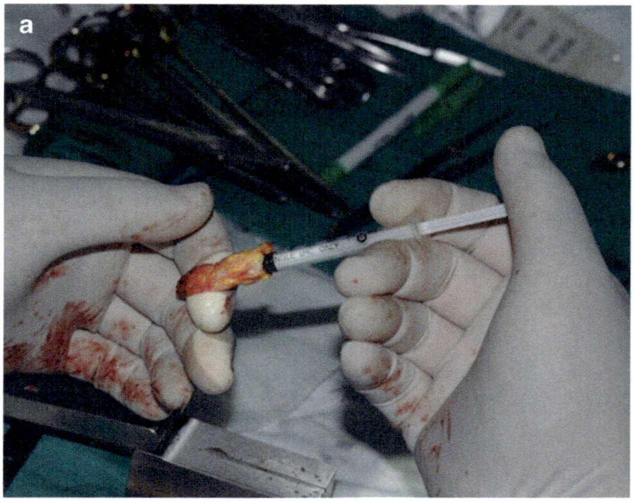

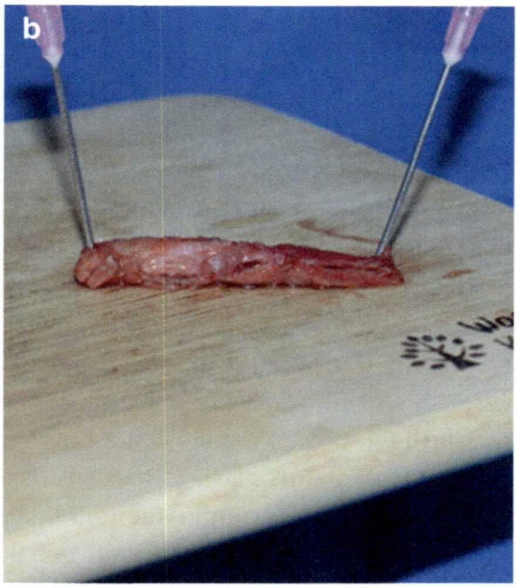

Fig. 6.10 Filling the diced cartilage inside the rolled SMF for more volume. (**a**) Use a 1 cc syringe to seal the SMF around the periphery, and then remove the syringe and apply the space. It is a useful method of filling. (**b**) Fill the cephalic portion more for the projection of Nasion

The absorption issue of autografts, including the dermis, will be covered in more detail in Chap. 7.

Harvest

The harvest is designed in the midline of the sacrum or just on the paramedian side. That is considered for a secondary harvest later.

Collect 20% longer and wider than the desired length, and keep in mind that contraction will occur immediately. The thickness is controlled using folding or molding by a triple layer. Usually, 50 mm-long and 40 mm-wide dermis yield a folded SDF of 8–9 mm wide graft. It is necessary to use a sufficient hydrodissection in the subepidermis and de-epithelization using a loop before detaching.

Septal Cartilage

The author does not use a unique method but collects septal quadrangular cartilage using a method already introduced in several textbooks. However, harvesting the septal cartilage should be determined by the priority of surgery

- The author tries not to perform SMR just because of the need for flat cartilage for the operation.
- Patients requiring septoplasty (deviated nose, hump nose, nasal obstruction) consider performing surgery only with autologous material.
- Dorsal alloplastic implant is a method of camouflage of the lower two-third of nose. Therefore, try to use it as a camouflage material.
- The nasal framework of the undersurface is better not to be destroyed.
- Putting an alloplastic implant on the top of the spreader graft, an invisible graft, if not for functional improvement, there is little evidence to do the spreader graft underneath the alloplastic implant.

The method of secondary septal surgery will be covered in detail in Chap. 11.

Rib Cartilage

Before accessing Dr. Toriumi's literature, the author used several levels of ribs. However, comparing the advantages and disadvantages of the fifth and sixth, and seventh ribs, it is advantageous to use the seventh rib for septal reconstruction because of the straightness and thickness [14]. The author entirely agrees with the explanation that the scar should no longer obligatorily match the inframammary fold if straighter rib cartilage can be obtained longer, and the risk of pneumothorax is low. It is also suitable for septal reconstruction because the upper and lower cortexes' inclusion causes less warping.

Cartilage pieces made of the only cortex are suitable for use in alar contour grafts, and the author thinks Dr. Toriumi's method is the best so far, and the evidence is sufficient. For the explanation of rib cartilage is mainly used in secondary septal surgery. It is recommended to look at Dr. Toriumi's many journals [15–17]. The authors' preferred technique for secondary septal surgery is also covered in Chap. 11.

References

1. Nyemb PM, Sankale A-A, Ndiaye L, NDiaye A, Gaye M. Morphometric study of the outer ear in young adults. Pan Afr Med J. 2014;19:355.
2. Hwang SM, Lim O, Hwang MK, Kim MW, Lee JS. The clinical analysis of the nasal septal cartilage by measurement using computed tomography. Arch Craniofac Surg. 2016;17(3):140–5.
3. Han K, Kim J, Son D, Park B. How to harvest the maximal amount of conchal cartilage grafts. J Plast Reconstr Aesthet Surg. 2008;61(12):1465–71.
4. Lan MY, Park JP, Jang YJ. Donor site morbidities resulting from conchal cartilage harvesting in rhinoplasty. J Laryngol Otol. 2017;131(6):529–33.
5. Echeverry A, Carvajal J, Medina E. Alternative technique for tip support in secondary rhinoplasty. Aesthet Surg J. 2006;26(6):662–8.
6. Sahin MS, Kasapoglu F, Demir UL, Ozmen OA, Coskun H, Basut O. Comparison of clinical results in nasal tip augmentation either via face to face or back to back technique with autogenous auricular conchal cartilage. J Craniofac Surg. 2015;26(7):2109–14.
7. Kridel RW, Scott BA, Foda HM. The tongue-in-groove technique in septorhinoplasty. A 10-year experience. Arch Facial Plast Surg. 1999;1(4):246–56; discussion 257–8.
8. Hwang N-H, Dhong E-S. Septal extension graft in Asian rhinoplasty. Facial Plast Surg Clin North Am. 2018;26(3):331–41.
9. Rabie AN, Chang J, Ibrahim AMS, Lee BT, Lin SJ. Use of Tragal cartilage grafts in rhinoplasty: an anatomic study and review of the literature. Ear Nose Throat J. 2015;94(4–5):E44–9.
10. Cochran CS, DeFatta RJ. Tragal cartilage grafts in rhinoplasty: a viable alternative in the graft-depleted patient. Otolaryngol Head Neck Surg. 2008;138(2):166–9.
11. Hong S-T, Kim D-W, Yoon E-S, Kim H-Y, Dhong E-S. Superficial mastoid fascia as an accessible donor for various augmentations in Asian rhinoplasty. J Plast Reconstr Aesthet Surg. 2012;65(8):1035–40.
12. Kim KY. Augmentation rhinoplasty using dermofat graft. J Korean Soc Aesthetic Plast Surg. 2001;5(1):33–40.
13. Hwang K, Kim DJ, Lee IJ. An anatomic comparison of the skin of five donor sites for dermal fat graft. Ann Plast Surg. 2001;46(3):327–31.
14. Toriumi DM. Dorsal augmentation using autologous costal cartilage or microfat-infused soft tissue augmentation. Facial Plast Surg. 2017;33(2):162–78.
15. Toriumi DM, Patel AB, DeRosa J. Correcting the short nose in revision rhinoplasty. Facial Plast Surg Clin North Am. 2006;14(4):343–55, vi.
16. Toriumi DM, Pero CD. Asian rhinoplasty. Clin Plast Surg. 2010;37(2):335–52.
17. Toriumi DM, Bared A. Revision of the surgically overshortened nose. Facial Plast Surg. 2012;28(4):407–16.

7 The Resorption: The Hurdle for Autogenous-Based Asian Rhinoplasty

Pearls

- Patients with too low nasion should consider using an alloplastic implant from the start.
- If the patient can wait for 12–18 months to complete the resorption, dorsal graft, including too low nasion can be grafted by autologous tissues.
- A consensus is needed between patients and doctors that the graft can be revised due to the resorption issues.
- Crushed cartilage has a significantly lower survival rate than diced cartilage. The resorption rate of diced cartilage is also high.
- Note that many methods of augmentation with micro-diced cartilage without molding can create a tremendous amount of scar tissue in unwanted areas.
- Hard scars made by micro-d iced cartilage injected without molding sometimes show a granuloma-like pattern.
- A dorsal graft of a single layer-superficial mastoid fascia is useful for obtaining a smooth dorsal line. The efficacy for augmentation is nothing more, nothing less than that.
- The long-term augmentation effect of rolled SMF is 1–2 mm. Its absorption should be considered more than 50%.
- The long-term augmentation effect of the rolled SDF in the same area is around 3 mm; the absorption rate is 40–50%.
- The effect of long-term augmentation of diced cartilage wrapped with SMF depends on the amount of packed cartilage, but the augmented amount should be planned with an absorption rate of 30–40%.

In Asian rhinoplasty, surgery without evidence or scientific concerns appears in many features: choosing alloplastic materials again in correcting the secondary problems resulted from previously applied alloplastic materials, applying functional spreader graft underneath ruthless thick silicone implants, harvesting conchal cartilage again in case of rib cartilage chosen as the major source of autogenous graft, and applying alloplastic materials with the belief that it will last forever.

In Asian rhinoplasty, many surgeons struggle in choosing the right autograft to get the best results.

"Resorption" is the unsolved, inextricable, imperative battle in performing "autogenous only" rhinoplasty, mostly when the grafts were applied as visible ones, and in the case of the patients' primary concern was dorsal augmentation. So the long-term results of autogenous grafts were analyzed out of 400 cases operated by the author. The categories are autogenous grafts applied on the nasal dorsum: diced cartilage only, rolled superficial mastoid fascia (SMF), diced cartilage wrapped with SMF,

Supplementary Information The online version of this chapter (https://doi.org/10.1007/978-981-16-0542-0_7) contains supplementary material, which is available to authorized users.

E.-S. Dhong, M.-W. Na, *Asian Septorhinoplasty*, https://doi.org/10.1007/978-981-16-0542-0_7

rolled sacral dermofat (SDF), and diced cartilage wrapped with rectus fascia. Autologous materials are preferred due to their high biocompatibility and low risk of infection and extrusion. However, these benefits should be balanced with concerns about graft absorption.

Moreover, in Asian rhinoplasty, which requires much dorsal augmentation, the projection from the nasal root to the tip is often the biggest goal of surgery. Therefore, the experiences of the authors below are critical in viewing Asian rhinoplasty objectively. The author prefers septorhinoplasty using the only autograft in patients who need septoplasty and have been treating patients with low nasion as an absolute indication of the alloplastic implant, so we are well aware that the largest hurdle of autograft is resorption.

7.1 Diced Cartilage

Diced Cartilage Vs. Crushed Cartilage

Crushed cartilage has a lower survival rate than diced cartilage, regardless of the amount [1]. In the author's experience, it can be found that the survival rate of crushed cartilage is very low. Even if it is troublesome, dicing the cartilage to a size of 0.5–1 mm can increase the survival of the tissue. For molding, hyaluronic acid can be sprayed for easy molding [2] (Fig. 7.1). However, the author uses Tisseel (Baxter Healthcare Corp., Deerfield, IL, USA) to mold and use it for small augmentation in the desired place. However, this use means to use the remnant without throwing it away. The authors experienced that most of these applications were absorbed. This meaning of remnant use is nothing more or less than wishing for augmentation of less than 1 mm or smoothing the dorsal profile.When micro-diced cartilage is applied without any molding or wrapping, enormous resorption and scar tissue will be encountered during revision. If a meaningful amount is needed, it is more effective to wrap it in soft tissue.

- Crushed cartilage has a significantly lower survival rate than diced cartilage.
- Diced cartilage molded with fIbrin glue is helpful for the affordable use of discarded cartilage.
- However, if meaningful augmentation is needed, wrapping it in soft tissue is good.
- Note that many methods of augmentation with micro-diced cartilage without wrapping can create a huge amount of scar tissue in unwanted areas.

Diced Cartilage Wrapped with Fascia

Probably this is one of the most used methods [3–5]. Wrapping in the deep temporal fascia is

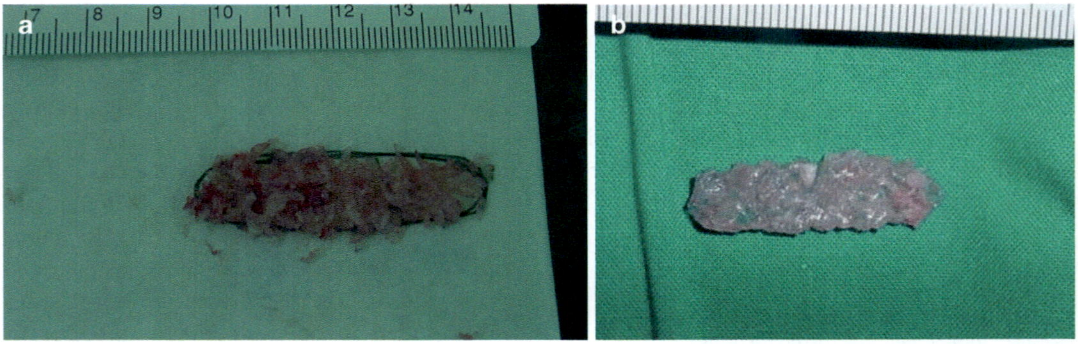

Fig. 7.1 Diced cartilage sprayed with Tisseel for molding. (**a**) Diced cartilage for the dorsal camouflage. (**b**) After applying the fibrin solution

less invading inflammatory cells than wrapping in Surgicel (Ethicon, Inc., a Johnson & Johnson company, Arlington, TX, USA), so more healthy cartilage survives [6]. The author does not prefer wrapping with Surgicel, either making an incision on the hairline during surgery. For soft tissue wrapping, superficial mastoid fascia is placed in a cartilage crusher and thinly bloomed using a mallet. Here, the author prefers the filling method using a 1 cc syringe (Chap. 6). Of course, when collecting costal cartilage, the preferred site is rectus fascia in a square shape for wrapping (Fig. 7.2).

7.2 Septal Cartilage

Septal cartilage is relatively used as strut, batten graft, and spreader graft. There is no worry about being absorbed because it is usually used as an invisible graft. The resorption is imperceptible because it is replaced by appropriate fibrous tissue. However, there are reports that the absorption rate is 12–50% in the past. Also, it is reported that even the spreader graft resorbed when its tension is severe and if it is crushed [7]. The anatomical graft or orthotopic graft does not resorb because the recipient site's remaining perichon-

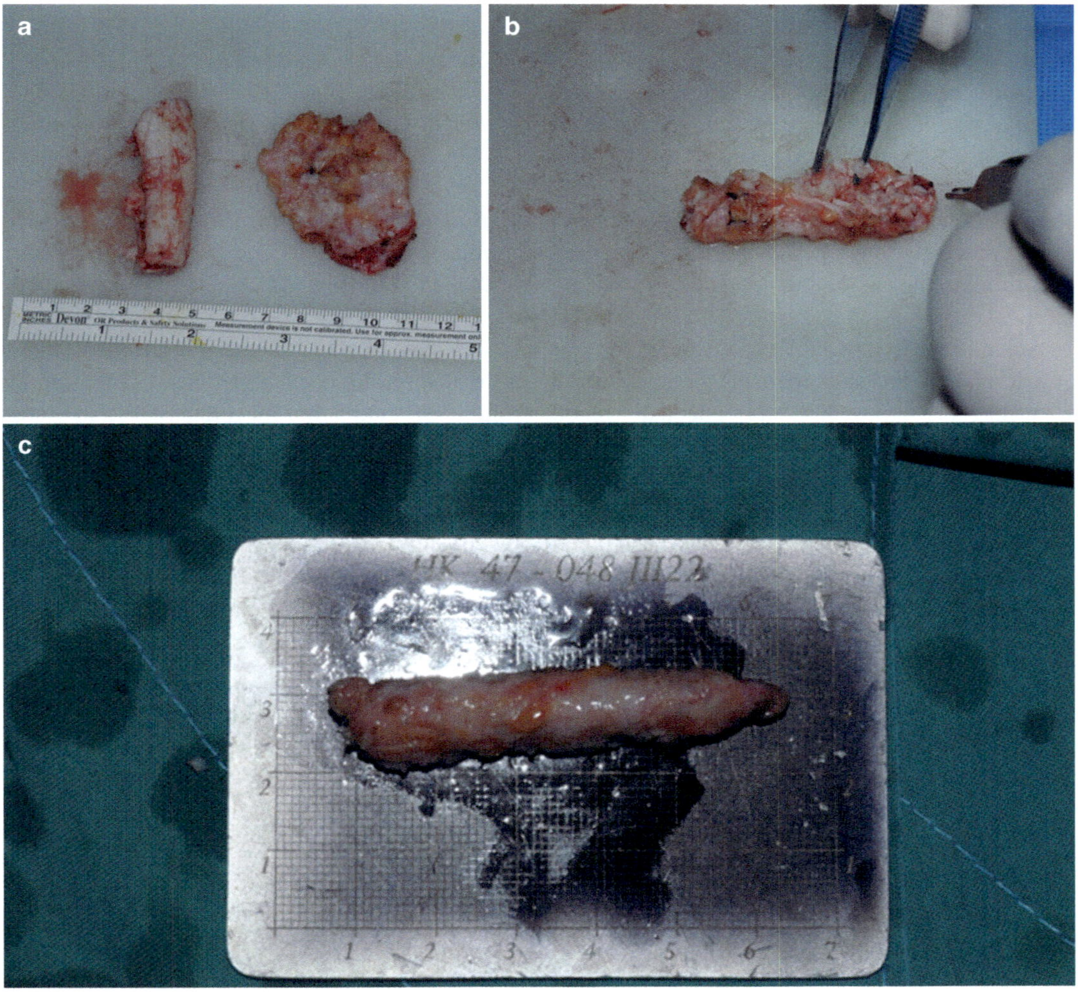

Fig. 7.2 Diced costal cartilage wrapped with rectus fascia. (**a**) Sixth rib and rectus fascia. (**b**) The remnant costal cartilages are diced and packed in the rectus fascia. (**c**) After molding for graft. (photo from other case)

drium provides an adequate blood supply. Septal cartilage cannot be harvested with perichondrium attached, so the orthotopic graft is more effective than the onlay graft.

7.3 Ear Cartilage

Like septal cartilage, ear cartilage is used in all types of rhinoplasty and is the primary choice of secondary rhinoplasty [8, 9]. In the case of secondary rhinoplasty, most of them are in SMR state, so cymba and cavum concha are the primary choices. If the septal L-strut is severely damaged and reconstruction of the nasal framework is not possible with ear cartilage, costal cartilage is used. At the time of the revision, it can be seen that most of the ear cartilages are alive, but the original size is a little smaller, and the shape of the margin is changed, indicating that resorption occurs. However, it is challenging to determine the absorption rate because it is impossible to know precisely how perichondrium was used according to the application method.

- Scientifically, it would be advantageous for survival, if the side with the perichondrium would be exposed to the adequate blood supply.
- In the author's study, when folded cymba concha is used for caudal septal extension graft, concave sides were coapted to face each other, so attaching the convex side's perichondrium would be advantageous for cartilage survival.

7.4 The Resorption Rate of Soft Tissues

The order below is from the lowest to the highest height of the target dorsum among the author's methods. There are six types of soft tissues that the author uses for dorsal enhancement. Other soft tissues include medial plantar dermis, axillary dermis, and groin dermofat graft, but each has too many disadvantages such as pain and hair-bearing, so they are not used anymore by the author. Of course, when surgery is planned with only ear cartilage, rectus fascia is not harvested only for dorsal augmentation. Rectus fascial is only used when costal cartilage is harvested.

- *Superficial Mastoid fascia (SMF)* [10].
- *Rolled SMF* (Fig. 7.3).
- *Rolled SMF filled with diced cartilage* (Fig. 7.4).
- *Sacral dermis-fat (SDF).*
- *Rolled Rectus Fascia filled with diced cartilage* (Fig. 7.2).
- *Rolled SDF* (Fig. 7.5).

In each case, the amount of targeted thickness after resorption is predicted as 1–1.5 mm for rolled SMF and 3 mm for rolled SDF, and preparations are made for surgery. The meaning of rolling is to make a tube shape by repairing both sides of the sheet and increasing the thickness twice. However, in the SDF case, due to the tissue's characteristics, the choice should be made whether placing the dermal portion inside (der-

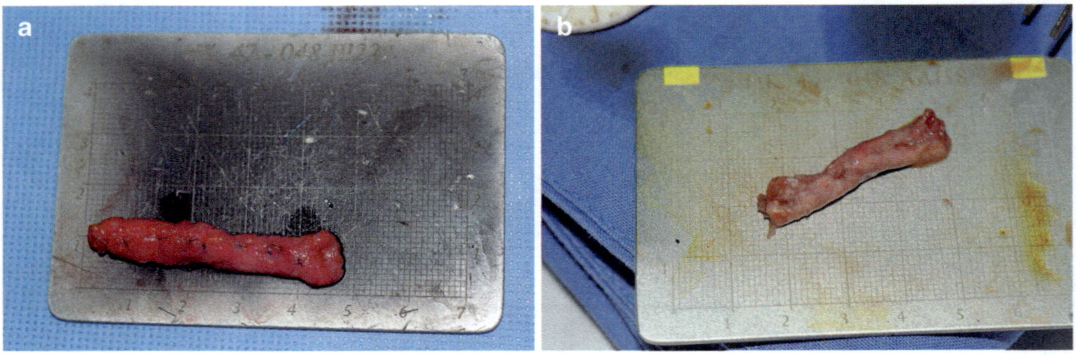

Fig. 7.3 Rolled superficial mastoid fascia. (**a**, **b**) Two different cases

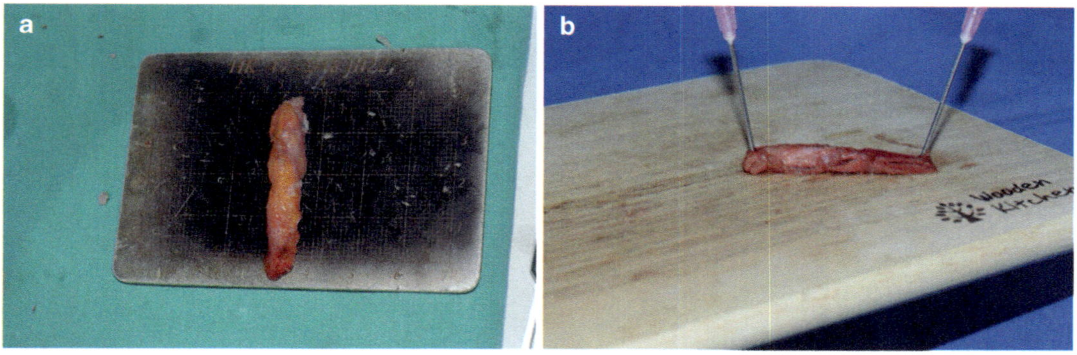

Fig. 7.4 Diced cartilage wrapped with superficial mastoid fascia. (**a**, **b**) Two different cases

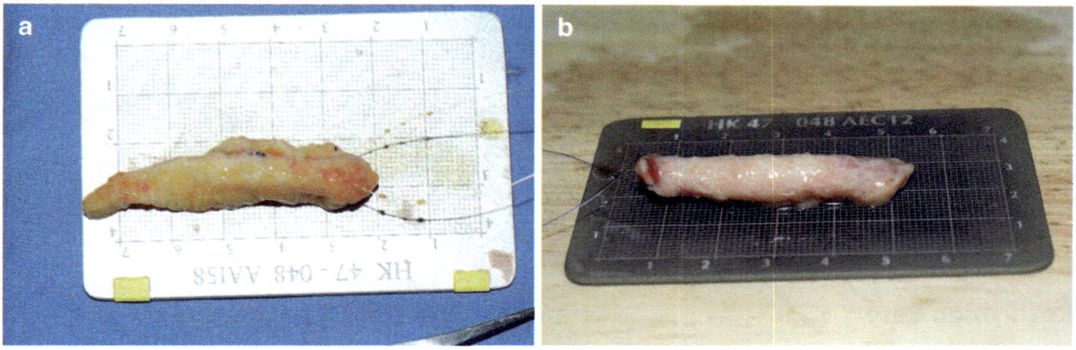

Fig. 7.5 Rolled sacral dermis-fat (SDF). (**a**, **b**) Two different cases

mis-in rolling) or outside (dermis-out rolling). The dermis-out rolling is mainly used when there is a puncture in the dorsal skin so that a uniform surface is to be placed directly under the skin and when to implement a more definite dorsal line (Video 7.1). If the remaining recipient site's skin is thin, the author selects the dermis-in rolling (fat-out rolling) technique to attenuate the graft's definition (Fig. 7.5a). Considering the dermal physiology, the dermis-out rolling, where the dermis layer contacts directly the recipient's surgical pocket, has a higher probability of rapid revascularization (Fig. 7.5b). However, since the bottom is nasal bone and the periosteum is mostly destroyed, some resorption cannot be prevented.

The dermal graft, which is located subcutaneously, is found to be hardly absorbed but rather survived at the revision surgery. The subcutaneous SDF graft is revised to move to a deeper location by elevating the nasal bone's periosteum. The demarcation is corrected by this method (Fig. 7.6).

It should be borne in mind that if the dorsal skin is too thin, the inserted SDF may be demarcated.

- Rolling method: In the case of concerning demarcation under the thin skin in reoperation, it is controlled by enrolling the thin fat layer outward (dermis-in rolling). If the subdermis of the dorsal skin is thick, it is good to use the dermis-out rolling.
- Since the dermal blood supply is critical to survival, it is suitable for the survival to use the dermis-out rolling.
- However, the author prefers to use only the dermal portion without including the fatty part due to resorption issues, and rarely uses the fatty portion.

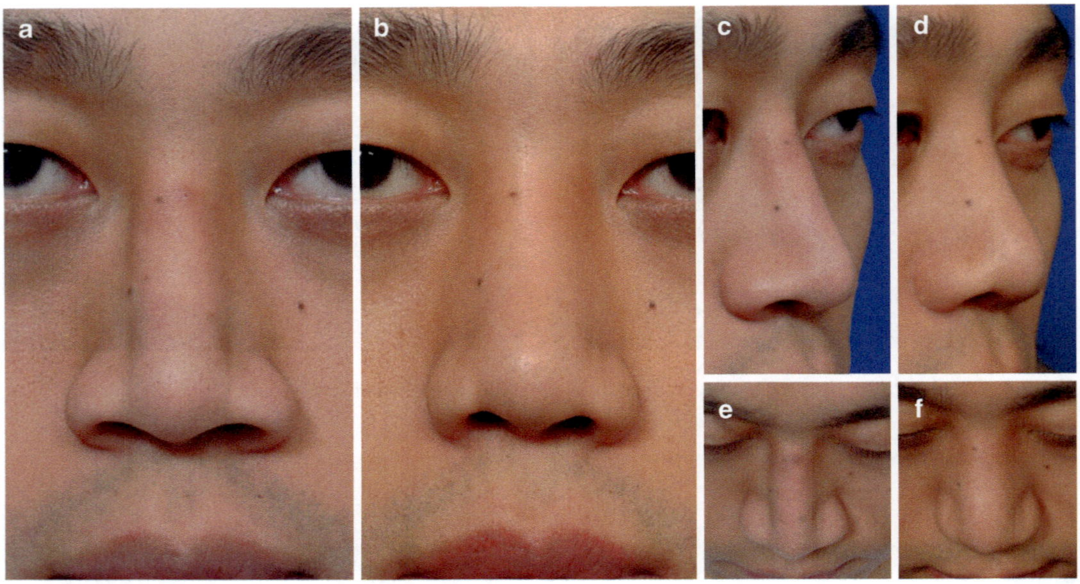

Fig. 7.6 A 34-year-old male patient underwent an SDF graft at another clinic. Demarcated SDF was corrected by changing the depth of the dissection plane from subcutaneous plane to subperiosteal plane. (**a**, **c**, **e**) Preoperative views, (**b**, **d**, **f**) Postoperative 1 year

Resorption Rate

Among the various types of autologous tissue recognition above, long-term results were obtained for the following three absorption rates. (Data in publishing, Plastic and reconstructive surgery 2021).

- ***Rolled SMF***
- ***Rolled SMF filled with diced cartilage***
- ***Rolled SDF***

One month after surgery was considered as the result of an immediate postoperative state, and the photo was used as a control. Postoperative photos of more than 1 year were used to compare as a long-term follow-up. We have recently published some of the research using two-dimensional photographs underneath three-dimensional photographs. Since a lot of past data is accumulated and written in a 2D photo, to analyze this photo objectively, two software MPS (Morpheus 3D Plastic Solution, Morpheus 3D scanner, Morpheus CO. Ltd., Seoul Korea,) and MDS (Morpheus 3D Dental Solution) was used for comparative analysis.

Usefulness of Standardized Two-Dimensional Photo Analysis

The author standardized the magnification using a baseline length adjustment for each photo. Anatomical proportions, including vertical height, were used for objective measurements: cheilion to the middle pupil line. The cheilion-mid pupil line was used as the basis for the calculation (Video 7.2). The magnification was adjusted by making each length equal. Bias in assessing the magnitude and direction of any differences found between 2D and 3D imaging software was evaluated statistically in many anthropometric points. The bias difference was calculated between the 2D and 3D imaging software measurements. For each landmark, the 3D imaging software yielded more extensive measurements on average. The average difference is 0.127 mm over the 2D imaging software. However, there were no significant differences between 2D and 3D imaging software. Therefore, it was possible to analyze past 2D pictures with modified MDS, and this standardization was possible according to this result.

How to Correct Yawing and Rolling in 2D Photographs

The author standardized the magnification using a baseline length adjustment for each photo. Anatomical proportions, including vertical height, were used for objective measurements: cheilion to the middle pupil line. The cheilion-mid pupil line was used as the basis for the calculation. To control yawing and rolling, the author standardized the two lengths of tragus-midpupil and tragus-cheilion line equal.

The Resorption Rate

To compare resorption rates, rhinion and 1/2 NR (the ½ of nasion–rhinion) projections were assessed.

In the author's surgical method, the cartilaginous dorsum and nasal tip projection were mainly projected using autogenous cartilage. The three types of autogenous grafts mentioned above were inserted from the nasal root to obtain a smooth dorsal line connected to caudally. As mentioned above, the dermal graft will survive better in the subcutaneous lower two-third of the nose, which is rich in blood supply, and it is difficult to compare the complexed surgical areas such as supratip and tip. Therefore, the author wanted to compare autologous tissue's absorption rate under the same conditions. The selected site was nasion and ½ NR (the midpoint between nasion and rhinion). Rhinion was defined here as the upper one-third point of nasion and tip defining point. All grafts were placed in the subperiosteal pocket. The results came out more than expected: "the vastness of the reabsorption."

The following is the resorption rate at 1/2NR, which is the bony dorsum's middle point among many data. If you are curious, refer to the author's journal to be published soon. It is a resorption rate expressed with a 95% confidence interval.

The resorption rate of rolled SMF at ½ NR: 50–70%.

In both three quarter and modified profile views, resorption rates were the highest and the most dramatic in the rolled SMF group: 54.8–72.8% (Figs. 7.7 and 7.8).

The resorption rate of rolled SMF filled with diced cartilage at ½ NR: 30–40%.

In both three quarter and modified profile views, The rolled SMF filled with diced cartilage showed the resorption rate as 27.3–43.3% (Figs. 7.9 and 7.10).

The resorption rate of rolled SDF at ½ NR: 40–50%.

In both three quarter and modified profile views, the rolled SD group showed the resorption rate as 37.1–51.2% (Figs. 7.11 and 7.12).

There were statistically significant resorption rate differences among the three autologous groups ($p < 0.001$).

This is a study of the upper bony dorsum's absorption rate, which is the most problematic in Asian surgery. The lowest absorption rate was SMF wrapped with diced cartilage grafted, and the highest absorption rate was rolled SMF. It is somewhat similar or different from the existing reports [11].

With the consensus among surgeons, SDF's absorption rate is thought to progress from one to one and a half years. The author also agrees that the more soft tissue graft contains, the higher the absorption rate. The more fatty tissue the graft contains, the higher the absorption rate, and absorption will proceed for more than 1 year.

- Crushed cartilage is almost completely absorbed when implanted in the nasion site.
- Diced cartilage is also absorbed, so the effect of augmentation is insignificant but remains more than crushed cartilage.
- A single-layer of SMF is useful for obtaining a smooth dorsal esthetic line at the rhinion.

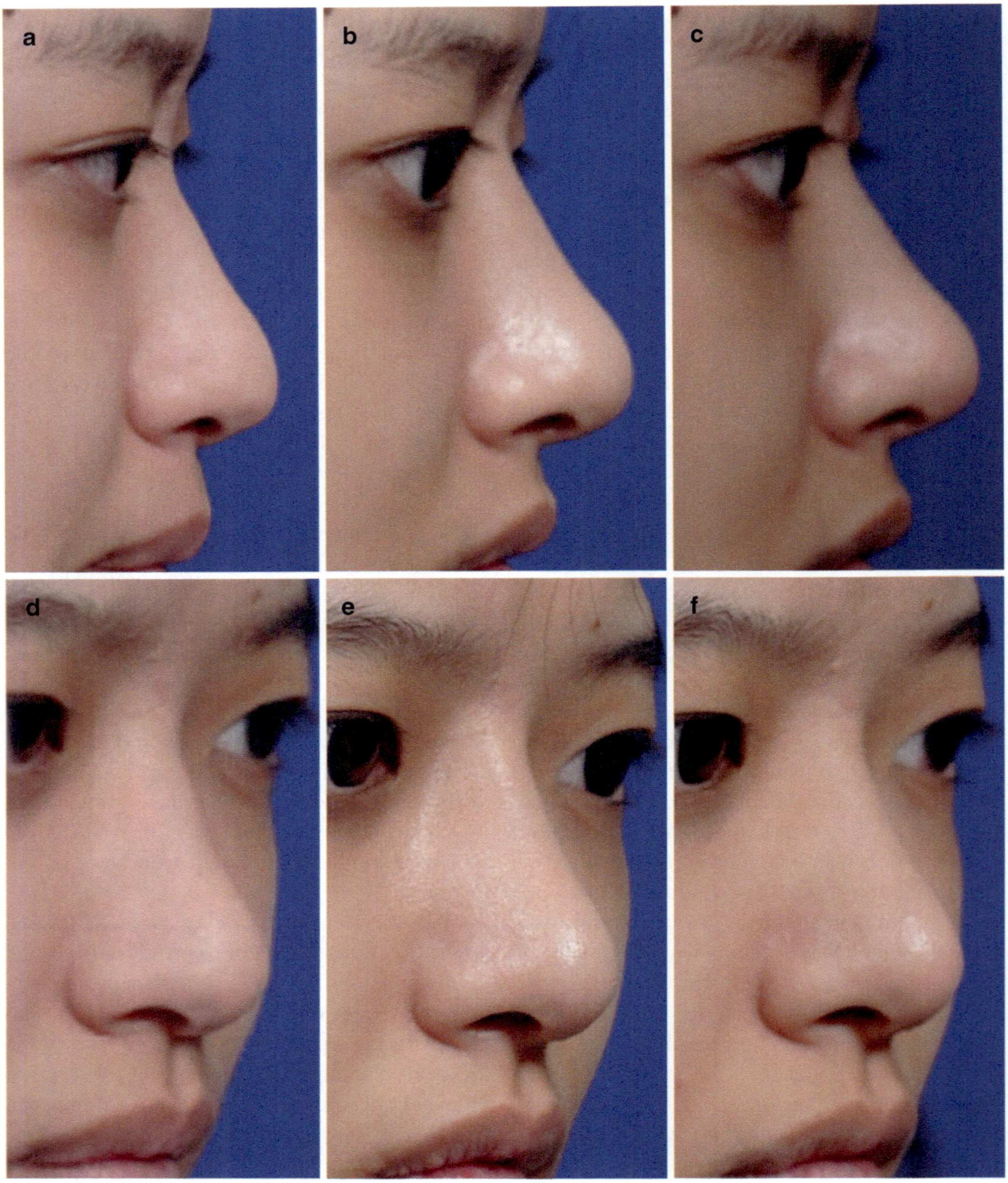

Fig. 7.7 Resorption of rolled superficial mastoid fascia (SMF). (**a**, **d**) Preoperative view. (**b**, **e**) Immediate postoperative view: postoperative 1 month. (**c**, **f**) Long-term postoperative view: 18 months postoperative

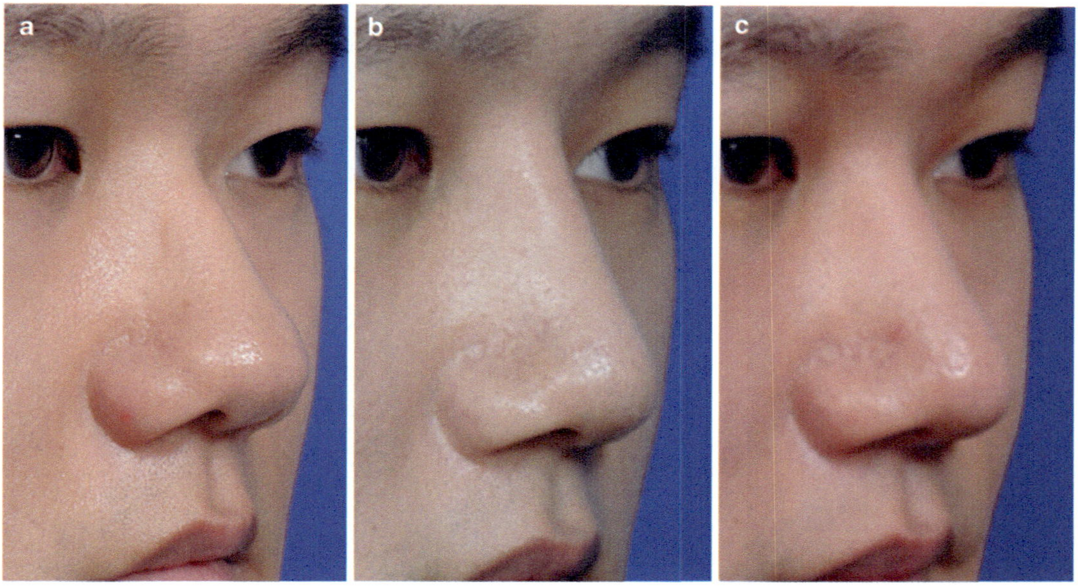

Fig. 7.8 Resorption of rolled superficial mastoid fascia (SMF). (**a**) Preoperative view. (**b**) Immediate postoperative view: postoperative 1 month. (**c**) Long-term postoperative view: 12 months postoperative

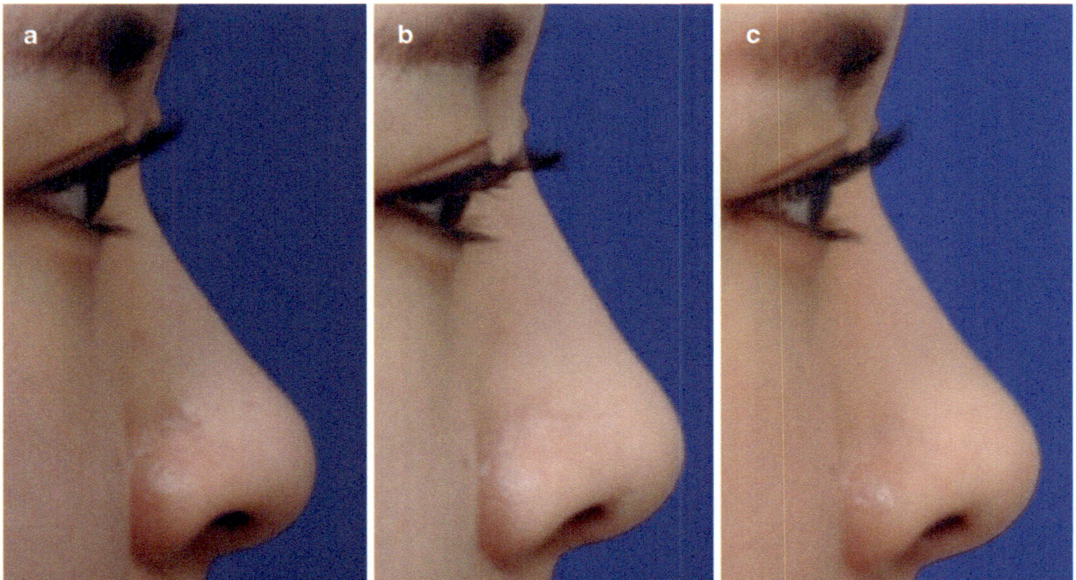

Fig. 7.9 Resorption of diced cartilage wrapped with rolled SMF. (**a, d**) Preoperative view. (**b, e**) Immediate postoperative view: postoperative 1 month. (**c, f**) Long-Term postoperative view: 14 months postoperative

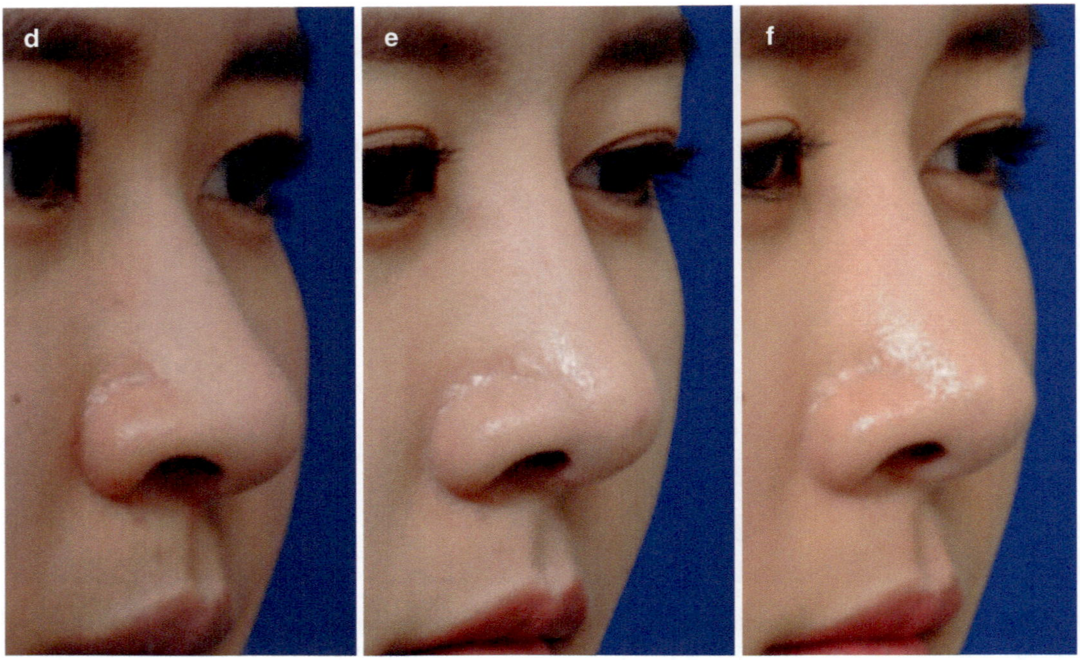

Fig. 7.9 (continued)

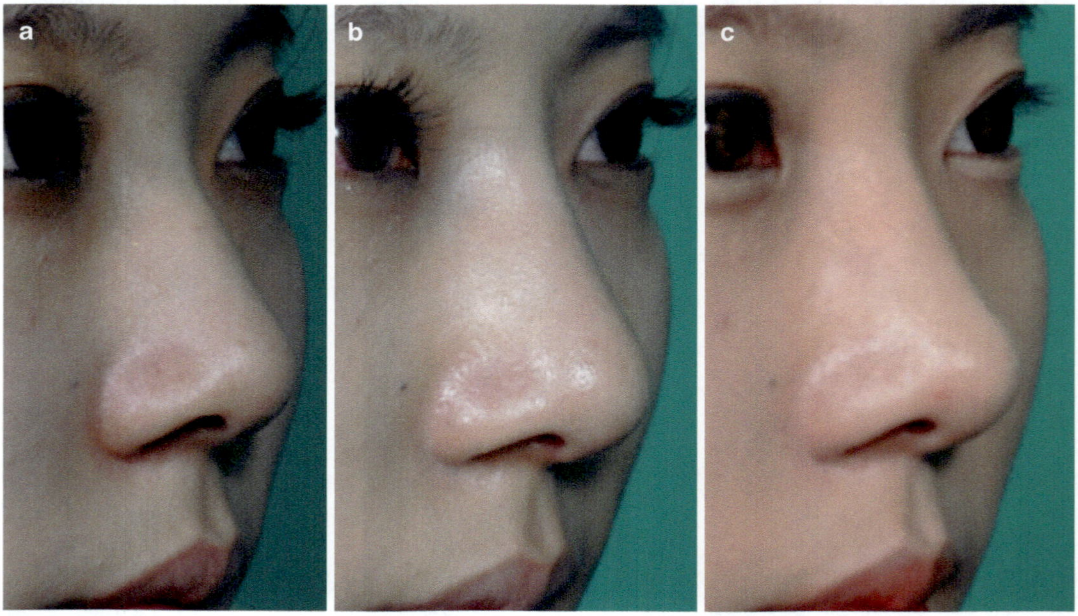

Fig. 7.10 Resorption of diced cartilage wrapped with rolled SMF. (**a**) Preoperative view. (**b**) Immediate postoperative view: postoperative fifth week. (**c**) Long-Term postoperative view: 12 months postoperative

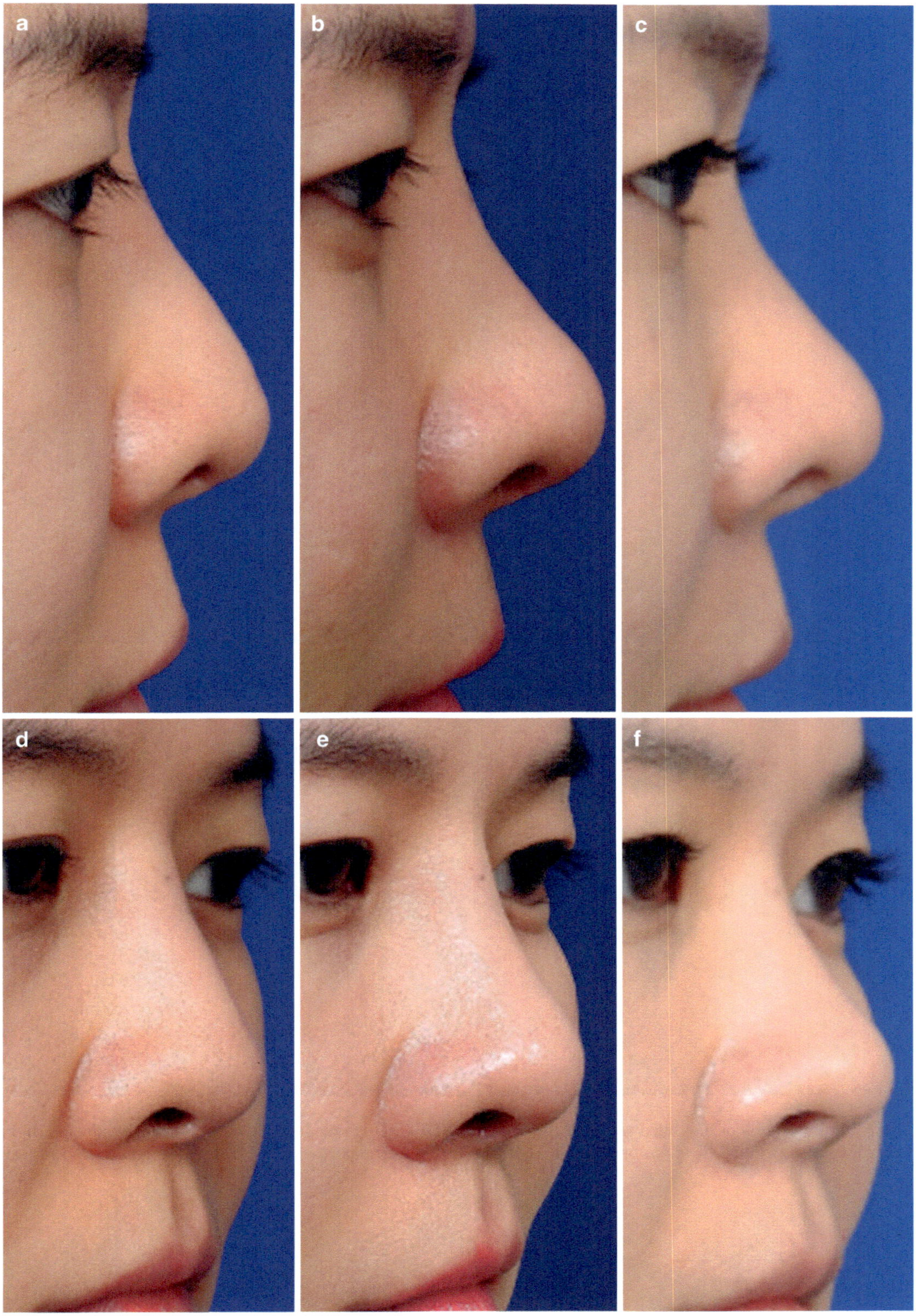

Fig. 7.11 Resorption of the rolled sacral dermis-fat graft (SDF). (**a**, **d**) Preoperative view with dorsal implant. (**b**, **e**) Immediate postoperative view: postoperative 1 month. (**c**, **f**) Long-Term postoperative view: 12 months postoperative

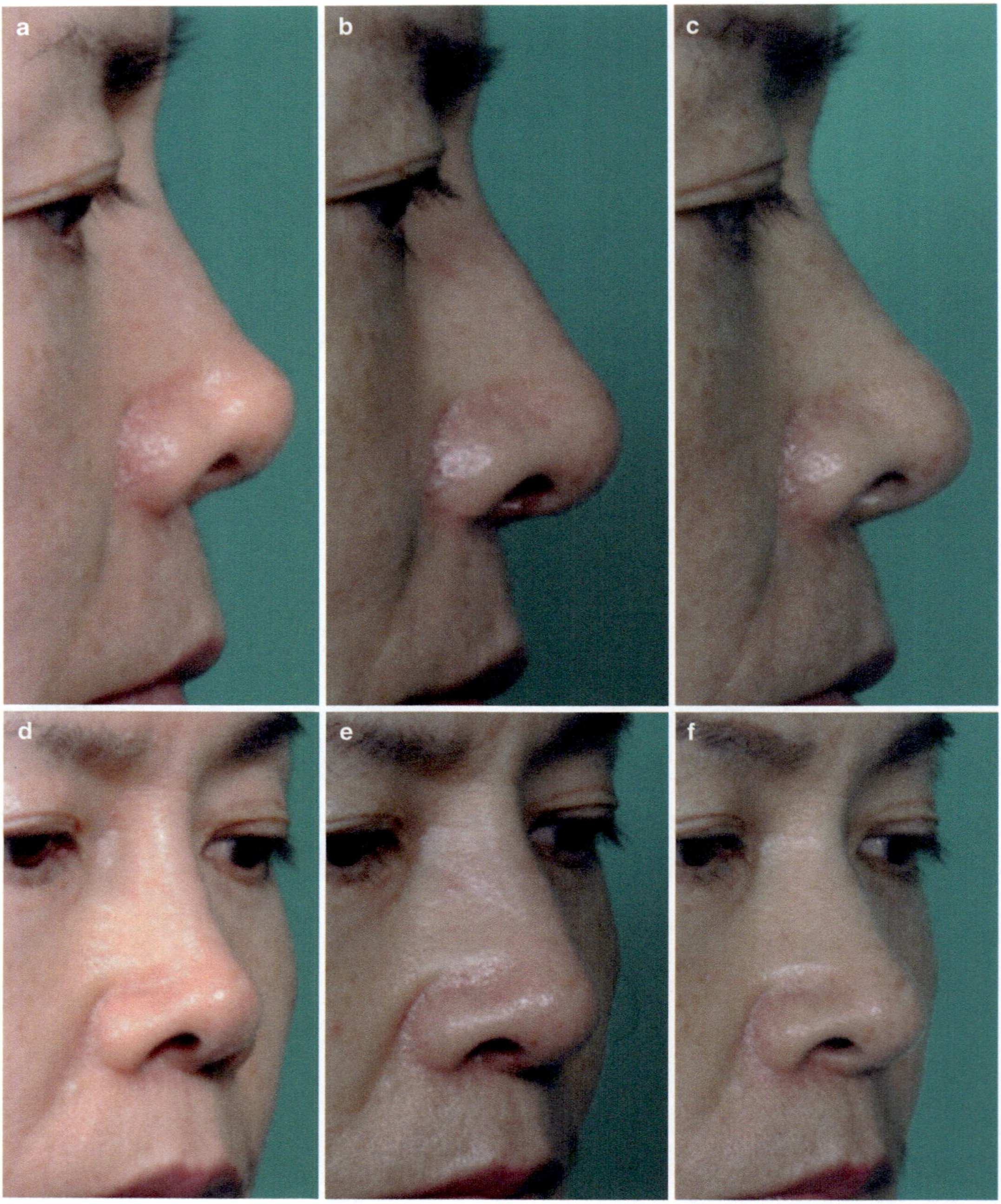

Fig. 7.12 Resorption of the rolled sacral dermis-fat graft (SDF). (**a**, **d**) Preoperative view with dorsal implant. (**b**, **e**) Immediate postoperative view: postoperative 1 month. (**c**, **f**) Long-Term postoperative view: 12 months postoperative

- Graft on the nasal bone is highly absorbed. Relatively where the perichondrium is a platform, the absorption is less.
- The long-term augmentation effect of rolled SMF is 1–2 mm in contact with bone in the bony portion of the nasion or below. Its absorption should be considered more than 50%.
- The long-term augmentation effect of the rolled SDF in the same area is approximately 3 mm. The absorption rate is regarded as 40–50%.
- The effect of long-term augmentation of diced cartilage wrapped with SMF depends on the amount of packed cartilage, but it should be planned with an absorption rate of 30–40%.

References

1. Cakmak O, Bircan S, Buyuklu F, Tuncer I, Dal T, Ozluoglu LN. Viability of crushed and diced cartilage grafts: a study in rabbits. Arch Facial Plast Surg. 2005;7(1):21–6.
2. Kazikdas KC, Ergur B, Tugyan K, Guneli E, Kaya D, Sahan M. Viability of crushed and diced cartilage grafts wrapped in oxidized regenerated cellulose and esterified hyaluronic acid: an experimental study. Laryngoscope. 2007;117(10):1728–34.
3. Daniel RK. Diced cartilage grafts in rhinoplasty surgery: current techniques and applications. Plast Reconstr Surg. 2008;122(6):1883–91.
4. Daniel RK, Calvert JW. Diced cartilage grafts in rhinoplasty surgery. Plast Reconstr Surg. 2004;113(7):2156–71.
5. Daniel RK. Rhinoplasty: dorsal grafts and the designer dorsum. Clin Plast Surg. 2010;37(2):293–300.
6. Brenner KA, McConnell MP, Evans GRD, Calvert JW. Survival of diced cartilage grafts: an experimental study. Plast Reconstr Surg. 2006;117(1):105–15.
7. Bujía J. Determination of the viability of crushed cartilage grafts: clinical implications for wound healing in nasal surgery. Ann Plast Surg. 1994;32(3):261–5.
8. Endo T, Nakayama Y, Ito Y. Augmentation rhinoplasty [Internet]. Plastic and Reconstructive Surgery. vol. 87; 1991. p 54–9. https://doi.org/10.1097/00006534-199101000-00010.
9. Toriumi DM. Augmentation rhinoplasty with autologous cartilage grafting [Internet]. Asian Facial Cosmetic Surgery. 2007. p. 229–52. https://doi.org/10.1016/b978-1-4160-0290-1.50026-x.
10. Hong S-T, Kim D-W, Yoon E-S, Kim H-Y, Dhong E-S. Superficial mastoid fascia as an accessible donor for various augmentations in Asian rhinoplasty. J Plast Reconstr Aesthet Surg. 2012;65(8):1035–40.
11. Kim H-K, Rhee SC. Augmentation rhinoplasty using a folded "pure" dermal graft [Internet]. J Craniofacial Surg. 2013;24:1758–62. https://doi.org/10.1097/scs.0b013e31828f1b5f.

Controlling Asian Tip: Tip Defining Point and Supratip Break

8

Pearls

- Asian LLC is fragile and does not have enough length, so it has limitations in making beautiful tips with its modifications.
- In many cases, the "tip tripod theory" cannot be applied. In primary rhinoplasty, the first step is to determine the position of the ideal sellion and the subnasale to determine the length of the nose accordingly.
- In secondary rhinoplasty, it is often necessary to first consider the tip position through tissue release and then perform the remaining procedures.
- Planning the tip defining point is the beginning of Asian rhinoplasty. The first step in determining the tip defining point is the interdomal suture.
- SEG has a disadvantage because the tip is tilted to one side when the nasal base is weak. Also, it is not easy to apply to secondary rhinoplasty.
- Floating type columella strut has a disadvantage. Its effect is not strong in Asian tip plasty because the amount of projection is small.
- The suture of the columella strut should be done in the area confined to the medial crura. The suture between the caudal margin of the middle crura breaks its own divergence.
- STB problems found in Asian rhinoplasty are related to alloplastic implants in many cases.
- The shield graft maintains the symmetry of the LLCs and the divergence of the middle crura and is useful for creating a tip-lobular angle.
- The anteriorly relocated high septum provides the necessary support for the positioning of the lateral crura, along with the correction of the saddle nose deformity.
- The high septal reconstruction is necessary to prevent STB deformity due to dorsal graft resorption, and STB expressed by the septum has less deformation in the long term.
- The onlay graft such as batten or derotation graft may cause convexity (supratip deformity) of STB.
- A lot of LLC's destruction or resorption is found in secondary surgery, and its strength is weak, making it difficult to obtain stability only with lateral crus. Methods such as lateral crural steal or lateral crural overlay are complicated.

Asian rhinoplasty is generally aimed into three purposes. These are lengthening the nose, enhancing the dorsum, and projecting the tip with tip plasty. Another classification uniquely exists in Asian rhinoplasty: primary vs. secondary rhinoplasty. As such, secondary rhinoplasty has an entirely different perspective. The tissue contracture is uniquely seen in Asian secondary rhinoplasty. Therefore, this chapter mainly describes general concepts, but

Supplementary Information The online version of this chapter (https://doi.org/10.1007/978-981-16-0542-0_8) contains supplementary material, which is available to authorized users.

E.-S. Dhong, M.-W. Na, *Asian Septorhinoplasty*, https://doi.org/10.1007/978-981-16-0542-0_8

we have included some pitfalls seen in the secondary nose at the end of each unit. The contracted nose will be covered again in Chaps. 11 and 12. For Asian rhinoplasty, most doctors will use a septal extension graft for extension and an alloplastic implant for augmentation. Most of the time, they will try nasal tip plasty with sutures and various grafts. Apart from that method, in this chapter, the author would like to talk about the consensus that is particularly problematic in Asian rhinoplasty or is the target of surgery. For Asians, it is difficult to obtain good results without a clear goal for the tip. The definition of the tip and soft triangle in the Western nose is clear, and the tip defining point has two highlights (Fig. 8.1). In many cases, the shape of the LLC can be observed from the external nose. Of course, some people have the same tip definition. However, a hypoplastic LLC with thick skin envelopes of Asian consists only of a smooth curve without tip definition (Fig. 8.2). It is challenging to make a beautiful tip that corresponds to the following content with a fragile LLC. The lateral crus is very short, and it is difficult to expect in East Asians that this follows Anderson's tip tripod theory [1]. Also, cartilaginous graft is required to make nasal frameworks and the tip. This is why Asian rhinoplasty has entirely different perspectives from Western one, which consisted of mainly reduction rhinoplasty. Also, a cartilaginous graft is required to make nasal frameworks and the tip.

8.1 Steps for Nasal Tip Plasty

In Asian primary rhinoplasty, the first step is to determine the position of the ideal sellion and the subnasale. That determines the total length, these two landmarks decide all. In other words, the first procedure is to decide the length with the starting point (golden point) of the nose. After that, the height of the tip is determined according to tissue resilience. Finally, the dorsal height is determined by various angles. If the nose's dorsal height is excessively projected, the tip projection will be insufficient if the tissue is not recruited. The tip projection exceeds the limit with excessive alloplastic material, causing a problem. In the case of secondary rhinoplasty, it is a little different. The resilience of the tip deteriorated. The amount of tip release determines the length of the nose.

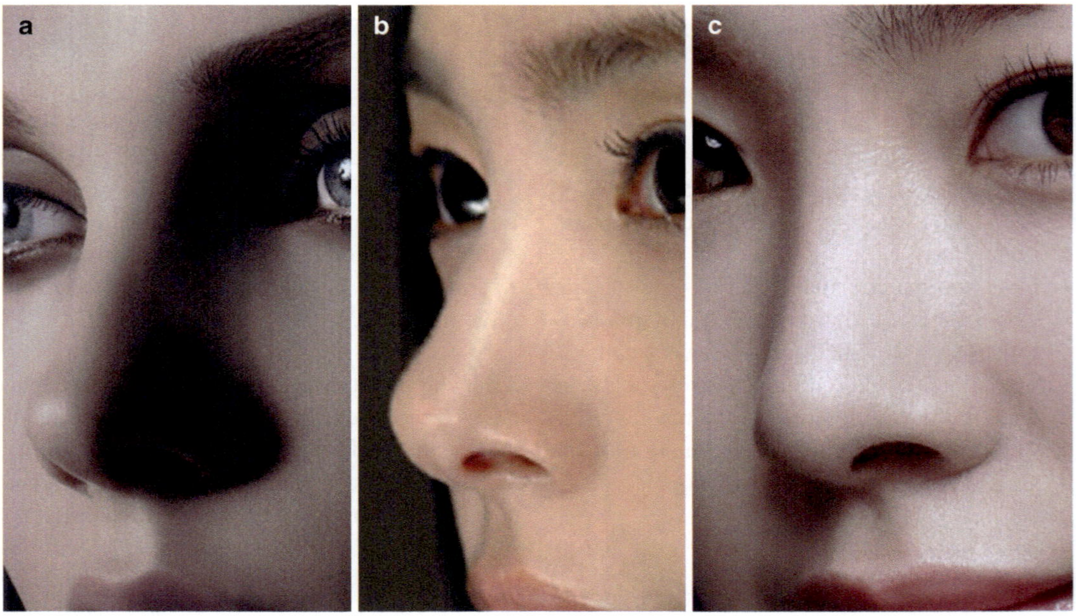

Fig. 8.1 Features of Asian nasal tip. (**a**) In Caucasian, you can find the highlight of a well-developed tip. (**b**) In the case of showing a well-developed tip definition in Asian. (**c**) Beautiful tip without definition seen in Asian

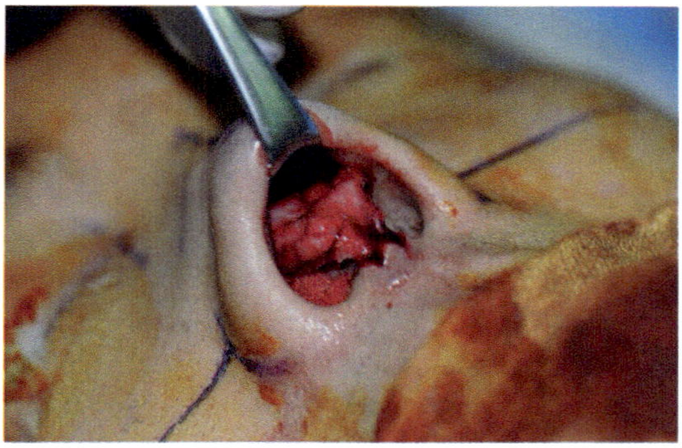

Fig. 8.2 Hypoplastic Asian nasal tip. It can be found that the development of middle crura, the medial crura is insufficient. If the cartilage is weak and subSMAS dissection proceeds, only the LLC, which is too fragile, will remain

The nose's height is automatically determined by the various ideal angles: columellolabial angle, tip-lobular angle, and nasofrontal angle. In other words, in secondary rhinoplasty, the tip position is considered first, and then performs the rest of the procedure. The amount of release determines the length of the nose and the amount of dorsal height. At this time, the modification of LLC is indispensable. In Asians, the middle crus is insufficiently developed, and the angle formed with the middle and medial crura is amorphous, so much effort is required in this part.

8.2 The Tip Defining Point

The tip defining point is the front most point of the tip projection made by two highlights of the middle crus's lateral border [2, 3]. It is the starting point of the tip plasty as the highlight of the tip of the Asian rhinoplasty. For a precise definition, a suture technique or graft is needed. If you have a weak LLC, it is difficult to obtain the desired definition with the suture technique. Tip plasty is started by the first interdomal suture on the cephalic border of the middle crus at the correct position of the tip lobule [4] (Fig. 8.3).

The tip defining point made by excessive transdomal suture applied to the lateral crus creates pinching deformity because the lateral crura and medial crural angles are too narrow. In this way, the physiology is damaged by the shape of the external nares. It can cause nasal obstruction and spoil the shape of the beautiful tip. The problem is that it also spoils the shape of the soft triangle, an essential part of the tip lobule esthetics. The following are the ways to project the tip defining point.

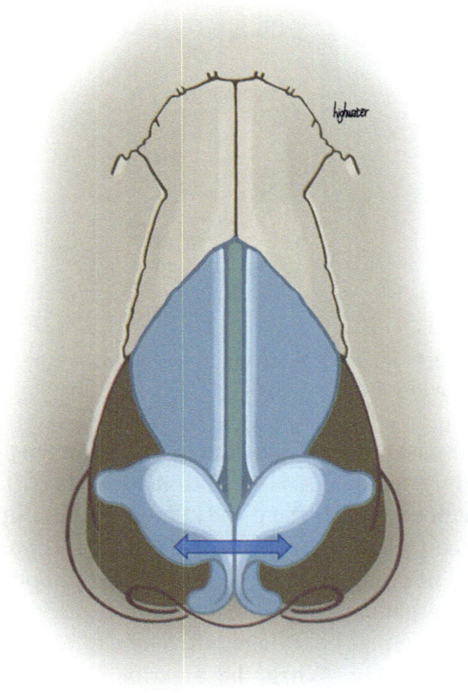

Fig. 8.3 The tip defining point: the distance between the lateral margin of caudal medial genu of middle crura

Septum-Dependent Tip Projection

A septal extension graft (SEG) is mostly used. When the caudal septum's projection is deficient, Dr. Byrd's SEG can help create a tip defining point more projected (Fig. 8.4). There are three types of SEG: direct type, batten type, and spreader type. In the author's case, the batten type is preferred, but the SEG starting from the middle of the caudal septum is not stable.

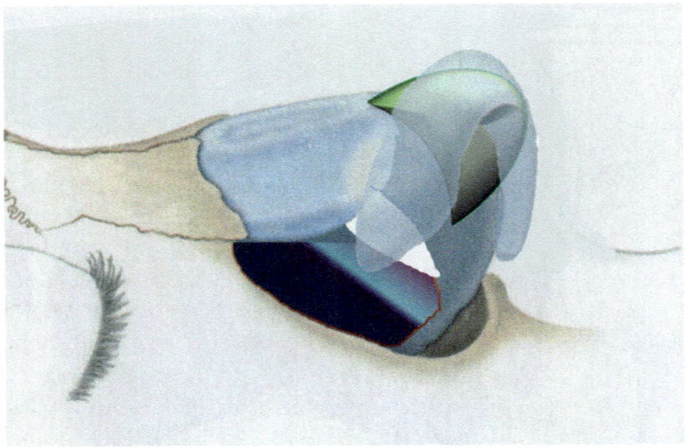

Fig. 8.4 Batten type septal extension graft: The most commonly found graft type

The nasal base constructed by ANS and the posterior septal angle is weak in many Asians. This method also has the disadvantage that the tip is tilted to one side when the nasal base is weak. It is not easy to apply to secondary rhinoplasty. Many patients underwent SMR, so there is no square type of cartilage left. The author prefers ear cartilage. When the anterior septal angle extending from the septum is directly connected to the interdomal suture, it is advantageous to place it in the cephalic portion of the middle crus when making the tip shape later. Multiple sutures in the intercrural position are performed for stability; however, the caudal border of the medial crus should be avoided (Fig. 8.5). It preserves the divergence of the medial genu on both sides of the middle crus and also preserves the divergence between the long axes of the lateral crus.

Septum-Independent Tip Projection

The representative one is the columellar strut. Floating type or fixed type can be used.

- The floating type has the disadvantage that its effect is inferior in Asian rhinoplasty because the amount of projection is small (Fig. 8.6).
- In the case of the fixed type, there is a disadvantage that a long length is required.

However, the biggest problem is that the caudal margin and repair of the medial crus or middle crus are required to obtain strong support, and the two divergence angles shown in Fig. 8.5 above are broken. When the caudal margin is coapted, the divergence of the medial genu disappears, and lateral crus is also caudally turned down. In other words, it is not easy to make beautiful infratip lobules or ideal soft triangles. For the beautiful infratip lobule, a columellolobular angle should be required, and it is difficult to make if the divergence of the middle genu is lost.

- The suture of the columella strut should be done in the area confined to the medial crura, and it is more ideal for repairing the mid-portion with the intercrural suture of the medial crura.

8.3 The Supratip Break: STB

Definition

Most Asian men want a straight dorsal line. In women, they want the subtle concavity of the part that transitions from the tip defining point to the dorsum. In the literature, the remaining convexity of this site is considered supratip deformity [5, 6]. In the primary patient, the deformity resulted from inadequate tip projection (pseudodeformation), over-projected caudal dorsum, and cephalically oriented LLC. In secondary patients, the anomaly was due to an under- or over-excised caudal dorsum, or a combination of some under the projected tip [7, 8].

From the tip defining point to STB, the subtle concavity is a part close to the straight line of lateral genu. The voluminous STB is made of the cephalic border of the lateral crus and subcutaneous fat. Convexity is worse in this area, but excessive concavity is also subject to patients' complaints. STB problems found in Asian rhinoplasty are related to alloplastic implants in many areas.

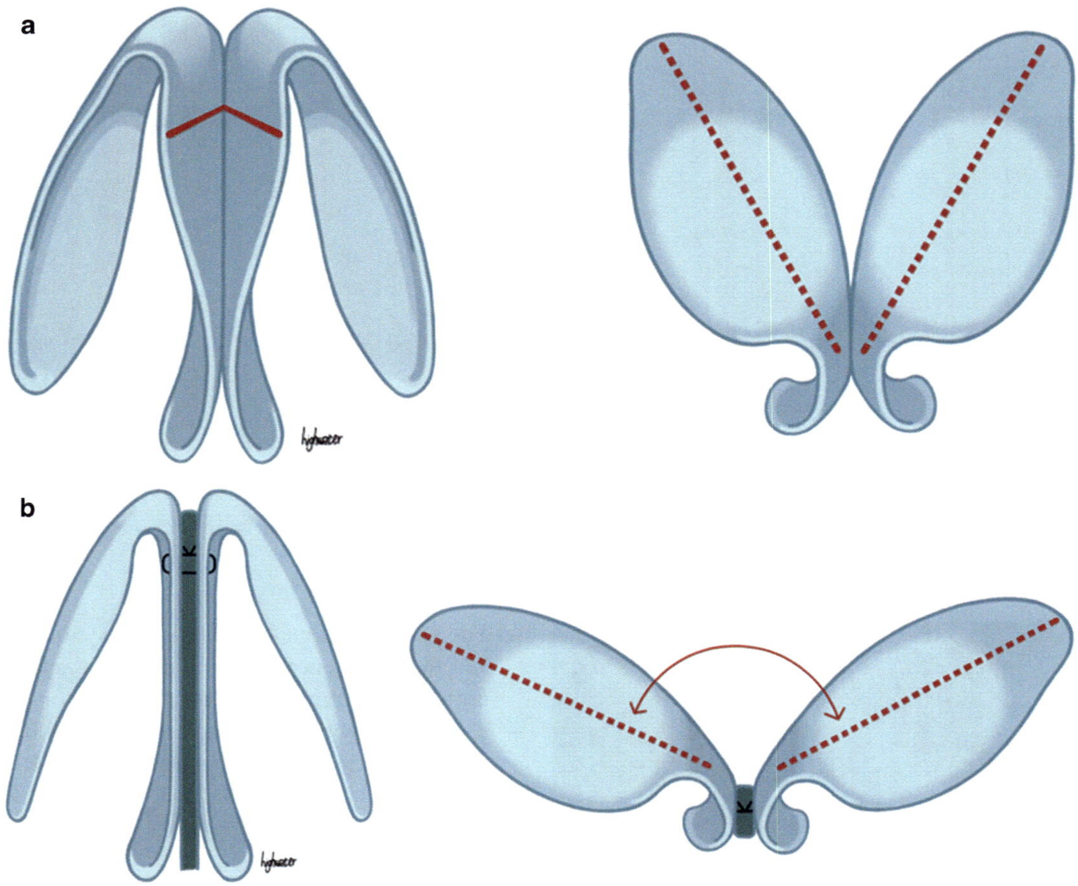

Fig. 8.5 Two divergences: middle crural divergence and the divergence of the long axis of lateral crura (**a**) Ideal feature. (**b**) The suture of the middle and medial crura's caudal margin resulted in a total break of beautiful angles. The long axis became obtuse

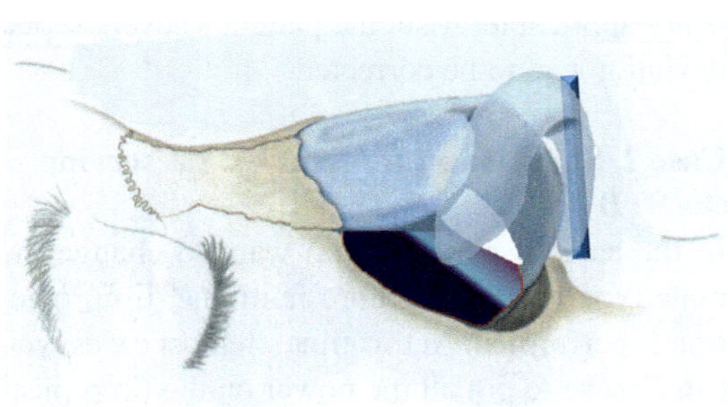

Fig. 8.6 Floating type columellar strut

8.4 My Strategy for Ideal STB in Primary Case

Case 1. Lateral Crural Deformity with Malposition

In the case of the following patients who complain of nasal obstruction with the address of nasal septal deviation, the long axis of the lateral crus is cephalically located intraoperatively, and the concavity of the STB is severely expressed because of the concavity of lateral crus (Video

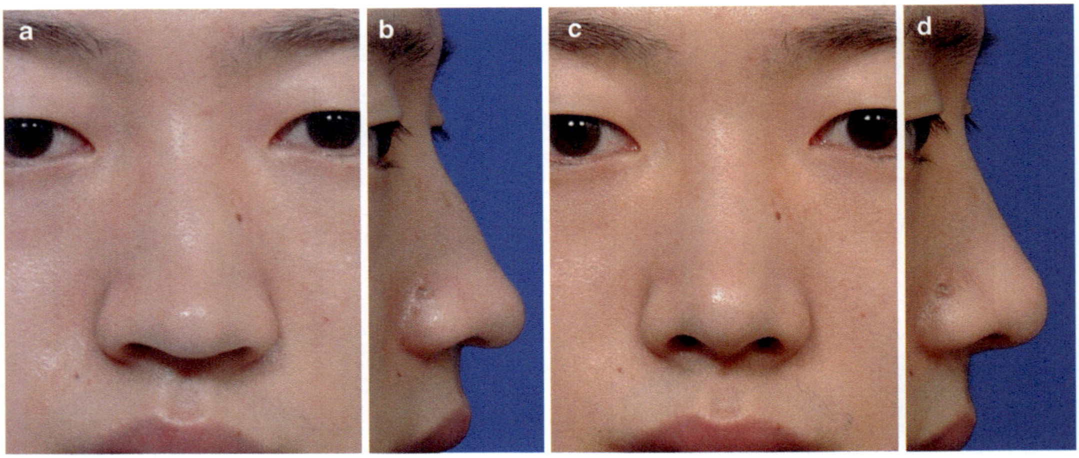

Fig. 8.7 Concave STB was corrected by lateral crural flattening and interdomal suture. And lateral crural spanning suture to the high septum after the anteriorly extended spreader graft. (**a**, **b**) Preoperative views. (**c**, **d**) Postoperative views

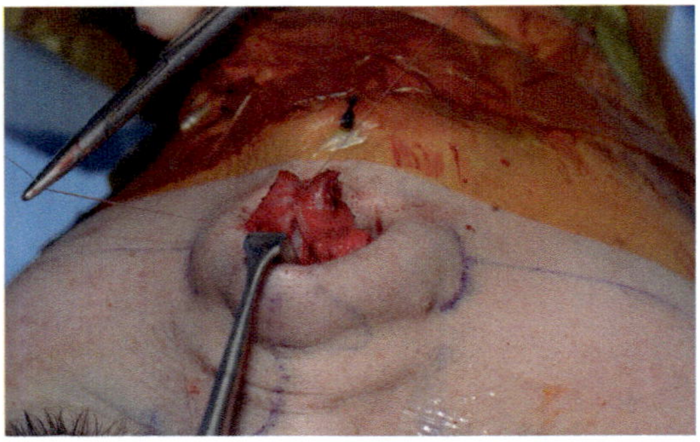

Fig. 8.8 After the key suture: the interdomal suture should be located at the cephalic portion of the middle crura

8.1). After correcting the mild hump by rasping, the lateral crus was fixed to the anteriorly extended high septum through the lateral crural spanning suture after lateral crural cephalic trim (Figs. 8.7 and 8.8).

Anterior septal reconstruction is required because fixation is required in relation to septum and LLC with lateral crural spanning suture. The septal L-strut extension will be discussed in detail later in Chap. 11 again. A shield graft was applied for the position along with the correction of the drooping of the tip.

- The shield graft maintains the tip's symmetry and the divergence of the middle crus and is useful for creating a tip-lobular angle.
- The anteriorly relocated high septum provides the necessary support to correct the lateral crus and correction of the saddle nose deformity.

Of course, the patient's saddle deformity and the concavity of the STB may be corrected using an appropriate alloplastic implant. However, in the patients' case, the augmentation of the bony dorsum is not indicated. If the skin is thin, this is not applicable. Also, the patient's severe septal deviation had to be corrected.

Case 2. Short Nasal Implant Vs. Preserving the STB

In the case of patients who want to change the male type nose to be more feminine, tip projection is performed. At this time, in most cases, you can choose to put all the power on the tip projection and camouflage the dorsum with an alloplastic material, but not using alloplastic material up to the tip is the consensus of the current Asian rhinoplasty. So many problems are caused by this short dorsal implant. These problems will be

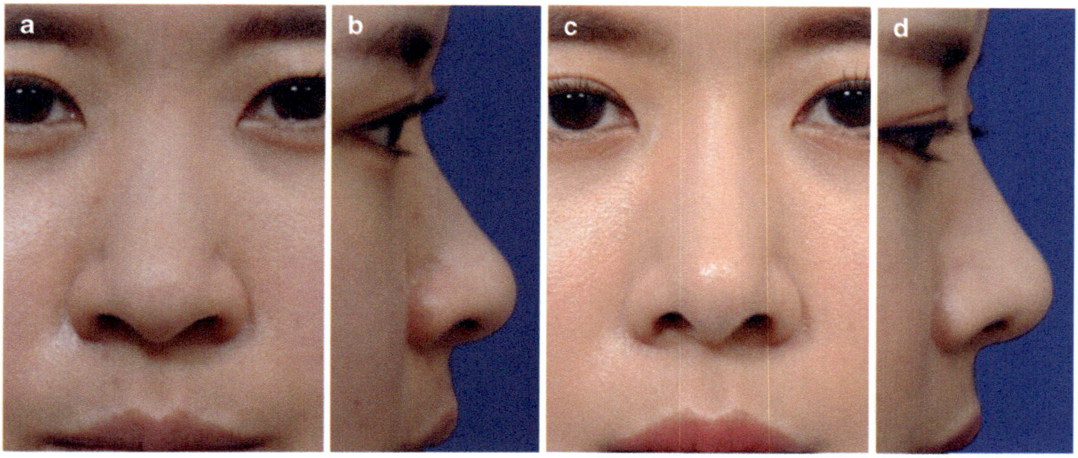

Fig. 8.9 Male type supratip bulbosity was corrected by lateral crural positioning with ideal divergence angles of LLC. Lateral crural spanning suture was applied to the high septum after the anteriorly extended spreader graft. (**a**, **b**) Preoperative views. (**c**, **d**) Postoperative views

covered in the secondary case below. In the case of using autograft without dorsal implant in the primary case, the abrupt concavity of STB can be found in the long term due to unwanted resorption, as mentioned in Chap. 7. The author recommends that the lower two-third nose is projected using cartilages as possible.

- The high septum reconstruction is required to prevent STB concavity due to resorption of dorsal graft, and supratip expressed by septum has long-term stability.
- The only graft method, such as derotation graft, may cause convexity (supratip deformity) and cause supratip deformity along with convexity. LLC, fixed to the high septum with tip projection, looks solid in the long term (Figs. 8.9 and 8.10).

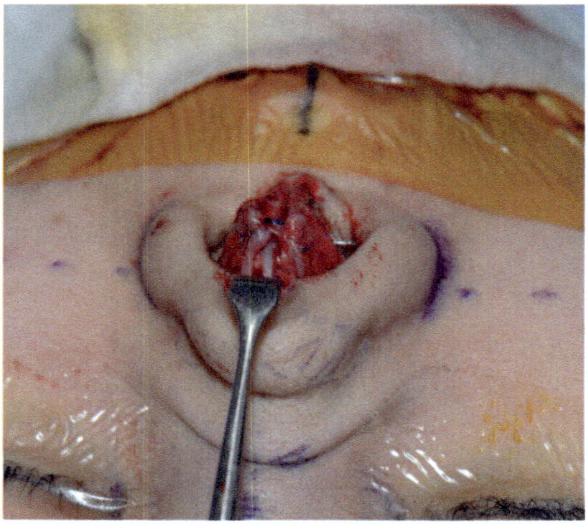

Fig. 8.10 Ideal LLC position with an apparent high septum at the supratip area

8.5 My Strategy for Restoring STB in Secondary Case

Case 1. Supratip Deformity Related to Secondary Tip Drooping

The loss of tip projection-support in the long term is the most common problem. The pseudodeformation caused by tip drooping is complicated, including scar underneath the implant, where the dead space existed between the alloplastic implant and the ULC platform (Fig. 8.11). In the case of profound tip projection, additional graft or implant molding is required to prepare for the dead space on the platform of ULC. However, the reason why the tip droops over time is complicated. The causes include loosening of suture, scar formation of applied cartilage, or the tendency of tension-loss due to depressor muscle and facial mimetic muscle (Fig. 8.12). However, most of the drooping is related to septum-non-

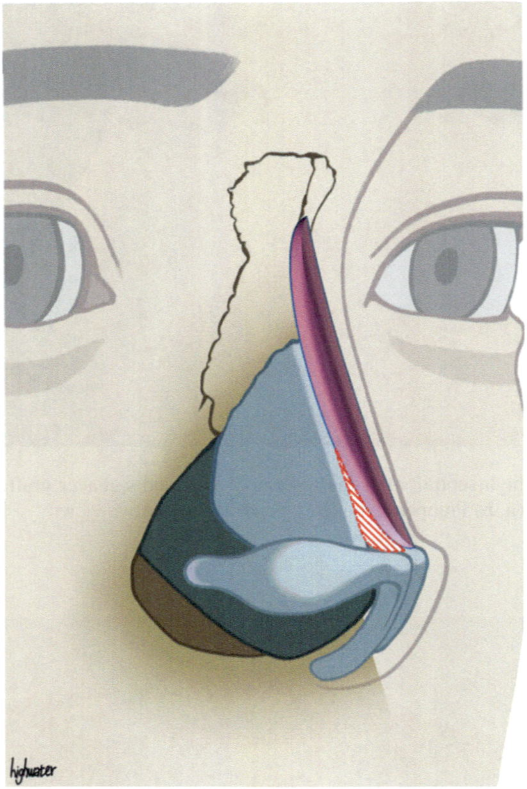

Fig. 8.11 Dead space under the alloplastic implant with the projected tip

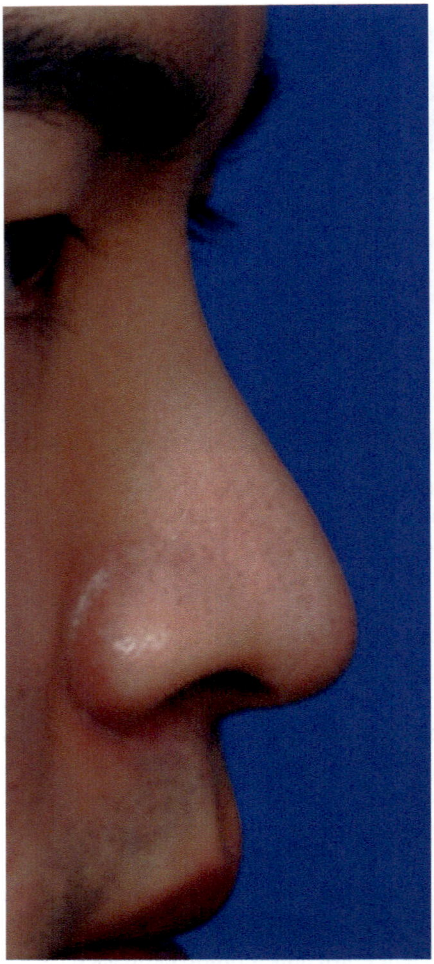

Fig. 8.12 Supratip deformity after the long-term tip drooping and dorsal silicone implant

dependency [9]. Also, there are cases where the long implant is not supported by the tip, and it is bent. Loss of tip projection-support in the long term is the most common problem. The pseudo-deformation caused by tip drooping due to this is very complicated, including scar formation underneath, such as the problem of the dead space underneath the alloplastic implant on the ULC platform (Fig. 8.11).

- Among the various methods for projecting drooped tips, LLC's own lateral crural stability method is not applicable in a secondary operation.
- A lot of LLC's destruction or resorption is found, and its strength is weak, making it difficult to obtain stability only with lateral crus (Fig. 8.13).

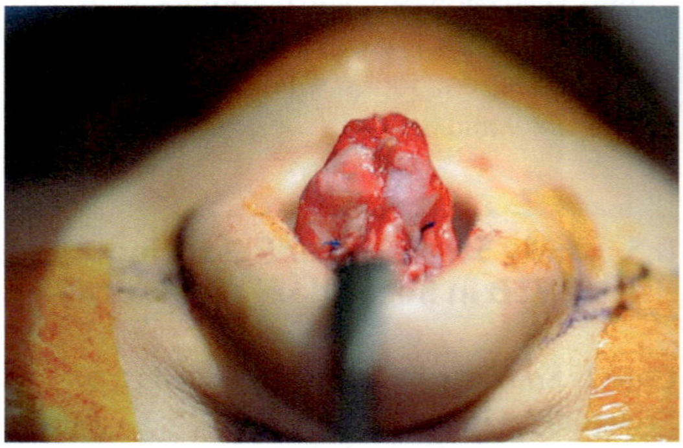

Fig. 8.13 Cartilage destruction at the right side

- Methods such as lateral crural steal or lateral crural overlay are not applicable [10].
- The author uses the lateral crural spanning suture for correcting STB as fixing the LLC to the high septum, even though it requires the reconstruction of the anterior septum. There are various reasons, the alloplastic material cannot be used, and the nasal function needs to be improved, the LLC cannot perform as much counter-clockwise rotation as desired, and the projection of the lower two-third of the nose is necessary without a dorsal graft.

Case 2. Supratip Deformity Related to Dorsal Implant

The causes of supratip deformity that can be caused by implants are diverse. The deformity of STB caused by the capsule problem caused by the dorsal implant is the most common, and it is caused by the formation of capsules and the failure of proper tip plasty without tip support. It is challenging to correct skin laxity made of capsules, and if this anterior capsulectomy cannot be completed thoroughly, the skin should naturally redrape by removing the capsule margin formed in the skin envelope with the capsulotomy in all directions (Figs. 8.14 and 8.15).

Case 3. Supratip Concavity Related to Autograft Resorption

This type is well found in patients who underwent autograft with dermis on the dorsum. The deformity occurs according to the dermis graft's resorption amount. Mainly, the dermis inserted in the bony dorsum tends to be absorbed more (Fig. 8.16 and Video 8.2). Since the findings underlying the deformity cannot be estimated using CT scan, the complex causes must be confirmed in the surgical field. Also, since the dermis graft also creates unwanted scars in the skin envelope, you must carefully score the skin flap undersurface for the dorsal skin envelope's natural redrape (Video 8.3).

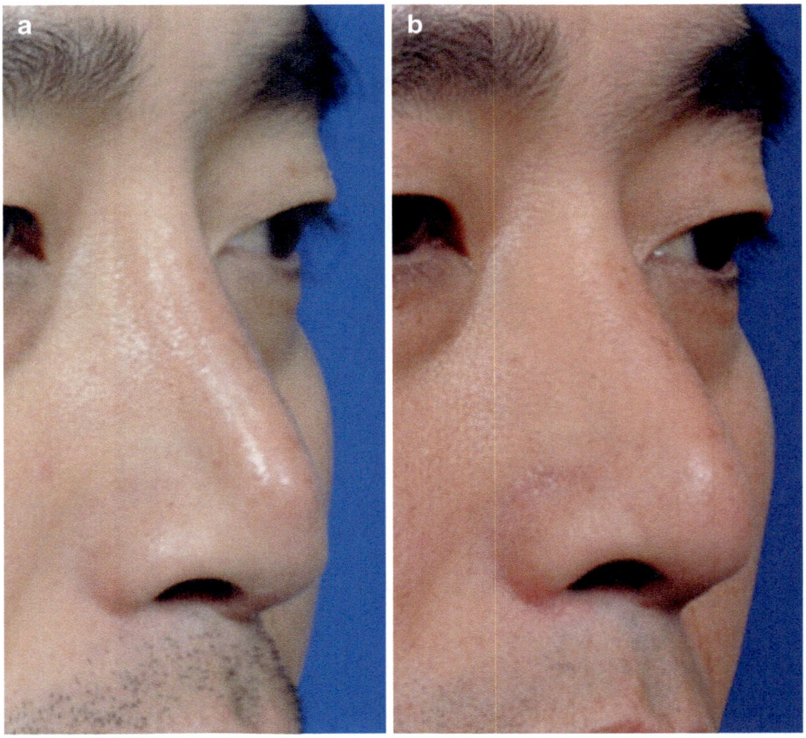

Fig. 8.14 Supratip deformity after the long-term result of Silicone implant: the skin pocket had a memory of bulbosity, so the capsular margin's scoring should be done for the redraping. (**a**) Preoperative view, (**b**) postoperative view

- Do not remove all of the previously applied cartilages. Try reusing them.
- The autologous cartilage applied with the shield graft can be used again as a middle and medial crus, and the cartilages do not need to be removed. Instead, it can be modified while attached as a reusable cartilage.
- Likewise, if there is no big problem with the septal extension graft, it is only necessary to preserve it and achieve the goal to achieve in the secondary operation.

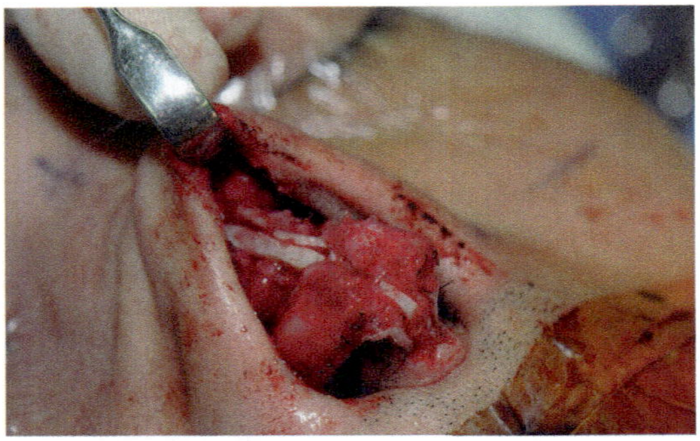

Fig. 8.15 L-strut reconstruction for the appropriate LLC positioning

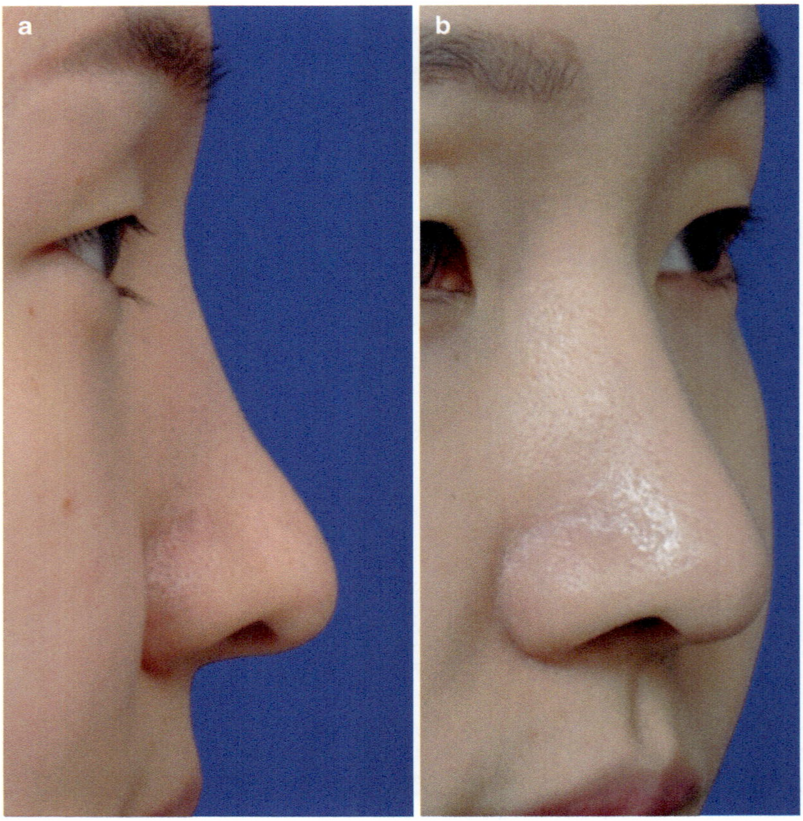

Fig. 8.16 Supratip deformity caused by irregular resorption of SDF. (**a**) Lateral view, the resorption at the bony dorsum is higher than the lower two-third. (**b**) Supratip deformity by SDF

References

1. Anderson JR. A reasoned approach to nasal base surgery. Arch Otolaryngol. 1984;110(6):349–58.
2. Toriumi DM. New concepts in nasal tip contouring. Arch Facial Plast Surg. 2006;8(3):156–85.
3. Toriumi DM, Checcone MA. New concepts in nasal tip contouring. Facial Plast Surg Clin North Am. 2009;17(1):55–90, vi.
4. Toriumi DM, Asher SA. Lateral crural repositioning for treatment of cephalic malposition. Facial Plast Surg Clin North Am. 2015;23(1):55–71.
5. Rohrich RJ, Liu JH. Defining the infratip lobule in rhinoplasty: anatomy, pathogenesis of abnormalities, and correction using an algorithmic approach. Plast Reconstr Surg. 2012;130(5):1148–58.
6. Oneal RM, Beil RJ Jr, Schlesinger J. Surgical anatomy of the nose. Otolaryngol Clin N Am. 1999;32(1):145–81.
7. Guyuron B, DeLuca L, Lash R. Supratip deformity: a closer look. Plast Reconstr Surg. 2000;105(3):1140–51; discussion 1152–3.
8. Sieber DA, Rohrich RJ. Finesse in nasal tip refinement. Plast Reconstr Surg. 2017;140(2):277e–86e.
9. Min HJ, Lee SB, Kim KS. A comparative analysis between primary and secondary nasal tip drooping. Ear Nose Throat J. 2019;11:145561319862222.
10. Foda HMT, Kridel RWH. Lateral crural steal and lateral crural overlay [Internet]. Arch Otolaryngol Head Neck Surg. 1999;125:1365. https://doi.org/10.1001/archotol.125.12.1365.

Controlling Asian Tip: Facet and Supra-Alar Groove

9

Pearls

- The soft triangle is not an object to be created but an object to be preserved.
- Since the soft triangle is made of soft tissue, it should be expressed by minimizing the dissection and reinforcing it with a structure supported behind it.
- The subdomal graft is a beneficial method in that it can obtain the desired dome angle along with the symmetry of the middle crura with a minimal amount of cartilage and secure the middle crural stability.
- The lateral crural strut graft has the most robust potency support since it can create the entire LLC angle by adjusting the lateral crus's position. However, most of the secondary operation requires the costal cartilage.
- In soft triangle correction, a resilient skin envelope is required to express the supportive graft to be considered in the primary rhinoplasty.
- Use the "sleeve-down" technique to recruit as much skin envelopes around the soft triangle as desired.
- After "sleeve-down," the nasal skin flap should be monitored well. Prostaglandin E1 and hyperbaric O_2 therapy is beneficial.
- For the definition of the supra-alar groove, the direct nasalis transverse and some complex mimetic muscles (partly LLSAN and LLS) is removed, if necessary, the fatty layer should be removed.

Supplementary Information The online version of this chapter (https://doi.org/10.1007/978-981-16-0542-0_9) contains supplementary material, which is available to authorized users.

The original version of this chapter was revised. The correction to this chapter can be found at https://doi.org/10.1007/978-981-16-0542-0_18

9.1 The "Facet"

Definition

Traditionally, facet refers to a soft triangle or soft tissue triangle. If you cut the jewel's spherical surface, you will have a beautiful surface, which is the only part of the nose that has such a surface. Just as a well-cut gemstone becomes a jewel, the soft triangle in the nose shows the beauty of the nose along with the infratip lobule (Fig. 9.1). In Western rhinoplasty, due to a well-developed LLC, the angles transferred to the middle crus [1] and well developed, so there is no big problem if these are well saved (Fig. 9.2). However, in Asian rhinoplasty, the creation of this part is challenging, and there are many reasons.

Due to the poor development of LLC, various angles of the middle crus are not well developed, the overlying skin is thick, making the inner structure difficult to express, and the amount of subcutaneous fatty tissue is thick. If the patient has a relatively voluminous tip, there is a percep-

E.-S. Dhong, M.-W. Na, *Asian Septorhinoplasty*, https://doi.org/10.1007/978-981-16-0542-0_9

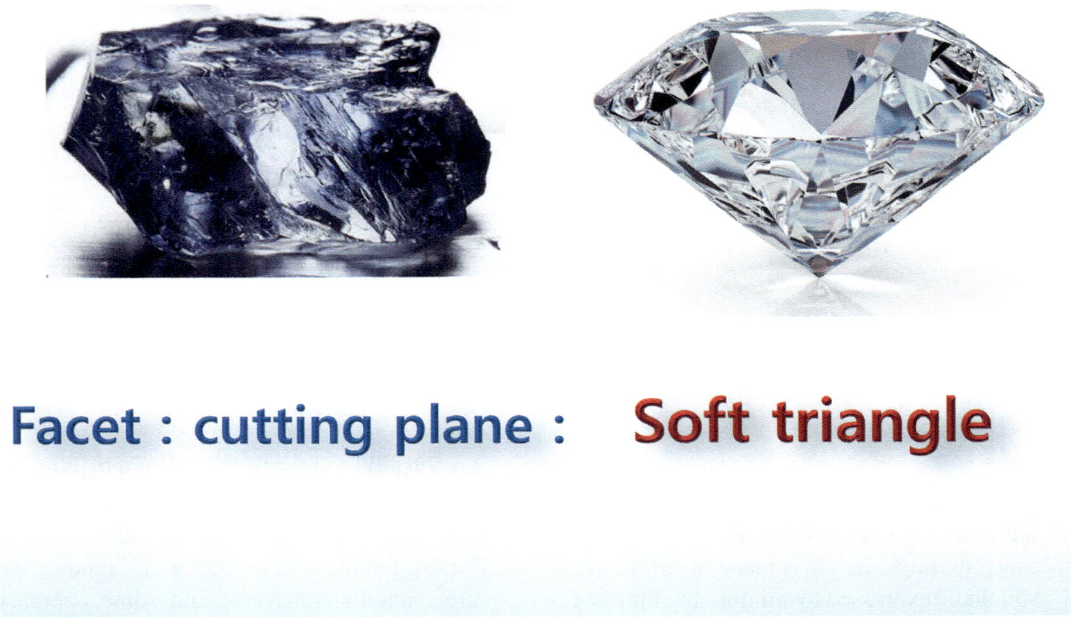

Fig. 9.1 Facet: This refers to a beautifully implemented surface by cutting an original stone and refers to a soft triangle

tion that it looks young and cute, but we need to know how to express the facet well to access the high-end result.

Anatomic Considerations

In a Cadaveric study, a study on the soft triangle revealed the safe zone for the incision. There are three zones in the soft triangle: muscle caudal to the lower lateral cartilages, an interval dermis-to-dermis contact area, and muscle interdigitating with dermis at the nostril rim [2]. Since the facet is the only body part that abut dermis to dermis, there is a characteristic that "pinch" comes well due to internal or external factors. The development of cartilage is poor, so in Asian rhinoplasty, the pinching deformity develops even though the marginal incision is well applied.

– If an implant or graft larger than the dissection pocket is contained, it may cause tension in the suture area.

According to the literature, several points are essential to preserve or make a soft triangle. First, precise marginal incision placement is the key factor. Second, LLC's internal support is needed. If existing LLCs do not have the support, various grafts can be applied, such as alar contour grafts, infratip lobular graft, and lateral crural strut graft are sufficient to create a beautiful facet. Avoiding undue tension and eradicating all dead space is indispensable during closure. Applying external supportive dressing is effective [3]. However, Asian rhinoplasty requires a graft to reinforce the weak middle crus.

Although less facet implementation is required than Western, not all patients have thicker skin. Another study categorized patients at risk of postoperative notching into three groups:

1. A narrow intermediate crus, which provided little or no caudal support
2. Adequate cartilage support but lengthy soft triangle skin
3. No anatomical problems of the soft triangle but had a wide middle crural angulation due to a cephalic orientation of the lateral crus

They believed that patients with cephalic positioning of the lateral crura are at the highest risk

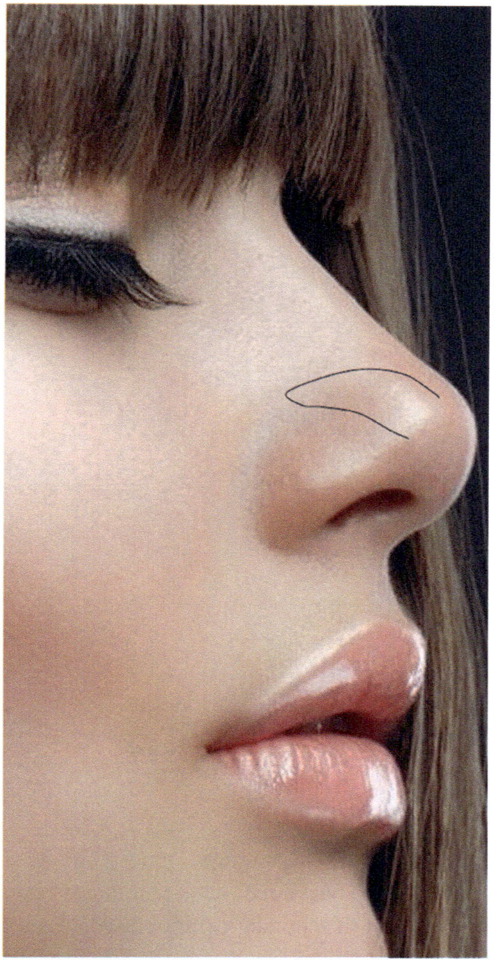

Fig. 9.2 Facet is an area of soft tissue with a unique structure under LLC's middle crura

of notching. Separating the intermediate crus cartilaginous structure from the overlying vestibular skin creates a space between two previously fused structures, causing wound healing and scarring. Moreover, they used an onlay filling graft for correction [4].

Asian primary rhinoplasty has the same problem, but with most problems, pinching is more likely to occur because the middle crus has less support. In addition to this, Asian secondary rhinoplasty must obtain the following surgical goals: (1) scar release, (2) secure soft triangle skin that can redrape, and (3) secure internal cartilaginous support. Ultimately, the supple skin's redrape is crucial because it is challenging to reconstruct after the scar is formed. Most of the alar rim graft does not affect the improvement, and it is common to correct the soft triangle along with the correction of alar retraction.

How to Preserve the Facet?

The most important thing is the correct infracartilaginous incision, also called marginal incision. Never use the rim incision. The rim incision is done only in direct ablation of the soft triangle in the cleft nose deformity (Fig. 9.3). If it is not a secondary operation, dissection of the soft triangle should be prohibited or it should be done very conservatively.

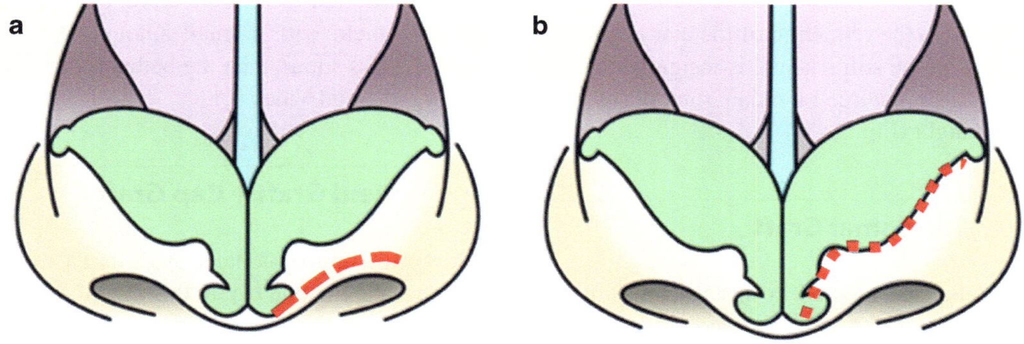

Fig. 9.3 The incision for preserving the facet must be an infracartilaginous (marginal) incision. Rim incision invades soft triangles. (a) Rim incision. (b) Infracartilaginous incision

- In many examples, soft triangles represent not objects to be created, but objects to be preserved.
- Since the soft triangle is literally made of soft tissue, it should be expressed by minimizing the dissection and reinforcing it with a structure that can support it.
- A drastic dissection can be attempted only in the secondary surgery, but the soft tissue that transitions to the alar ridges must be protected.
- In the primary and secondary surgery, the incision should be an infracartilaginous incision.
- Excessive suture tension should be avoided.

How to Create a Beautiful Soft Triangle?

As has been introduced in many other articles, the caudal support of the lateral and medial genu of the middle and lateral crus is the most important, and the corresponding sufficient skin redrape is a crucial factor. It is a subtle part that should not be too excessive or too small [1].

Among the various types of grafts that can support lateral crura, you should choose the method well depending on whether the cartilage amount is sufficient or insufficient. Below are some methods the author uses to create a beautiful angle.

9.2 Alar Rim Graft [5]

It helps solve the retraction of the alar ridge, but the effect on the soft triangle is insignificant due to the graft's nature. In Asian rhinoplasty, the effect is slight (Fig. 9.4).

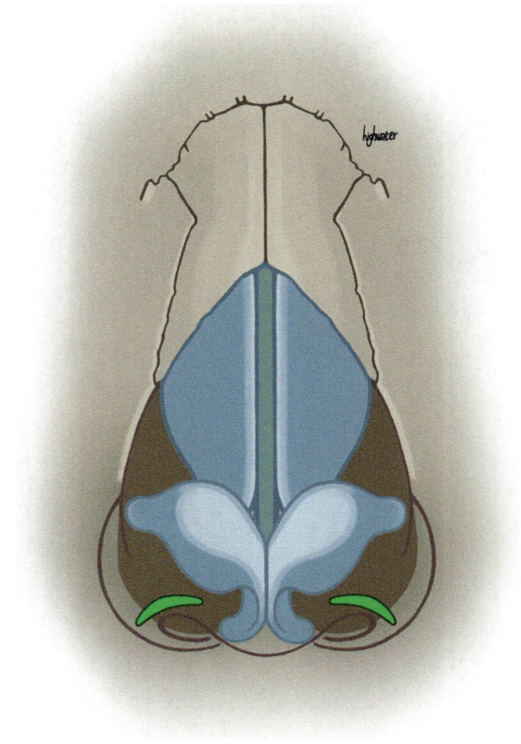

Fig. 9.4 Alar rim graft

9.3 Subdomal Graft

It is a beneficial method in that it is possible to obtain the desired dome angle and the symmetry of the middle crura with a minimal amount of cartilage and secure the middle crural stability [6, 7].

- The authors prefer this method as it is a situation where surgery with a small amount of cartilage is always required unless the costal cartilage is harvested. This technique is possible even in secondary rhinoplasty with a lot of LLC damage.

The author prefers subdomal graft because it has the advantage of natural coaptation of the cephalic portion of the middle crura, direct symmetry alignment with a small amount of cartilage, and a less suture than the batten type onlay graft (Fig. 9.5 and Video 9.1).

9.4 Shield Graft + Cap Graft

Shield graft using tip-lobular angle is an excellent supportive method [8]. In this way, the divergence of the middle crura can be saved. Moreover, simultaneously, the shape of the lobule can be created. The shape of the medial crura and symmetric LLCs can be created. To make a more sturdy middle crus, you can use an anatomic graft or cap graft on the top to reinforce the middle

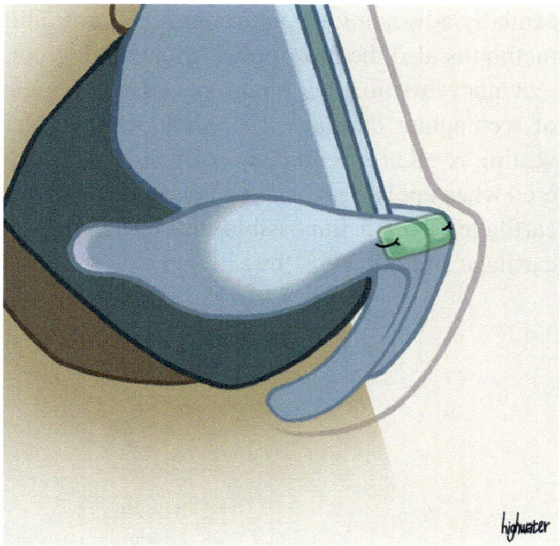

Fig. 9.5 Subdomal graft

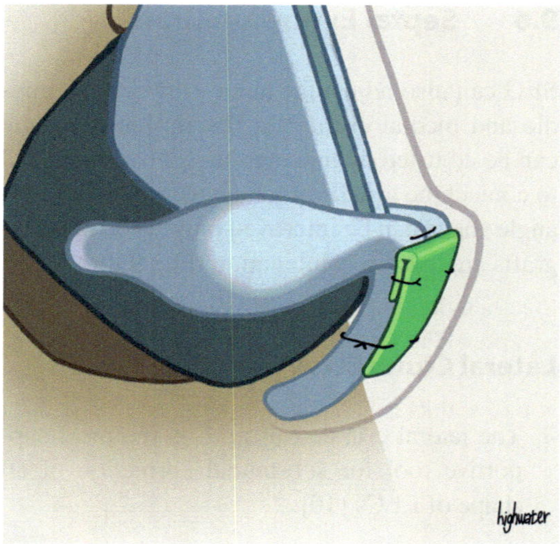

Fig. 9.6 Shield graft, the figure expresses the double-layered graft at the upper side. It is common to apply one layer

crural support. However, without the caudal septal support, this graft alone cannot achieve tip projection, even more so when the lateral crus's strength is weak. This graft is for ideal shaping of facet and lobule rather than tip projection (Fig. 9.6 and Video 9.1).

9.5 Middle Crural Extension Graft

This method can be used when applying the double-layered conchal cartilage. If the double-layered concha position is used as a columella strut or caudal septal strut, it can be used as a method for reinforcing the middle crura by extending it from the columella strut to the middle crura. It can be used to reinforce the middle crus. It is difficult to apply with the septal cartilage (Fig. 9.7).

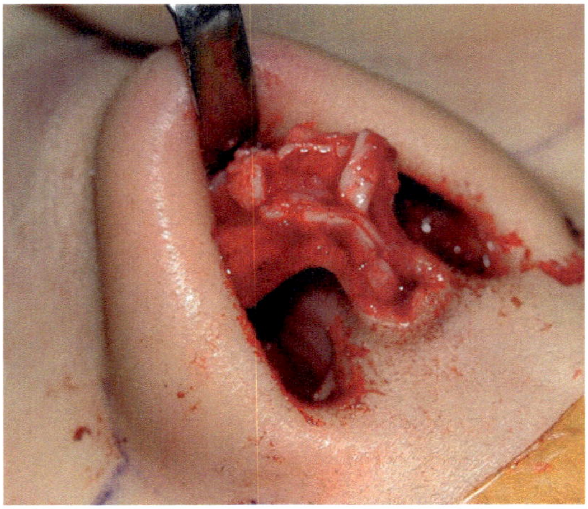

Fig. 9.7 Midcrural extension graft: Middle small rim of double conchal cartilage

9.6 Septal Extension Graft

SEG can also adjust the angle between the middle and medial crura [9]. The tip-lobular angle can be adjusted by making the SEG's caudal end to contact the middle crura. However, the soft triangle shape can be improved only when other tip grafts are used in combination (Fig. 9.8).

Lateral Crural Strut Graft

– The lateral crural strut graft is the most supportive tool for substantial correction of all shape of LLCs [10].

Therefore, there is an effect of changing the dome angle by adjusting the lateral crura and caudally advancing the entire middle crura. This method is also the most powerful method to correct alar retraction, but it requires a large amount of rectangular cartilage, so costal cartilage harvesting is often essential, so it should be considered when applying to Asian rhinoplasty. Conchal cartilage is often impossible due to the lack of cartilage strength (Fig. 9.9).

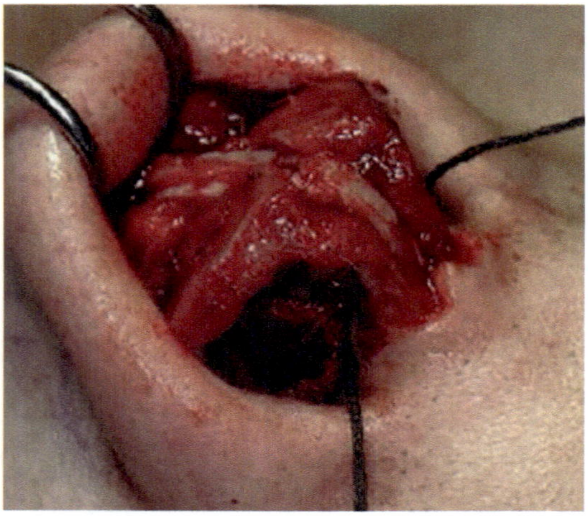

Fig. 9.8 Septal extension graft reaches to the middle crura modifying the tip-lobular angle

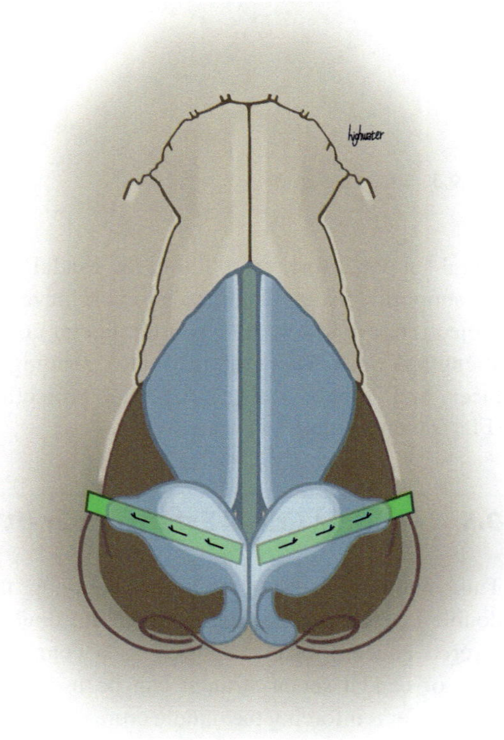

Fig. 9.9 Lateral crural strut graft

Case Study 1: Underdeveloped Middle Crura in Primary Rhinoplasty

A 20-year-old female patient was referred to the author with septal deviation and a small nose. The middle crus was underdeveloped, and the lower two-third of the nose was hypoplastic. The tip was supple and soft when the author pressed it. After structural graft, such as the caudal septal extension graft, the middle crura was reconstructed with shield graft and midcrural extension graft (Fig. 9.10).

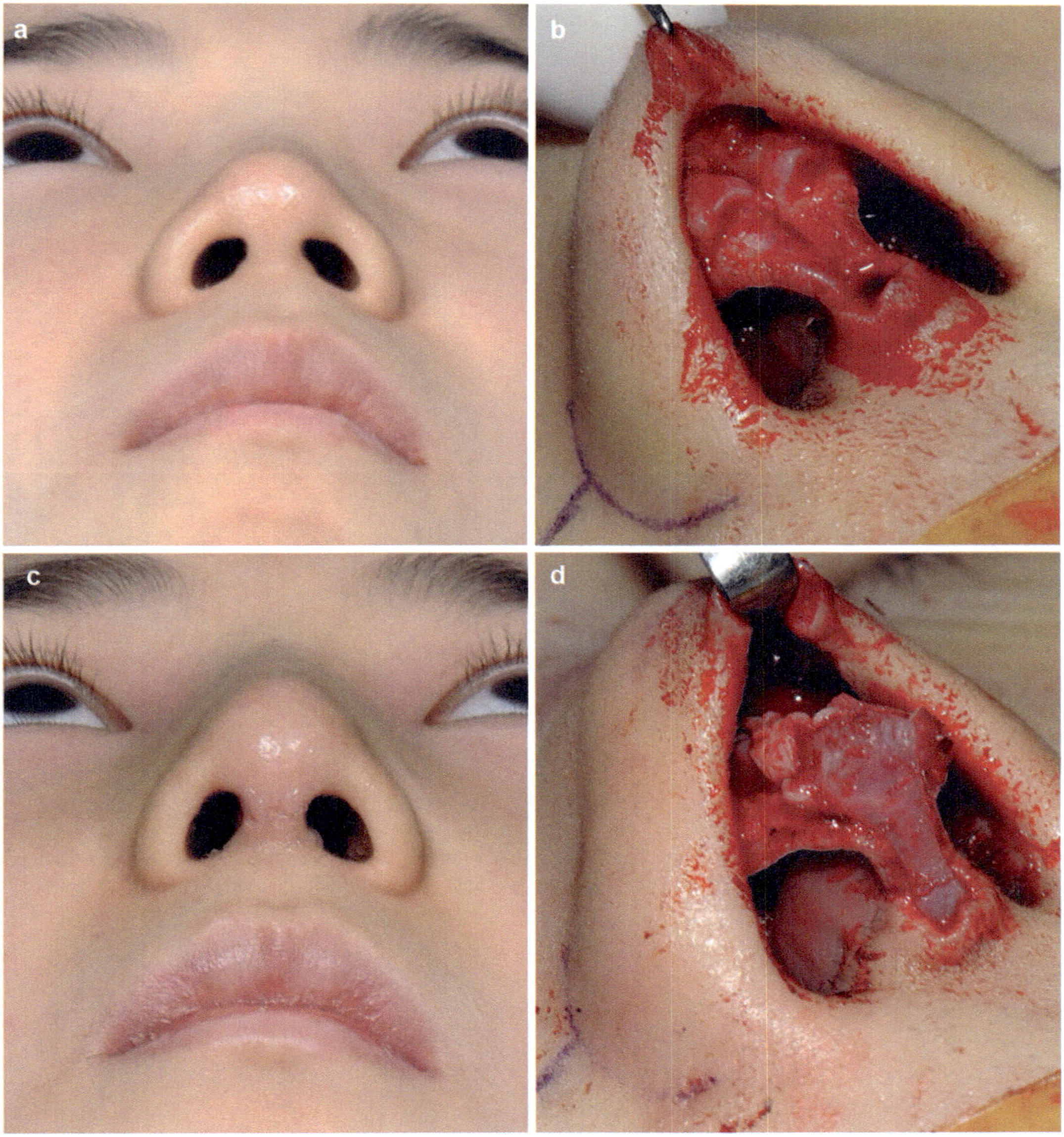

Fig. 9.10 Underdeveloped middle crura in primary rhinoplasty: reconstructed with midcrural extension graft and a shield graft. (**a**) Preoperative view. (**b**) Before the grafts. (**c**) Postoperative view. (**d**) Before closure

Case Study 2: Tortuous Middle Crura in Primary Rhinoplasty

A 19-year-old female patient was referred with a septal deviation with a mild hump nose. Cymba concha and SMF were needed to project tortuous middle crus and undeveloped medial crus. First, a septal L-strut extension graft was performed on the structural framework, a middle crural extension graft and a shield graft were applied to the tip using a concha, and an onlay graft was performed using the remaining SMF. After 2 years of long-term postoperative follow-up, a large part of the resorption of SMF was seen, but the overall balance was not broken (Figs. 9.11 and 9.12).

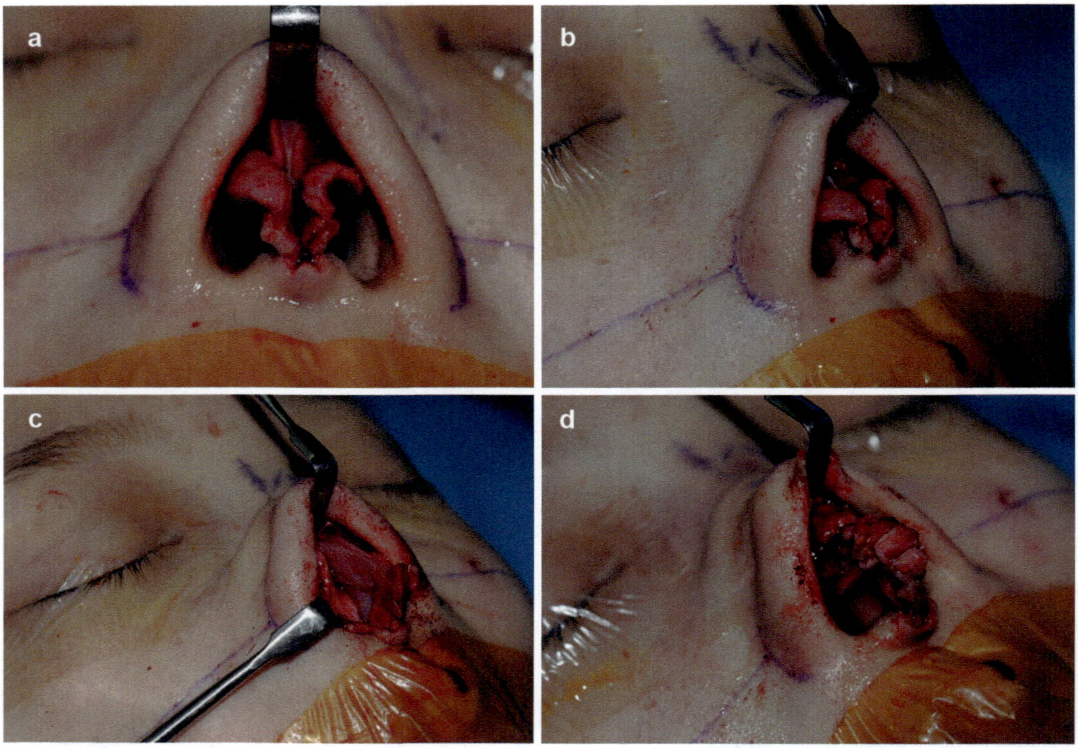

Fig. 9.11 Tortuous middle crura in primary rhinoplasty: Septal L-strut extension graft, shield graft, and a tip onlay graft using SMF (**a**, **b**) Intraoperative view before the grafts. (**c**) Septal L-strut extension graft. (**d**) Tip onlay graft

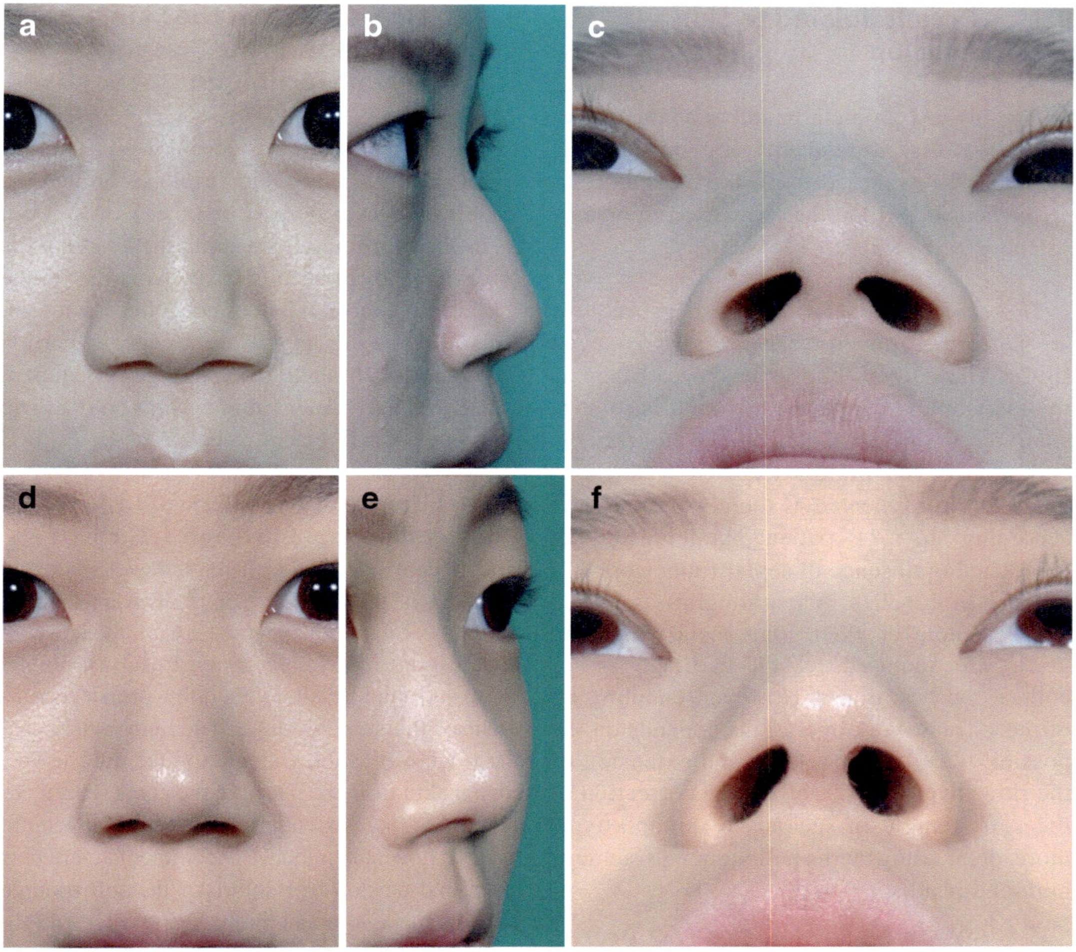

Fig. 9.12 Tortuous middle crura in primary rhinoplasty. (**a**–**c**) Preoperative views. (**d**–**f**) Postoperative view

9.7 Pitfalls Related to Skin Envelop

– The biggest problem in soft triangle correction is that a resilient skin envelope is required to succeed in all the techniques to be considered in the primary rhinoplasty above.

In secondary operation, these procedures are performed on the scar bed and damaged LLCs. The author chooses costal cartilage as the last choice. The biggest reason is to consider the hardness of the tip. Of course, the author uses and prefers the costal cartilage. However, it is selected as the next best option according to (1) patient preference, (2) destructed or absence of septal framework, (3) absence of conchas. When allografts are used at the septum or when long septal extension grafts are required, costal cartilage is, of course, the best donor. However, enabling all of these framework operations depends on the possibility of proper release and extension of the skin envelope. Therefore, the correction of the soft triangle in secondary rhinoplasty is more demanding and challenging to achieve high-end results.

9.8 How to Recruit the Skin Envelope?: The "Sleeve-Down" Technique

– The author uses the "sleeve-down" technique to recruit as many skin envelopes around the soft triangle as desired. In other words, it is a method for forcibly lowering the length of the envelope by dissecting the undersurface of the skin. Of course, if it does not come down well, bold scoring or release of the cephalic portion of the soft triangle or alar ridge is required. Here, electrocauterization using a colorado tip is used or a 15 blade scalpel is used.

Case 1: Unilateral Hypoplasia of LLC, Primary Pinching of Left Soft Triangle
The patient's left LLC is underdeveloped, and pinching of the left soft triangle is found preoperatively. Rebuild the devoid LLC on the left with batten graft (anatomic reconstruction), domal graft, and shield graft do not allow proper recruitment of the skin envelope. The author dissected the ridge of the soft triangle to take out the vestibular skin from the inside of the nares. This technique is like extending the sleeve's length: "sleeve-down technique." The immediate effect is seen, and tension-free suture of the soft triangle must be made to maintain the shape (Fig. 9.13).

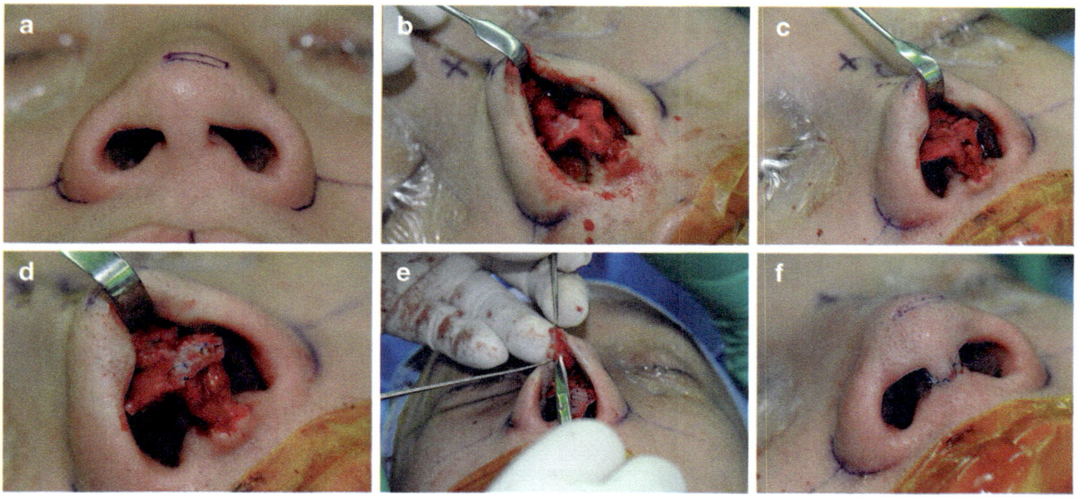

Fig. 9.13 Unilateral hypoplasia of LLC, primary pinching of the left soft triangle. (**a**) Preoperative basal view. (**b**) Intraoperative view, Lt side LLC is underdeveloped, and middle and medial crura are also hypoplastic. (**c**) Lt. LLC batten graft (anatomic reconstruction). (**d**) Domal graft (cap graft) for hypoplastic middle crura. (**e**) Sleeve-down technique after applying a short shield graft. (**f**) Immediate postoperative view

Case 2: Skin Envelope Shortage in Secondary Rhinoplasty

A 24-year-old female underwent septorhinoplasty twice using silicone and Medpor. All alloplastic materials had been removed 2 years before visiting the author. The pinching of the soft triangles on both sides was the most problematic, and septal collapse accompanied. Septal L-strut extension graft (SLEG) was performed with cymba and cavum conchas, and tip and dorsum were grafted using SDF. The shape of the soft triangle improved 2 years postoperatively.

It is more difficult to dissect the entire hard scars. As shown in Fig. 9.15, the "sleeve-down" technique may induce a temporary vascular compromise, and check for marginal bleeding. Efforts should be made to preserve the subdermal plexus as much as possible (Figs. 9.14 and 9.15).

– After "sleeve-down," the nasal tip flap should be monitored well. Prostaglandin E1, which is helpful for flap physiology, should be administered, and hyperbaric O_2 therapy, if possible.

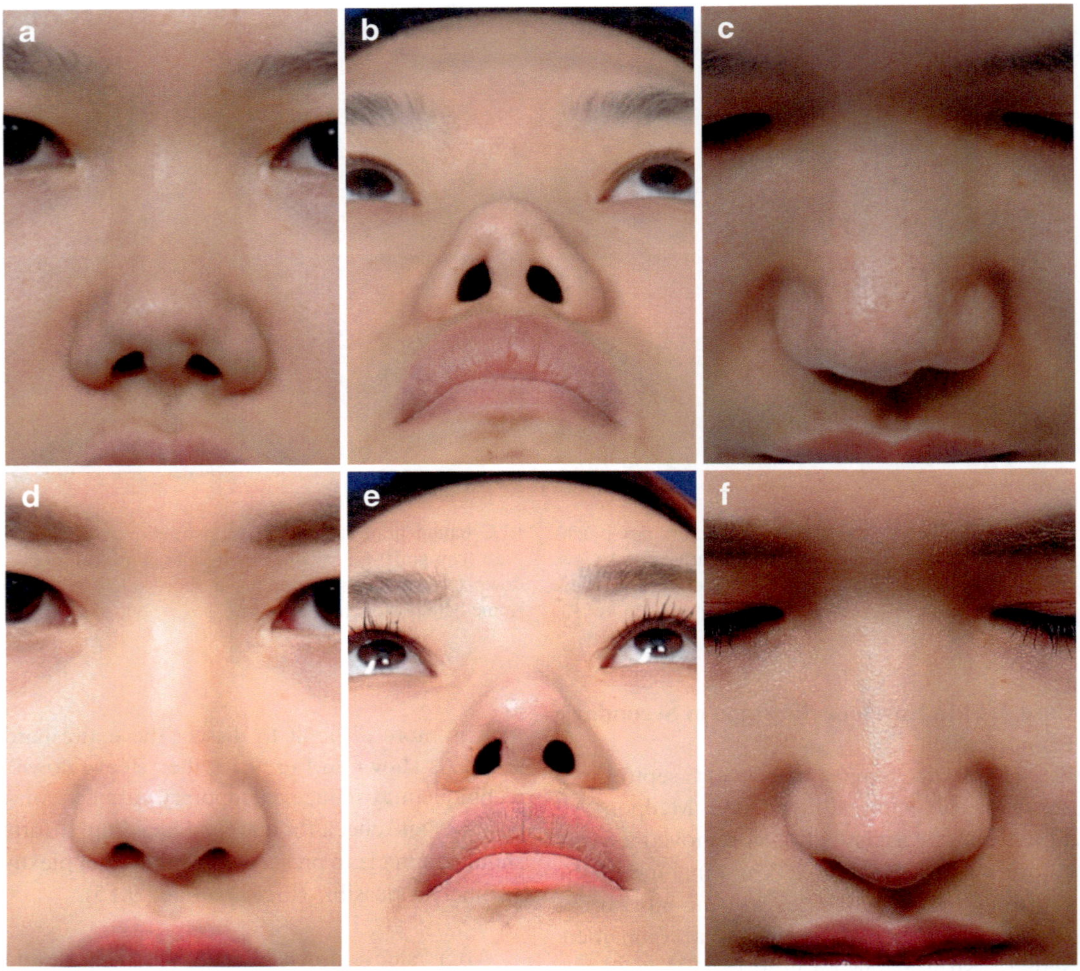

Fig. 9.14 Deformity of the soft triangle after removal of alloplastic materials. (**a–c**) Preoperative views. (**d–f**) Long-term postoperative view

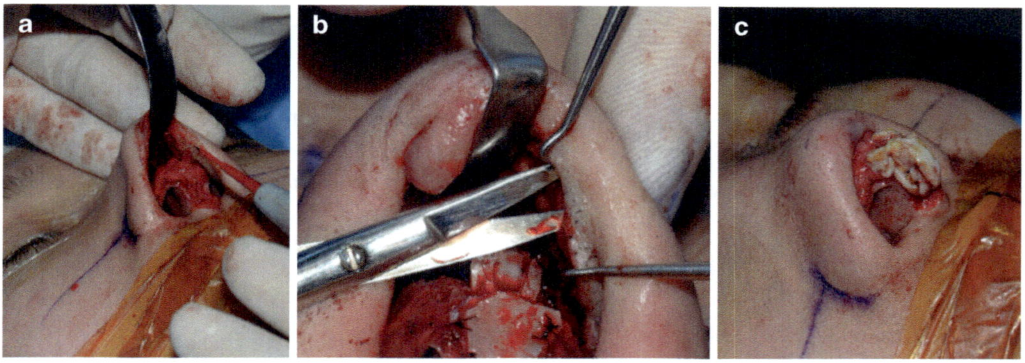

Fig. 9.15 Sleeve-down technique. (**a**) Using a fine tip of electrocauterization. (**b**) Using sharp scissors. (**c**) After the "sleeve-down," a proper amount of soft tissue should be applied

9.9 How to Reduce the Soft Triangle

When correcting the difference in the amount of soft tissue of external nares in the correction of cleft lip and nose deformity, alar rim incision is applied, or the vestibular skin is directly excised. The most reliable method is to do as many dome-lining removals as desired, and when repairing, the soft triangle skin enters the inside of the vestibule, and the total amount is reduced [11]. It is crucial never to apply direct incision to soft triangles. It is safe to remove the dome lining using the rim incision first, creating the excessive lining to be excised, which is the gap between the rim incision and the future marginal incision to be repaired (Fig. 9.16).

- Apply the rim incision first, when repairing, perform the marginal incision again. The lining removed will be the gap between two incisions, so the rim incision's position is decided by the amount to be removed.

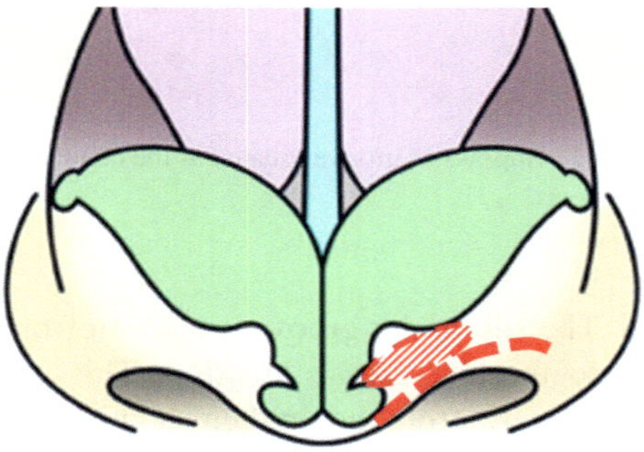

Fig. 9.16 The domal lining removal for reducing the soft triangle; the gap between the rim incision and the marginal incision is excised

9.10 The Supra-Alar Groove

Western rhinoplasty is relatively not much interested in this area. However, especially for Asian males with very thick skin envelopes, proper grooving of this area should be consid-

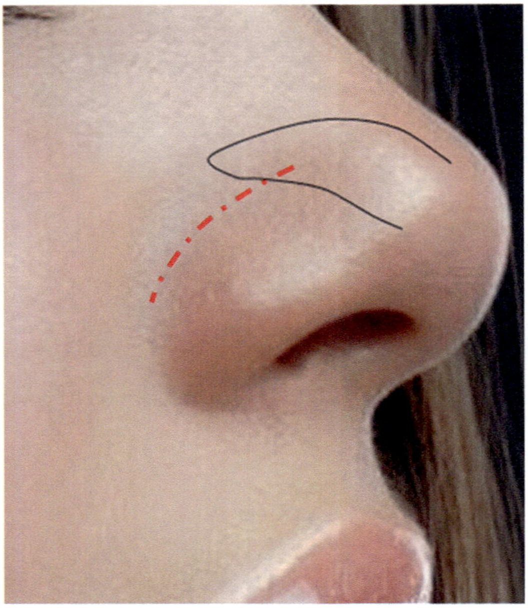

Fig. 9.17 Supra-alar groove located at the caudal area of LLC

ered. The supra-alar groove is smooth from the STB to the alar crease junction. This groove vaguely starts from the tip then shows a definite end to the alar crease junction. The shape of the lateral crus depends on the degree of cephalic rotation, but the groove is usually located at the caudal margin of the lateral crus (Fig. 9.17). This groove is intermingled with the deep levator labii superioris alaeque nasi (LLSAN) when it exists between the dilator naris vestibulars and the vertical fibers of the dilator naris anterior.

Therefore, there are several ways to sharpen this groove.

- reduce the volume of the lateral cartilage with a cephalic trim.
- make the lateral crura flat by reducing the convexity.
- reduce the soft tissue directly at that location.

How to Reduce the Bulbosity and Create the Supra-Alar Groove?

There is a method for removing the direct nasalis transverse and its alar parts from the dissected flap. The involved mimetic muscles (partly LLSAN and LLS) on the top can be removed, and if necessary, the subcutaneous fatty layer on the top is removed. Of course, it is essential to do a supra-alar stitch or firm compression dressing to eliminate dead space after removing this area. However, the dissection should be cautiously performed monitoring the vascularity and compression sore.

Case Studies: Reducing Bulbosity and Creating Supra-Alar Groove

In the case of male patients with parenthesis deformity (Fig. 9.18) and another male patient with very thick skin underwent the soft tissue reduction. When the definition of the supra-alar groove is insufficient the direct soft tissue excision can be done to reduce bulbosity (Figs. 9.19 and 9.20). However, care should be taken not to make the flap too thin, and it is necessary to check whether the pressure sore when applying the compression dressing.

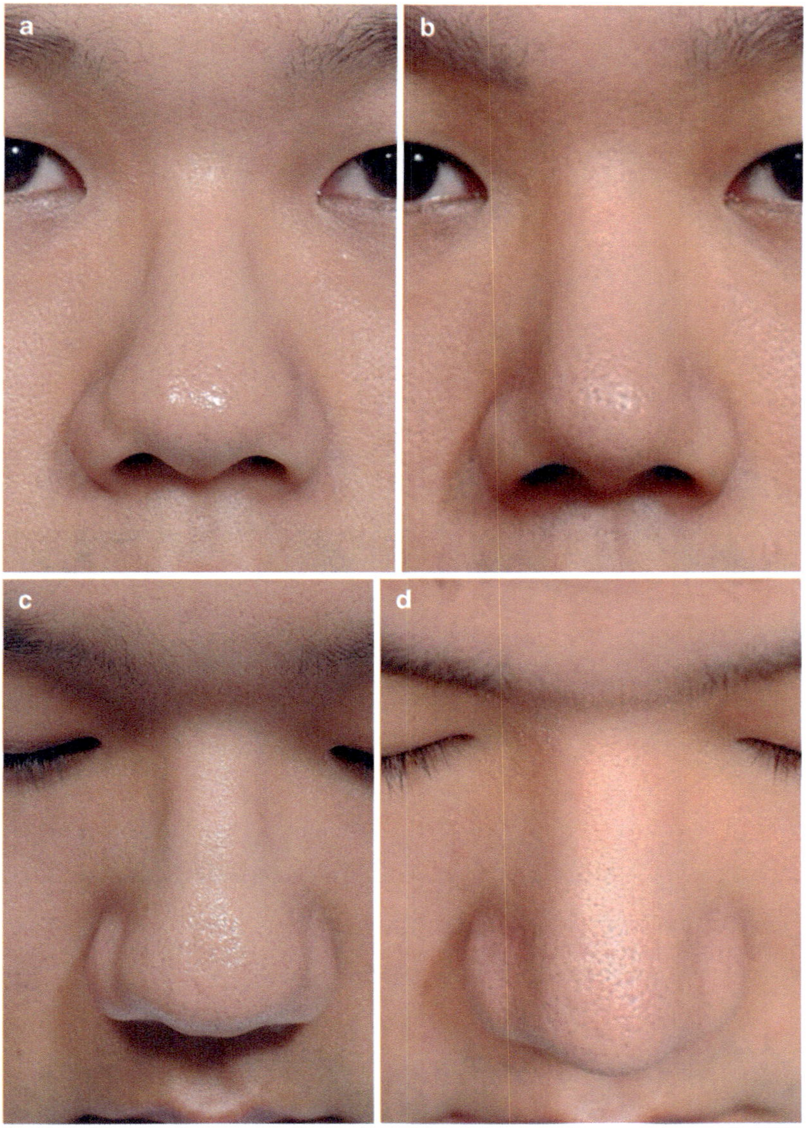

Fig. 9.18 Creating the definition of the supra-alar groove in a bulbous tip with a parenthesis deformity. (**a**, **b**) Pre- and postoperative AP views. (**c**, **d**) Pre- and postoperative bird's eye views

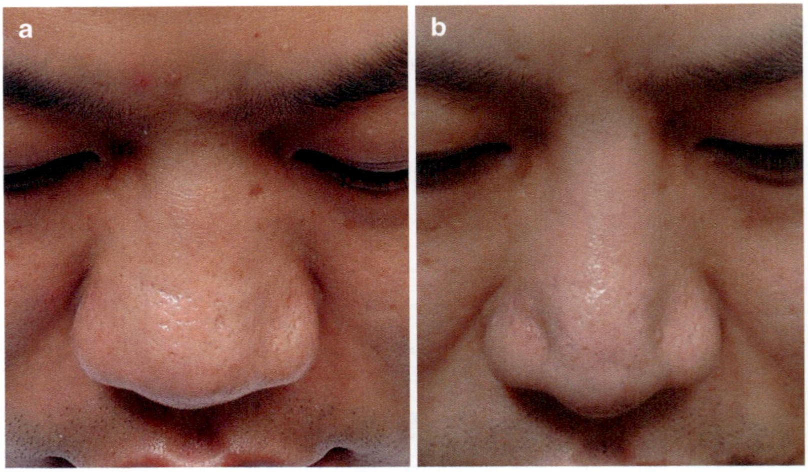

Fig. 9.19 Creating the supra-alar groove's definition in a bulbous tip with a thick skin. (**a**) Preoperative bird's eye view. (**b**) Postoperative bird's eye view

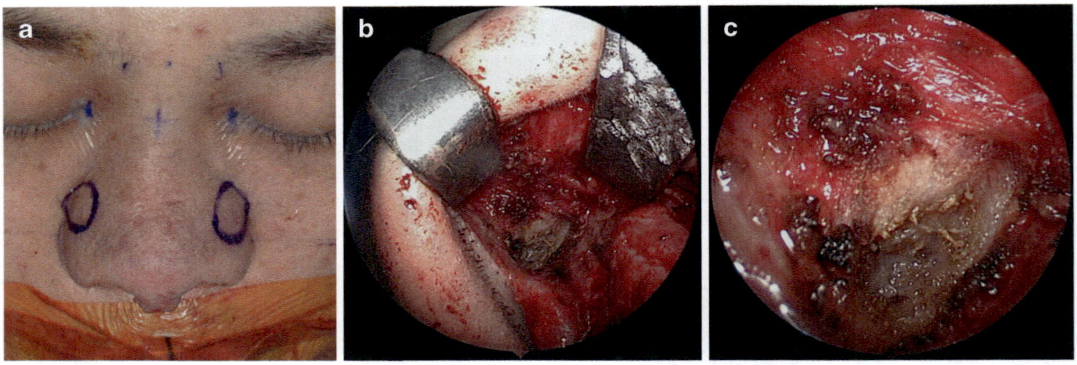

Fig. 9.20 Creating the definition of the supra-alar groove by excision of soft tissue and the muscles. (**a**) Preoperative design for excising the LLSAN and LLS. (**b**) Muscles are detached and removed. (**c**) Dermal exposure after removing the subcutaneous fat

References

1. Toriumi DM. New concepts in nasal tip contouring. Arch Facial Plast Surg. 2006;8(3):156–85.
2. Ali-Salaam P, Kashgarian M, Persing J. The soft triangle revisited. Plast Reconstr Surg. 2002;110(1):14–6.
3. Campbell CF, Pezeshk RA, Basci DS, Scheuer JF, Sieber DA, Rohrich RJ. Preventing soft-tissue triangle collapse in modern rhinoplasty. Plast Reconstr Surg. 2017;140(1):33e–42e.
4. Kayabasoglu G, Nacar A. The soft triangle: an often neglected area in rhinoplasty. Aesthet Plast Surg. 2015;39(5):659–66.
5. Fomon S, Bell JW, Berger EL, Goldman IB, Neivert H, Schattner A. New approach to ventral deflections of the nasal septum [Internet]. Arch Otolaryngol Head Neck Surg. 1951;54:356–66. https://doi.org/10.1001/archotol.1951.03750100018003.
6. Guyuron B, Poggi JT, Michelow BJ. The subdomal graft. Plast Reconstr Surg. 2004;113(3):1037–40; discussion 1041–3.
7. Guyuron B. Rhinoplasty: expert consult premium edition—enhanced online features and print. Elsevier Health Sciences; 2012. 468 p.
8. Sheen JH. Finesse in rhinoplasty. In: Symposium on corrective rhinoplasty. CV Mosby; 1976. p. 263.
9. Byrd HS, Andochick S, Copit S, Walton KG. Septal extension grafts: a method of controlling tip projection shape. Plast Reconstr Surg. 1997;100(4):999–1010.
10. Gunter JP, Friedman RM. Lateral crural strut graft: technique and clinical applications in rhinoplasty. Plast Reconstr Surg. 1997;99(4):943–52; discussion 953–5.
11. Guyuron B, Ghavami A, Wishnek SM. Components of the short nostril. Plast Reconstr Surg. 2005;116(5):1517–24.

10 Controlling Asian Tip: Infratip Lobule and ACR

Pearls

- Unlike Western classification, Asian infratip lobules can be divided into tortious middle crus, hypoplastic middle crus, asymmetric middle crus, mixed type, and secondary cases.
- Suppose the infratip lobule's shape cannot be obtained even after the interdomal suture is appropriate in the cephalic portion of the medial genu. In that case, subtle convexity can be made with a spacer graft or lobule graft.
- Most of the operations of Asian rhinoplasty are focused on enhancing the central component, the longitudinal axis of the septum, and the lengthening of the lateral component, including the alar, has received less attention.
- Extensive nasal lengthening is an operation that simultaneously causes hanging columellar and alar retraction.
- Misconfiguration of the tip-defining point ruins the entire ACR relationship.
- In the case of not harvesting costal cartilage, cartilage consumption for lengthening, and projection of the central component results in insufficient cartilage in modifying the lateral component, making this procedure impossible.
- Even a less developed LLC can solve alar retraction with proper positioning if the lateral crural spanning suture (LCSS) can be fixed to the high septum.
- If the high septum cannot be fixed, there is a method for attaching it to the septum by performing an alar spreader graft or a lateral crural spanning graft for the LLC positioning.
- The most effective method for correcting alar retraction is the lateral crural strut graft (LCSG) method.
- The method of alar base reduction does not help the practical lifting of the alar crease.
- Direct alar lift methods include resectioning the alar vestibule or detaching the alar depressor muscle. However, direct vestibular excision is more effective.
- The authors apply the LCSG method using costal cartilage, which requires total elevation from the LLC's lower mucosa in secondary rhinoplasty.

10.1 The Infratip Lobule

Definition

Infratip lobule refers to the voluminous convexity created by the middle crura descending from the tip-defining point. This angle is changed to the columello-lobular angle and transferred to the nasal base. When viewed from the side, it is an important volume that influences the entire nose's shape because it overlaps the alar base and the alar ridge above it. The tip-defining point and the lower middle crura's normal divergence are essential factors that determine the infratip lobule (Fig. 10.1).

E.-S. Dhong, M.-W. Na, *Asian Septorhinoplasty*, https://doi.org/10.1007/978-981-16-0542-0_10

Anatomic Considerations

A gentle convexity from the columella breakpoint to pronasale is created when the appropriate middle crural divergency is formed by the cephalic portions of the medial genu touching each other at the cephalic point; this is where the ideal interdomal suture located. The transition of the medial genu to the lateral genu of the middle crura is the domal segment. The lobular segment starts from the medial genu of the middle crura to the medial crura. The infratip lobule volume is adjusted by the angle formed by the left and right medial genu of the middle crura. Therefore, when the middle crus's caudal margin is repaired, the natural angle that creates the infratip lobule is lost. Instead, it is necessary to open a divergent angle with an appropriate shield graft (Fig. 10.2).

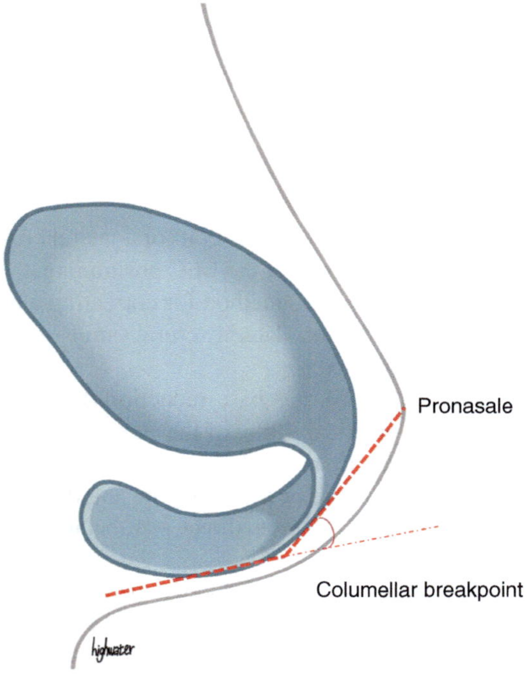

Fig. 10.1 The columello-lobular angle starts from the columellar breakpoint to pronasale

In the ideal nose, the nostril apices coincide with the midpoint of the infratip lobule. The anatomical abnormalities of the infratip lobule were divided into intrinsic and extrinsic factors, and each surgical method was well described [1].

In the Asian nose, the author has never seen a case of middle crus too wide or middle crus too long. It would be right to do an Asian classification differently. The author classified the following three intrinsic factors. However, note that in the case of hypoplastic patients, lateral crus, as well as their medial crus, are hypoplastic. It is correct to classify problematic middle crus into the following five categories (Fig. 10.3).

- tortious middle crus
- hypoplastic middle crus
- asymmetric middle crus

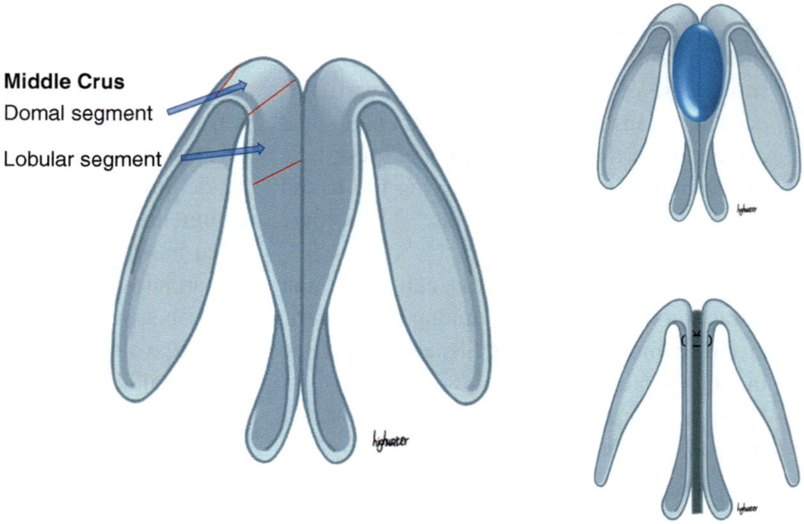

Fig. 10.2 The ideal middle crus: The lobular segment is from the middle crus' medial genu to the middle-medial crural junction. For the lobular volume, a spacer is grafted to maintain the middle crura's horizontal divergence. A columellar strut may ruin this divergence

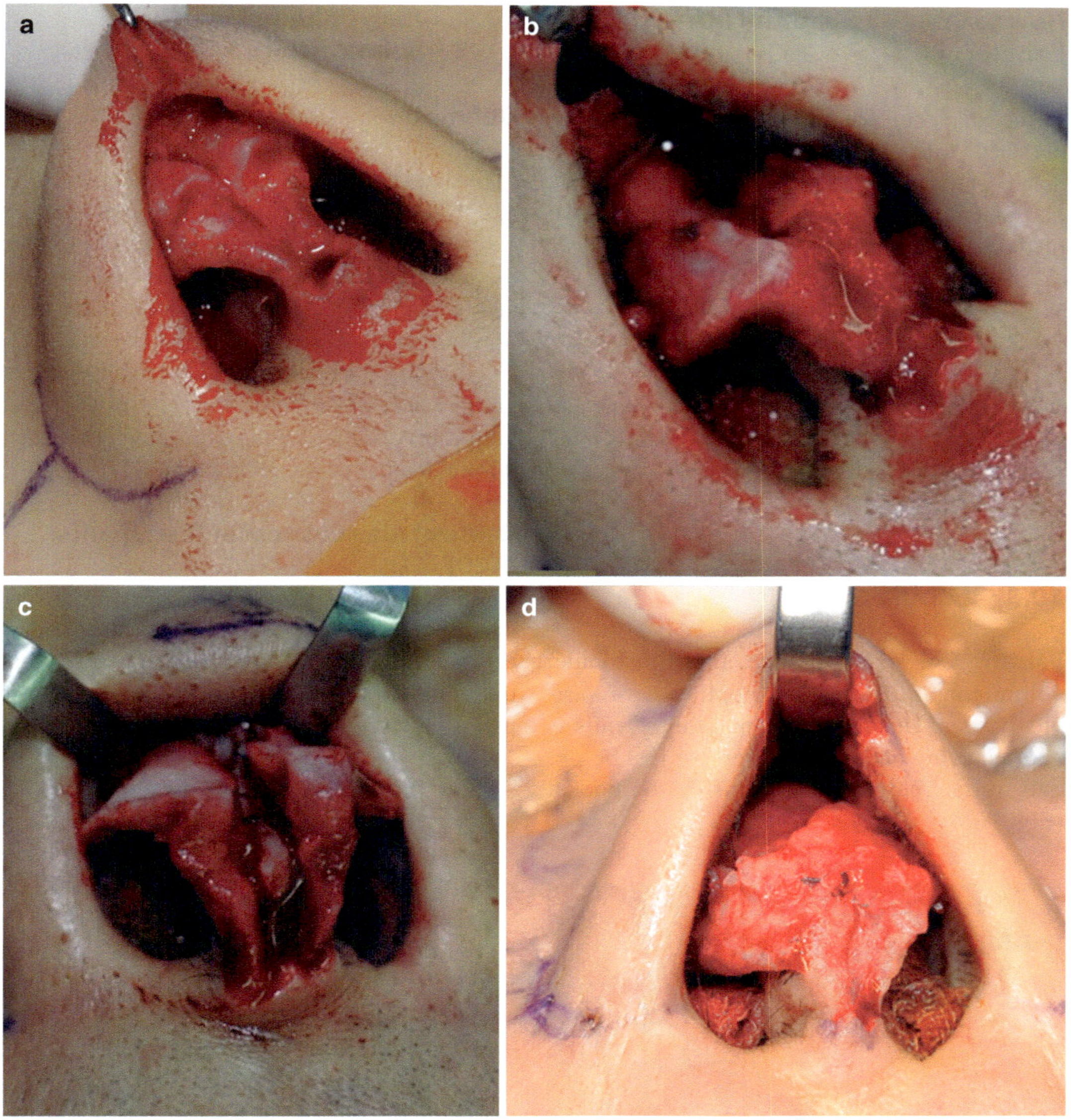

Fig. 10.3 The classification of middle crura in Asians (**a**) Hypoplastic middle crura. (**b**) Mixed type. Asymmetric + Lt. hypoplastic middle crura (**c**) Tortious middle crura. (**d**) Secondary case

– mixed type
– secondary case

The reason that the secondary case is specifically classified is that it shows different characteristics from the primary. The secondary alar-columellar discrepancy requires another level of surgery. It requires many cartilage grafts that must create something from nothing. The classification and method below were based on the primary nose. Since the secondary nose is often a total-tip-reconstruction, it is a task that requires thorough analysis and preparation of vast autogenous materials.

How to Create a Beautiful Infratip Lobule?

If the shape of the infratip lobule cannot be obtained even after the above-mentioned interdomal suture is done correctly in the cephalic portion of the medial genu, the following two methods can be used.

10.2 Spacer Graft

A spacer graft is applied between the middle and medial crura to open the divergence between the medial genu; A shield graft keeps the gap as a spacer graft (Fig. 10.2).

10.3 Lobule Graft

For the convexity of the infratip lobule, voluminous grafts can be applied with various tissues. Usually, the remaining dermis is applied using one or two layers, or just before closure, a free graft is put inside the pocket (Fig. 10.4).

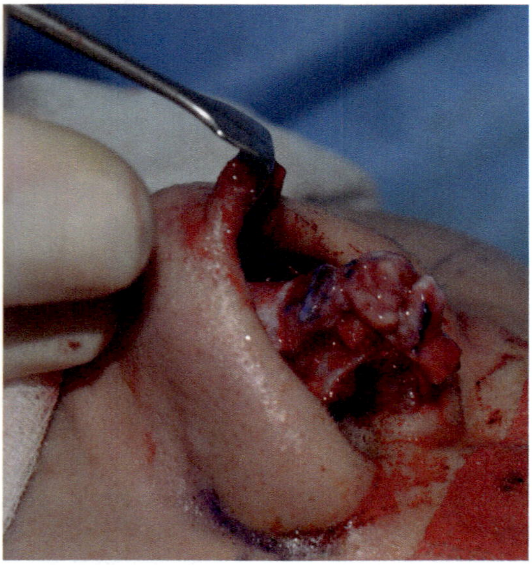

Fig. 10.4 Lobule graft using SDF remnant

10.4 Alar-Columellar Relationship: ACR

Definition

In the lateral view, the nostril's apex comes in the middle between the tip-defining point and the columellar breakpoint. The relationship between the columellar and alar is divided into hanging and retraction with the ideal alar-columellar relationship as 2 mm of columellar show [2] (Fig. 10.5). Moreover, the study concluded that graft is needed for retraction, and resection or graft is needed for hanging depending on whether it is columellar or alar (Fig. 10.6).

Cause of Alar-Columellar Discrepancy (ACD)

In Asian rhinoplasty, the cause of ACD is very complicated. Projecting the tip and extending the entire nose is defined as the operation of the central component, while the operation of the alar part is the lateral component.

- Most Asian rhinoplasty focused on enhancing the central component, which is the septum's longitudinal axis. The lengthening of the lateral component, including the alar, has received less attention.
- Extensive nasal lengthening is an operation that simultaneously causes hanging columellar and alar retraction.
- Misconfiguration of the tip-defining point ruins the entire ACR relationship.
- The wrong resting angle in the LLC's horizontal relationship will spoil the overall alar ridge's shape.

Case Study 1

A 20-year-old woman visited the author with septal deviation and a small nose. The septal deviation was corrected by swing-door procedure, and a septal extension graft was performed using conchas. The low nasion was augmented using a dorsal 3.5 mm silicone, and as shown in the picture, the length of the central component

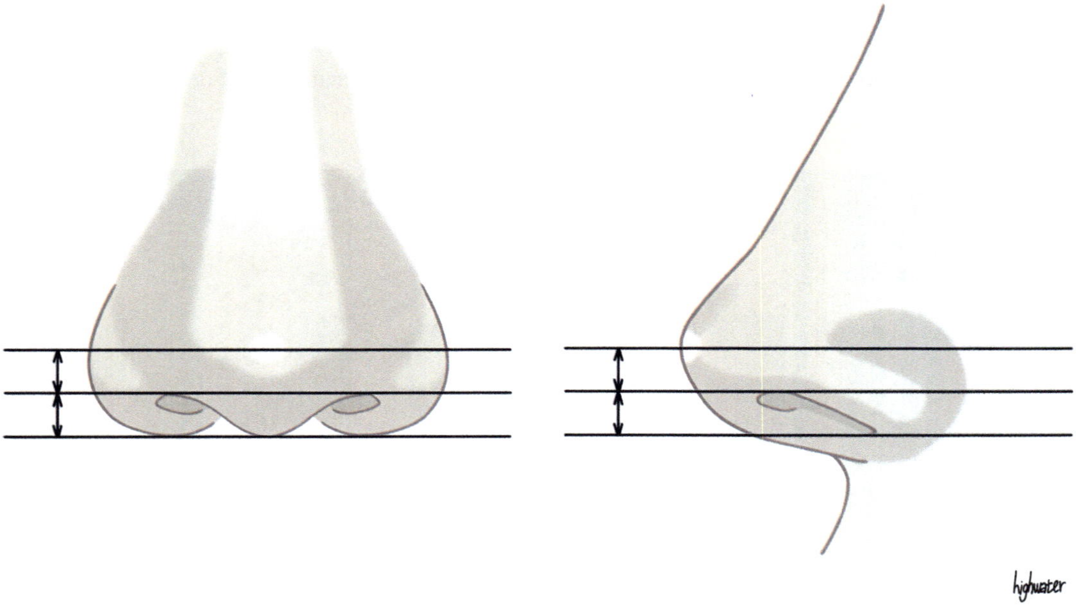

Fig. 10.5 The ideal alar rim starts at the half distance between the columellar-lobular angle and the tip-defining point [2]

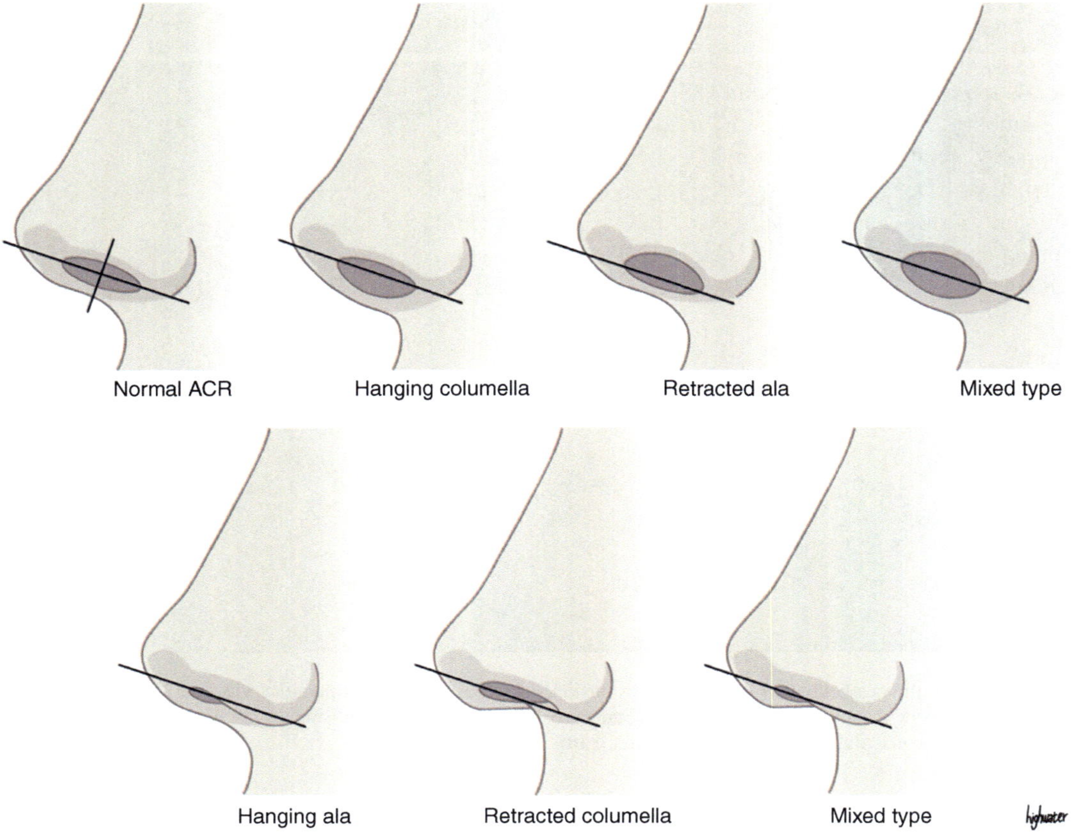

Fig. 10.6 Various types of ACR: The retraction vs. hanging [2]

was extended, and the dorsum was augmented, but there was no extension of the lateral component. There was no complaint from the patient after the operation, but the alar retraction became obvious, and the hanging of the columella appeared more than 2 mm (Fig. 10.7).

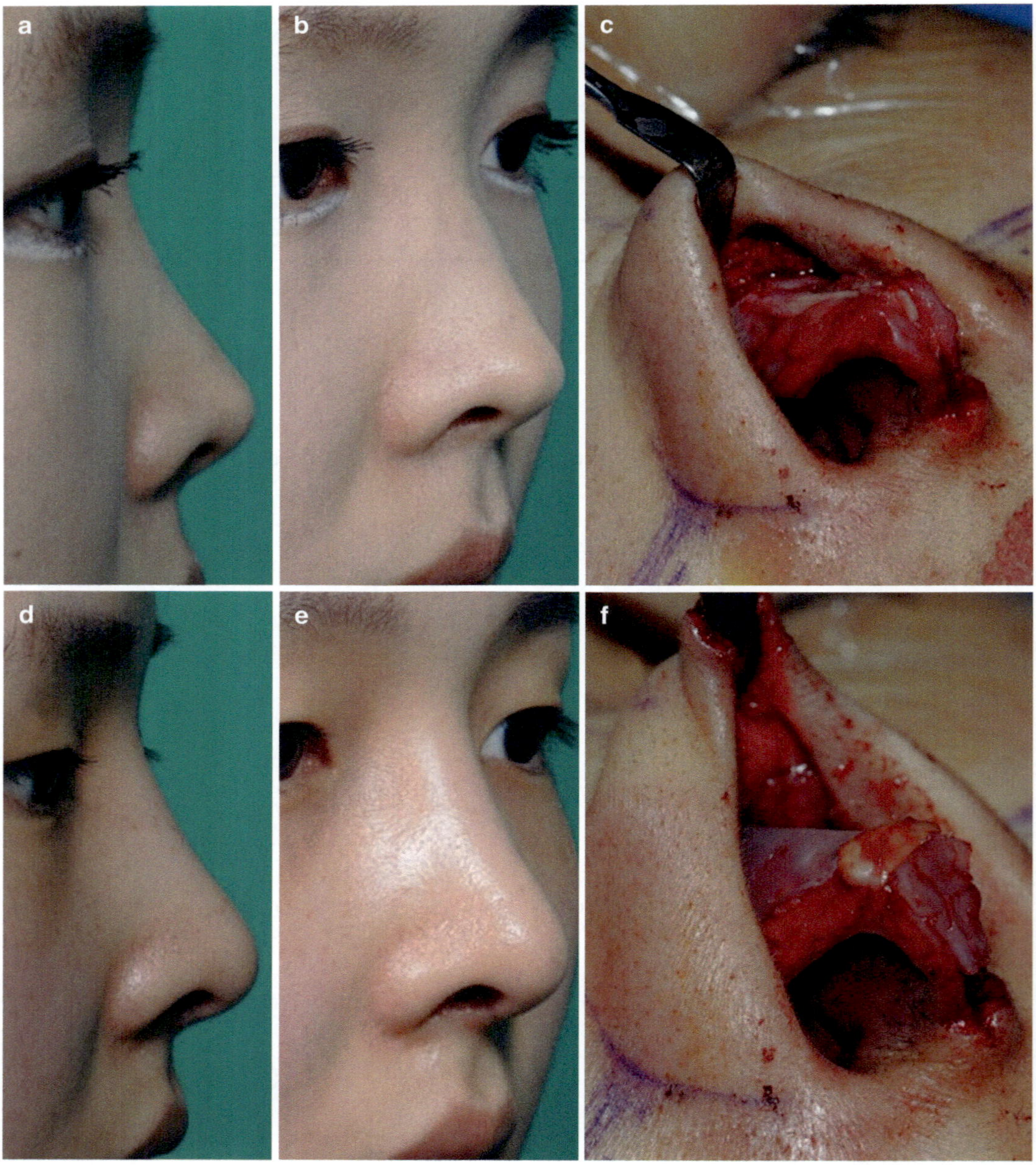

Fig. 10.7 With the perspective of ACR, septal extension graft may aggravate the alar retraction. (**a**, **b**) Preoperative views. (**c**) After the septal extension graft using ear cartilages. (**d**, **e**) Postoperative views. (**f**) Before closure, 3.5 mm silicone and shield graft were applied

- However, the cartilage was insufficient, and costal cartilage was not in the plan for modifying the lateral component, and firm slices of cartilages are indispensable.

Case Study 2

A 50-year-old male visited the author with the chief complaint of alar retraction seen from the front. Since he did not want any type of rhinoplasty, a composite graft from cavum concha for vestibular lining improved the alar retraction (Fig. 10.8).

Central Component Vs. Lateral Component Discrepancy

As shown in the above-mentioned two cases, ACR cannot be improved only by preoperative planning. Modifying ACR after lengthening the central component is required. It is necessary to consider the lateral component of ULC and LLC together after the nasal lengthening, including tip projection and caudal septal extension. In case study 1, a lateral crural strut graft would have been needed because of the underdeveloped LLCs. This would have required the costal cartilage, and the patient may have refused the surgery after being explained. Unlike secondary rhinoplasty, there are many limitations to recommending ribs as donors in Asian primary rhinoplasty.

Strategy for Lateral Component Extension

In primary rhinoplasty, since most of the harvested cartilages are spent in the central component, there are many restrictions on lowering the lateral component. The following methods are selected accordingly.

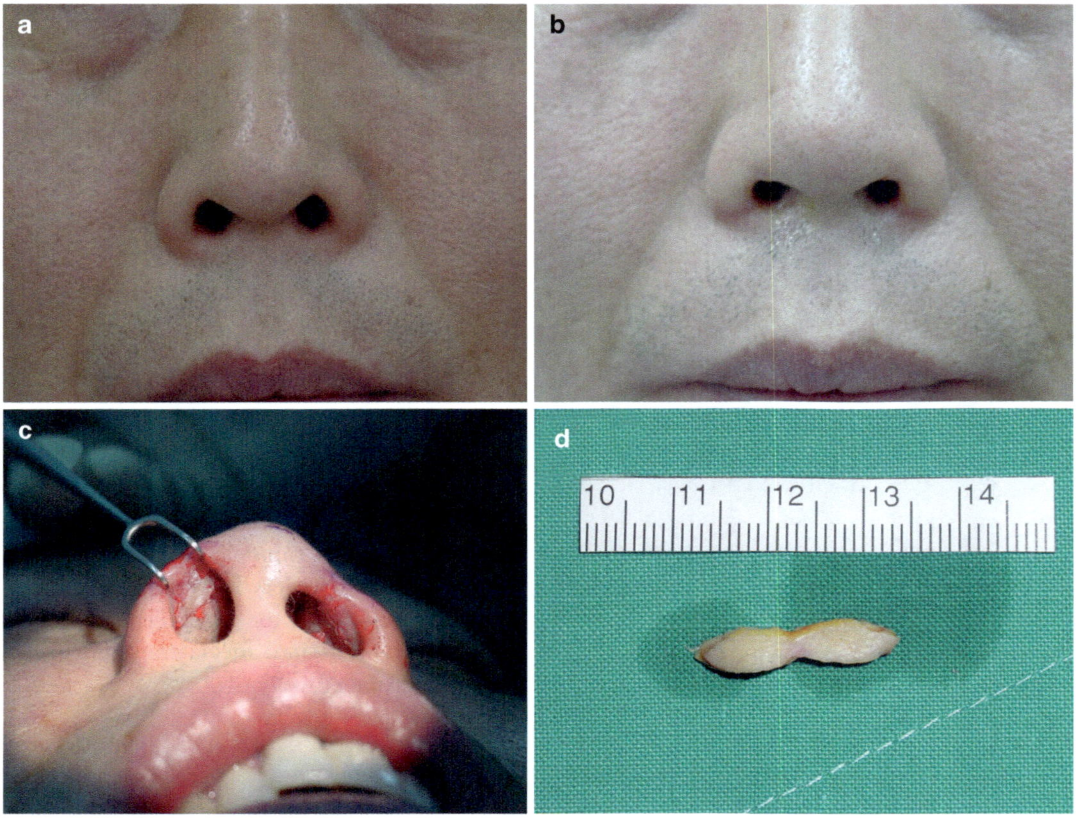

Fig. 10.8 Composite graft for the retracted alar. (**a**) Preoperative AP view. (**b**) Postoperative AP view. (**c**) Intraoperative basal view. (**d**) The composite graft was harvested from the right posterior ear

10.5 Lowering LLC by Lateral Crural Spanning Suture (LCSS)

Doing LCSS only between LLCs does not affect the position. It must be able to penetrate the high septum and lower the LLC to the desired location. LCSS can be used for reducing the bulbosity of the tip. However, LCSS is useful in the LLC positioning. If the high septum cannot be coapted together, this method will not lower the total LLC complex (Fig. 10.9). This method does not affect lowering the LLC as much as desired, but the author thinks it is a method that does not worsen the alar retraction.

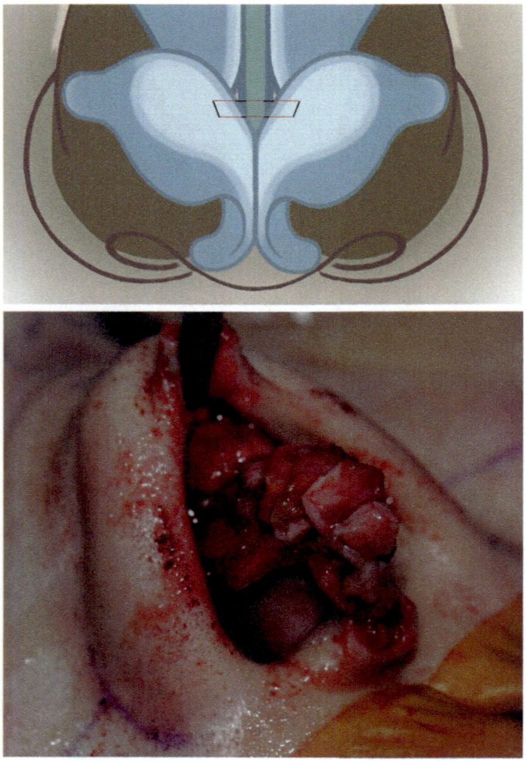

Fig. 10.9 Positioning LLC only by lateral crural spanning suture is not enough for the lowering. It is not recommended to graft excessive central components like the photo

10.6 Alar Batten Graft: Alar Extension Graft

A method was introduced to locate the nostrils downwardly applying batten graft in contact with the LLC's caudal margin [3, 4]. The entire LLC can also be lowered by performing batten graft on the scroll area at the boundary between LLC and ULC. This procedure was initially developed as surgery for internal valve collapse [5, 6]. The authors do not prefer this method because the amount of cartilage used here is too high. If the surgery of the lateral component is the main procedure, you can try. The author does not use it because of the stability issue, and the retracted alar margin does not come down in this way as much as wanted.

10.7 Camouflage of Retracted Alar Ridge

The alar rim graft and the composite graft of nasal lining introduced above is a method for improving retraction by redraping the alar ridge without moving LLC and can be used for mild alar retraction (Fig. 10.8).

10.8 Lateral Crural Strut Graft (LCSG)

The most potent LLC lowering method is LCSG [7]. It has been introduced in the literature for a long time modifying secondary rhinoplasty using costal cartilage. It can be applied as an alar contour graft according to its position [8]. However, in Asian rhinoplasty, where the central component's surgery is prioritized, it is difficult to apply due to the lack of cartilage. It is not easy to insert into the lateral side pocket with ear cartilage.

How to Recruit the Skin Envelope?: The "Sleeve-Down" Technique

- The author uses the "sleeve-down" technique to recruit skin envelopes around the alar ridge as desired.

In other words, it is a method for forcibly lowering the length of the envelope by dissecting the undersurface of the skin. Of course, if it does not come down well, bold scoring or release is needed. Electrocauterization using a colorado tip is beneficial or a 15 blade scalpel is used. These methods are the same as how to make beautiful facets in Chap. 9.

Strategy for Lifting the Alar Base: Alar Lift

Often the alar base reduction (excising the nostril sill and lateral alar base) makes the alar hanging more severe and the tip projection decreased [9].

Although the alar flaring is improved, there is no change in the alar crease junction's vertical position (Fig. 10.10). Therefore, along with alar base reduction, the vestibule skin's vertical amount should be excised and sealed in any way. Several methods are introduced, but the author prefers performing vertical wedge resection of the medial vestibule sill for reducing its internal nasal lining. If the base is not raised vertically, reducing the lateral alar flap's vestibule does not affect the alar position. Direct levator plication can be applied by dissection of the lateral sill [10].

Although the supra-alar groove's modification is described in Chap. 9, the author agrees that the alar position's vertical changed by dissecting the mimetic muscles near the alar. More simply, the elevation of the alar crease junction of 2 mm is possible even by plicating the basal cutting plane after resection of the vestibular skin. However, compared to the central component, the lateral component is affected more by facial mimetic muscles, so the effect of muscle repair is limited, and the effect will be more significant only when the vestibular lining is removed.

Case Study
A 32-year-old woman was referred to the author with nasal septal deviation, tip under projection, and alar flaring. However, a nostril sill was seen from the front, and alar retraction was accompanied. The above-mentioned method was used. The central component was extended and projected by the caudal septal extension with folded cymba concha, and an onlay graft with SMF was performed on the dorsum. Afterward, the vertical reduction of the sill was 2.5 mm during the alar base resection. It can be found that the alar crease junction was lifted after surgery (Figs. 10.11 and 10.12).

Strategy for Achieving the Ideal Resting Angle of LLC

One of the critical factors determining the alar ridge's shape is the angle between the LLC and ULC in the resting state. The left and right LLCs' symmetry can be balanced by adjusting this angle and creating an ideal alar ridge. It has been reported that 100 is the ideal angle between ULC and LLC, but Asian is different from the Western nose, so it would be correct to view this resting angle more obtuse [11] (Fig. 10.13).

Correction of Alar-Columellar Discrepancy (ACD) in Primary Rhinoplasty

The retraction is corrected by increasing with graft, and the hanging is corrected by direct excision. Below is a strategy that considers the central component and the lateral component. The ideal ACR is 1–2 mm of the columellar show below the long axis of the nostril. However, it is better to apply a more conservative amount in Asian [2].

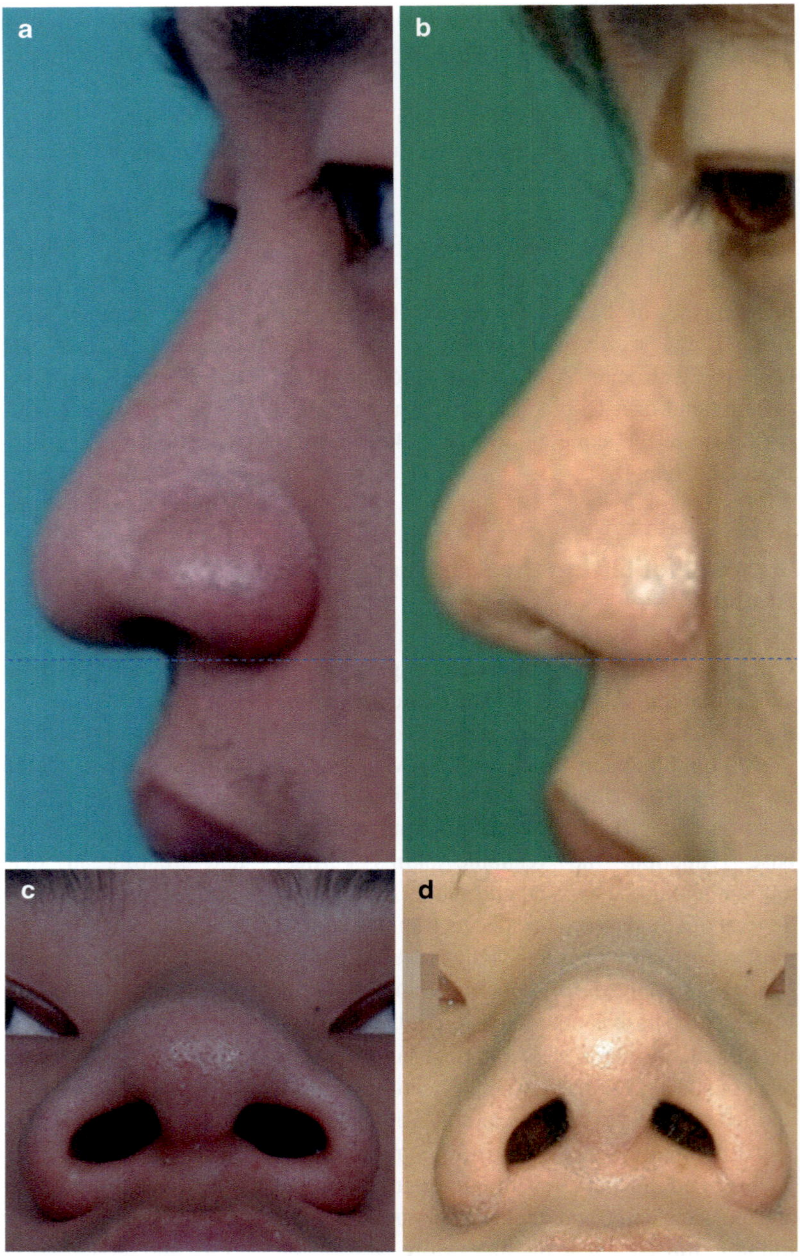

Fig. 10.10 Alar base reduction does not improve the alar hanging. (**a**, **c**) Preoperative views. (**b**, **d**) Postoperative views. Although the alar flaring is improved, there is no change in the alar crease junction's vertical position

Small Nose: Short Septum + Alar Retraction

The small nose is commonly seen in Asian, and it can be said that most LLCs are underdeveloped. Therefore, an excessive increase in the central component can worsen alar retraction (Fig. 10.7).

- Even an underdeveloped LLC can solve alar retraction with proper positioning if the lateral crural spanning suture can be fixed to the high septum.
- If it cannot be fixed to the high septum, there is a method for attaching it to the septum by performing an alar spreader graft or lateral crural spanning graft for the LLC positioning [12]

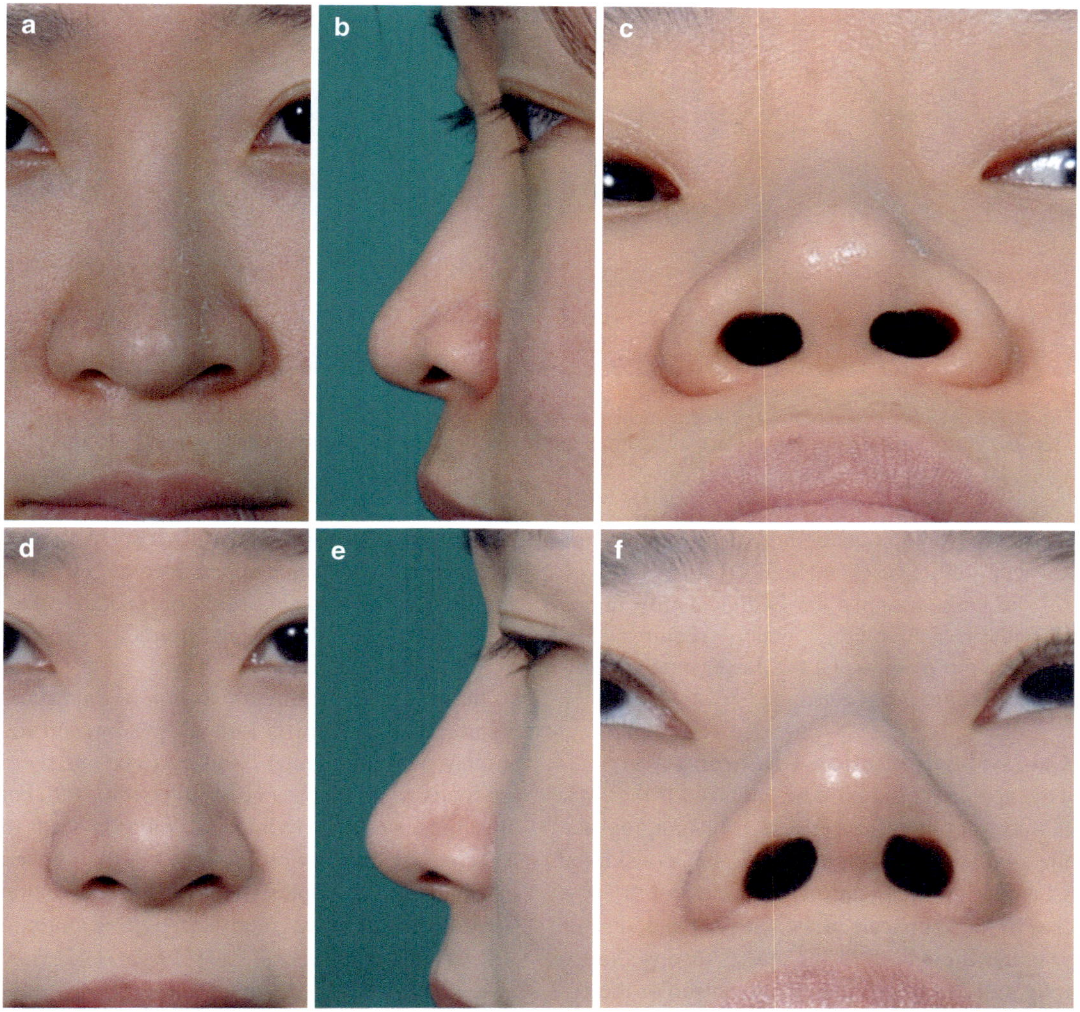

Fig. 10.11 Alar base reduction with vertical vestibular excision. (**a**–**c**) Preoperative views. (**d**–**f**) Postoperative views. Septoplasty, caudal septal extension using folded cymba, dorsal SMF graft, and alar base reduction with vertical lift was performed

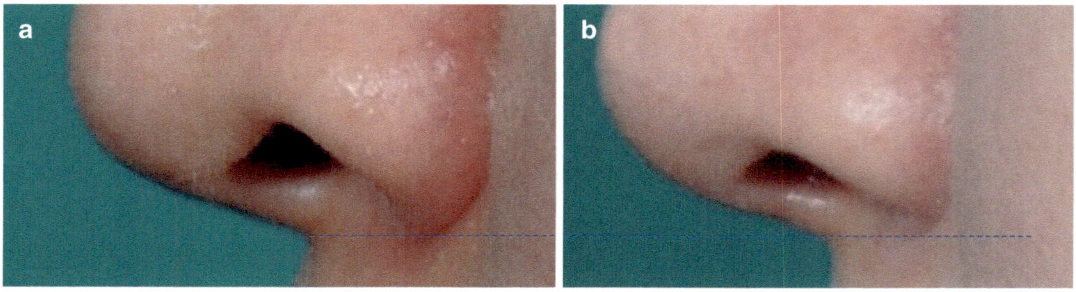

Fig. 10.12 Lateral views show improvement of alar retraction and vertical lift of alar crease junction. (**a**) Preoperative view. (**b**) Postoperative view

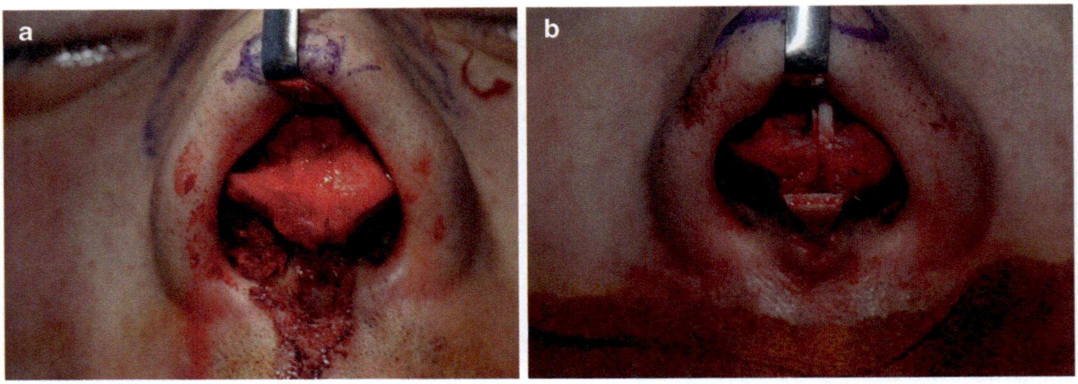

Fig. 10.13 The correction of the asymmetric resting angle between ULC and LLC. (**a**) A secondary case. Preoperative view. (**b**) Postoperative view. The costal cartilage was applied for the L-strut reconstruction and shield grafting

- The most effective method is the lateral crural strut graft (LCSG) method [7] (Fig. 9.9).
- The authors apply the LCSG mainly in secondary rhinoplasty, which requires total elevation from the LLC's lower mucosa when harvesting costal cartilage.

Columella Retraction + Hanging Alar

This appearance should be analyzed if the cause is due to columellar retraction or hanging alar, the entire nasal tip should be considered. Considering the position of the tip and the position of the subnasale, the priority is to determine whether the length of the entire nose is short or long and determine the ideal position of the columellar accordingly. The central component determines whether the alar is hanging or not. While considering ACR, the disharmony that cannot be solved by the central compart must be modified by a reduction in the lateral component.

- The method of alar base reduction does not help the practical lifting of the alar crease.
- Direct alar lift methods include resecting the alar vestibule or plicating the alar levator muscle.
- ACR is improved by increasing the tip projection and nasal length in most Asians.

Hanging Columella + Alar Retraction

Asian patients with this appearance are rare. For the hanging columella, first the caudal septal margin is removed then alar retraction is corrected with the LLC modification.

In most patients, direct excision of the caudal membranous septum is rare. Depending on the amount of quadrangular cartilage to be cut, there are times when mucosa needs to be removed, but most mucosa can be redraped. If mucosa needs to be removed, transfixion incision can be applied like Western rhinoplasty. However, transfixion incision is the most rarely used procedure in Asian rhinoplasty.

References

1. Rohrich RJ, Liu JH. Defining the infratip lobule in rhinoplasty: anatomy, pathogenesis of abnormalities, and correction using an algorithmic approach. Plast Reconstr Surg. 2012;130(5):1148–58.
2. Gunter JP, Rohrich RJ, Friedman RM. Classification and correction of alar-columellar discrepancies in rhinoplasty. Plast Reconstr Surg. 1996;97(3):643–8.
3. Toriumi DM. New concepts in nasal tip contouring. Arch Facial Plast Surg. 2006;8(3):156–85.
4. Kim HS, Roh SG. The alar extension graft for retracted ala. J Korean Soc Plast Reconstr Surg. 2009;36(1):66–74.
5. Cervelli V, Spallone D, Bottini JD, Silvi E, Gentile P, Curcio B, et al. Alar batten cartilage graft: treatment

of internal and external nasal valve collapse. Aesthetic Plast Surg. 2009;33(4):625–34.
6. Toriumi DM, Josen J, Weinberger M, Tardy ME Jr. Use of alar batten grafts for correction of nasal valve collapse. Arch Otolaryngol Head Neck Surg. 1997;123(8):802–8.
7. Gunter JP, Friedman RM. Lateral crural strut graft: technique and clinical applications in rhinoplasty. Plast Reconstr Surg. 1997;99(4):943–52; discussion 953–5.
8. Cochran CS, Sieber DA. Extended alar contour grafts: an evolution of the lateral crural strut graft technique in rhinoplasty. Plast Reconstr Surg. 2017;140(4):559e–67e.
9. Guyuron B. Dynamic interplays during rhinoplasty. Clin Plast Surg. 1996;23(2):223–31.
10. Taş S. The alignment of the nose in rhinoplasty: fix down concept. Plast Reconstr Surg. 2020;145(2):378–89.
11. Çakir B, Doğan T, Öreroğlu AR, Daniel RK. Rhinoplasty: surface aesthetics and surgical techniques. Aesthet Surg J. 2013;33(3):363–75.
12. Gunter JP, Rohrich RJ. Correction of the pinched nasal tip with alar spreader grafts. Plast Reconstr Surg. 1992;90(5):821–9.

Correction of the Short Secondary Nose: Dissection and the Framework Reconstruction

11

Pearls

- There is no rationale for using an alloplastic implant again that solves the complication caused by the alloplastic implant itself.
- The only way to secure the secondary surgery safe would be using autografts. Allografts are also unsafe substitutes.
- The addition of low concentration Hyaluronidase (50–100 unit/mL) is advantageous for a hardened scar.
- If a dorsal alloplastic implant is present, the capsulectomy range should be determined during surgery because the scar tissue around it causes the contracture.
- Depending on the thickness of the dorsal skin flap and the likelihood of compromise, you should decide whether to perform an anterior capsulectomy or not.
- If the skin is too thin to maintain vascularity, anterior capsulectomy may not be performed. At this time, it should be noted that the dorsal skin flap may not be released sufficiently.
- The posterior capsule should be removed entirely. Be careful not to communicate with the nasal cavity.
- The most crucial procedure in a short nose correction is the LLC positioning and the dorsal skin repair without tension.
- An appropriate amount of autologous cartilage should be prepared for the septal L-strut extension graft.
- In most secondary cases, there may no longer be existing septal and concha cartilages. The rib cartilage is the best and definitive source for septal reconstruction.
- The septal L-strut extension graft can be applied using folded cymba concha and folded cavum concha in most Asians.
- Dissecting the septum may be impossible in cases where the mucoperichondrium had been destroyed.
- There is severe destruction where the Medpor was applied at the septum as a spreader or septal extension graft.
- If there is severe destruction at the keystone area, stable fixation between the caudal nasal bone and the anterior grafts is needed after drill holes are made. The same principle applies to the ANS area.
- This method is applied to the septal extension graft applied to the anterior septum and the caudal septal extension graft applied to the caudal septum.

Supplementary Information The online version of this chapter (https://doi.org/10.1007/978-981-16-0542-0_11) contains supplementary material, which is available to authorized users.

E.-S. Dhong, M.-W. Na, *Asian Septorhinoplasty*, https://doi.org/10.1007/978-981-16-0542-0_11

11.1 The Secondary Rhinoplasty in Asians

A short nose is one of the biggest challenges in Asian rhinoplasty. If Asian rhinoplasty is mainly divided into two, it can be divided into primary rhinoplasty and secondary rhinoplasty. If you do secondary rhinoplasty with the strategy of primary rhinoplasty, you will be frustrated. The method of directly elongating the septum resolved the shortness and complemented the central nasal area and allowed for the next steps in the lateral side of the lower two-third of the nose.

Alloplastic Implant with SRP: Is it Safe?

There have been many reports on complication rates, such as infection in surgery using alloplastic implants, but there are few detailed studies on inflammation/infection, which cause short nose deformity. There will be a clear difference depending on the simultaneous septal surgery, only one study reported that 13.8% of 695 patients who used silicone implants had contractures requiring correction [1]. This is different from the standpoint of infection or inflammation. It can be seen as a high rate of contracture.

The septal surgery makes a considerable difference when the infection involves.

It involves two big problems. Structurally, it causes the nasal framework's collapse and chronic soft tissue contracture.

Technically, separating the upper lateral cartilage (ULC) from the anterior septum is the preferred procedure when applying septal extension grafts and spreader grafts. The mucosa area is completely separated from the nasal cavity and is well preserved, but even without communication between the incised pocket and the nasal cavity, it may not be safe to place the allogeneic implant on the widely detached platform. If an acute infection occurs after surgery, the infection around the implant can spread to the deep space, causing a severe intraseptal abscess. Most people with severe infections, whether acute or chronic develop nasal shortening due to destruction of the septal skeleton and soft tissues. Even if the capsules around the allogeneic implant are safe, the question of longevity remains. Gravity forces the homologous implant to continuously compress the platform below by adding pressure on the surrounding soft tissue (Chap. 1). Salvaging an infected nose after septorhinoplasty is entirely different from that of a relatively simple rhinoplasty. In the case of SSI or delayed infection (late-onset inflammation), the infectious soft tissue, including the capsule, can be completely excised and irrigated to save the nose. However, if the septum was dissected and grafted, nasal support may be lost, and moderate to severe malformations may remain even after complete eradication of the septal abscess (Fig. 11.1).

Bacterial biofilms result in chronic refractory inflammation and impending extraction of allogeneic implants. Further studies are needed for the growth of the mucin-producing cells or new proliferation of the endothelium. Post-inflammatory contracture is similar to breast capsular contracture. A dense layer of avascular connective tissue is formed by the aggregation of monocytes and severe fibroblasts around the capsule.

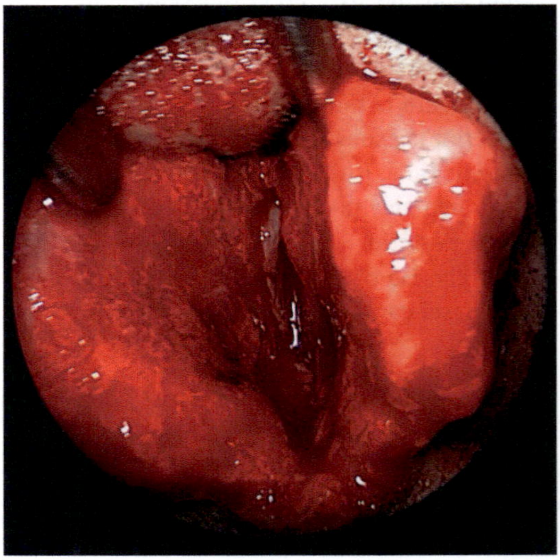

Fig. 11.1 Destruction of remaining septal cartilage after the septal abscess

- There is no rationale for using an alloplastic implant again that solves the complication caused by the alloplastic implant itself.
- The only way to secure the secondary surgery safe would be using autografts. Allografts are also unsafe substitutes.

Specific Considerations of Secondary Surgery

The biggest obstacle to surgery is that it is difficult to excise the scar tissue in detail. There is no accurate dissection plane in many cases, and if all scars are removed, a vast amount of volume is lost. All scars need to be removed when it is directly gripping the framework, and longitudinal release is not possible without release. After the scar removal, the remaining ULC and LLC's destruction or resorption can be observed (Fig. 11.2).

The Dissection

It can be said that more than 70% of the operation time is spent on proper dissection. The more complicated the dissection is, the more sharp instruments are needed, but many hard scars even do not cut well by a scalpel. Especially, such a stone-like scar is the multilayered alloderm. Sometimes the dissection is performed using a colorado microdissection tip of electrocautery.

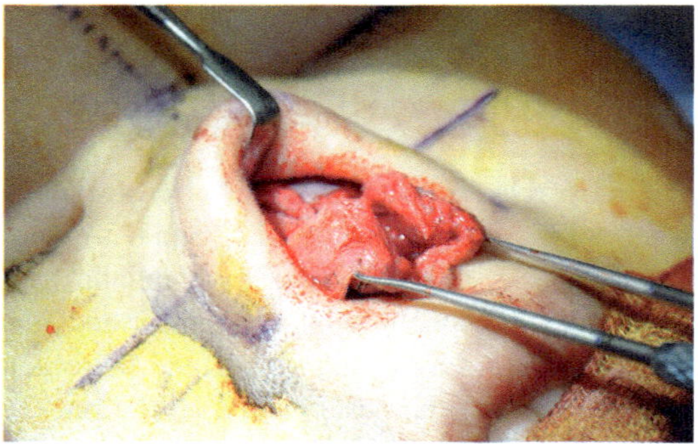

Fig. 11.2 After the scar removal, the remaining LLC's destruction was found with multiple non-absorbable sutures

- The addition of low concentration Hyaluronidase (50–100 unit/mL) is advantageous for a hard scar. This method has been used since the 1950s [2].

Its advantages are local anesthetics mixed with epinephrine quickly enter hard scar tissue; temporarily hydrodissection is facilitated; swelling caused by local anesthetics is reduced. The disadvantage is that if the pharmacological effect is maintained until the end of the surgery, it makes the thickness of the soft tissue thinner than its actual size. So the thin envelope induces overgraft more than needed. However, there are more advantages than disadvantages in dealing with hard tissues. There are cases where all of the following dissections should be performed in nine areas where severe contracture is involved. Below one to three are methods for releasing dorsal skin flaps, and the rest are methods for releasing nasal frameworks (Fig. 11.3).

- The dissection plane is the presumed sub-SMAS. However, it will be a subcutaneous plane in most secondary operations.
- If a dorsal alloplastic implant is present, the capsulectomy range should be determined during surgery because the scar tissue around it causes the contracture.
- Depending on the thickness of the dorsal skin flap and the likelihood of compromise, you should decide whether to perform an anterior capsulectomy or not.
- If the skin is too thin to maintain vascularity, anterior capsulectomy may not be performed. At this time, it should be noted that the dorsal skin flap may not be released sufficiently.
- The posterior capsule should be removed entirely. Be careful not to communicate with the nasal cavity.
- When doing the posterior capsulectomy, it is often necessary to remove all the scars, leaving only a thin intranasal mucosa.
- The most important point in a short nose correction is the LLC positioning and the dorsal skin repair without tension.

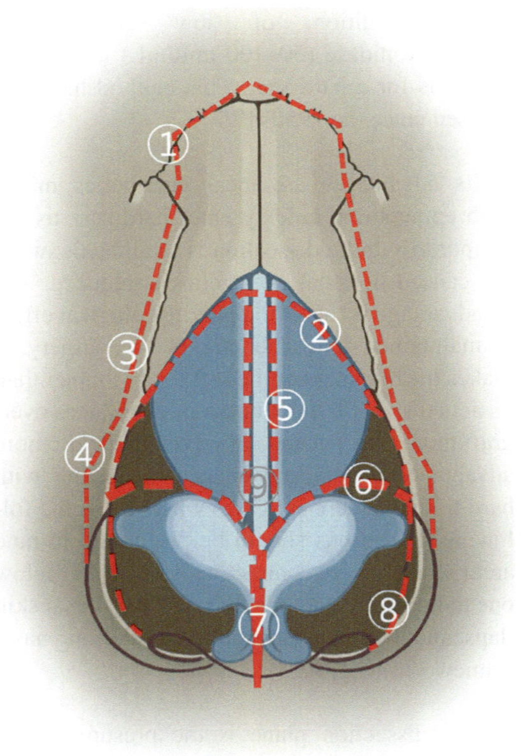

Fig. 11.3 Schematic of releasing areas in severe contracture. (1) Dissection of nasal sidewall and root. (2) Dissection between nasal bone and ULC. (3) Dissection between skin flap from the maxillary process. (4) Dissection between sidewall and maxilla. (5) Dissection between the septum and ULC. (6) Dissection between ULC and LLC (scroll area). (7) Dissection between LLC and LLC. (8) Dissection between LLC and pyriform aperture. (9) Secondary septal dissection

Dissection Above Nasal Sidewall and Root

All bone attachments of the cephalo-lateral portion of the skin flap should be released. Lateral release requires releasing part of the transverse nasalis muscle and part of the bone attachment of LLSAN. For a large amount of skin flaps to be caudally redraped, nasal root release is often essential. Temporarily, the medial canthal skin may be pulled downwardly, but this phenomenon does not cause the deformation later. The medial canthal tendon is not severed, so the mongoloid slant normalizes when swelling disappears.

Dissection Between Nasal Bone and ULC

Detaching the periosteum under the caudal nasal bone and detaching the upper part of the ULC is performed simultaneously. After dissecting this part, much release does not occur. However, since the longitudinal capsule is usually present on the top of this area, there are cases where the posterior capsule must be removed, and this area must also be released (Video 11.1).

Dissection Between Skin Flap from Maxillary Process

Like the pyriform aperture below, this part's dissection is necessary for the release and caudal extension of lateral components, including LLC.

Dissection Between Sidewall and Maxilla

It is often necessary to release the skin flap right up to the side of the LLC. Here, massive bleeding can be encountered and should be cauterized well. If you plan to do a lateral crural strut graft on this area, space should be preserved to insert the strut with partial detachment rather than complete detach.

Dissection Between Septum and ULC

This dissection must go through to reconstruct the septal framework. Care must be taken not to expose the nasal cavity. Likewise, since the strongest contracture exists in the posterior capsule area, this area must be released.

Dissection Between ULC and LLC (Scroll Area)

The most release occurs here. The scroll area is where LLC is overriding the ULC, and it is essential to release this part after the cephalic trim completely. If cephalic trim is not performed, it is challenging to release accurately, and there is a risk of exposing the nasal cavity. If you put the freer elevator in the nasal cavity and release the scroll area above, you can prevent mucosal tear and preserve mucosa as much as possible and release this area. Here you can get an extra length of 2–3 mm (Video 11.2).

Dissection Between LLC and LLC

Dissection is performed along the midline between the LLCs on both sides to find the caudal septum.

Because alloplastic material is usually contained in this area, it is often difficult to dissect. Besides, there are many cases where the middle crura's scarring is severe, or the medial crus on one side is lost. The priority is to find the caudal septum first along the midline and find the subperichondrial plane of the caudal septum. Then, if necessary, the mucoperichondrium is preserved, and the surrounding scar tissue is removed. In some cases, it may be necessary to release the perichondrium, leaving the mucosa only. Loss of mucosa in this area can cause SSI later, and in most cases, cartilage graft on the caudal septum is required, so if mucosa laceration occurs in the membranous septum, it needs to be repaired.

Dissection Between LLC and Pyriform Aperture

Pyriform ligament must be released in connection with the scar above. However, most patients' contracture rarely occurs here because this area is far from the implants and contains abundant muscles underneath.

Secondary Septal Dissection

The elevation of the bilateral septal mucosal flap has little effect on the release in the longitudinal or anterior direction. The septal mucosa to which perichondrium is attached does not have much elasticity, and this flap after infection does not stretch well. Secondary dissection of the previous SMR site is not recommended, but the dissection is possible if the dissection plane has accurately proceeded in the previous surgery.

Postoperative Re-scarring

After successful surgery, unwanted scar tissue may develop again. When the dorsal skin flap remains thin, or if a scoring incision is put on the dermal flap's undersurface, an intractable dermal scar is formed. If dermis graft was applied to the dorsum previously, more severe scar tissue might be encountered. Before redraping the dorsal skin at the end of the surgery, the author prefers to inject diluted Kenalog into the subdermis. Kenalog is effective in preventing swelling after surgery and reducing subdermal scarring (Video 11.3).

11.2 Camouflage or Restoring the Framework?

- The most important factor of planning secondary septorhinoplasty is soft tissue resilience.
- A cantilever graft can be applied to camouflage without septal surgery.
- If there is a functional problem, that is, nasal obstruction, septal surgery needs to be done.
- The cantilever graft is safe if the septal perforation is located in the anterior-caudal septum.

Specific Considerations in Septal Surgery in Asians

Septal cartilage in Asians tends to be smaller than in Caucasians. The average area of septal cartilage in Koreans was reported to be 8.18 cm^2 for men and 7.36 cm^2 for women [3].

For Koreans, the amount of septal cartilage collected was usually insufficient for various graft use. Therefore, additional cartilage grafts such as the concha and costal cartilage should be considered before surgery [4]. The septal cartilage is thinner in Asian, and submucosal resection of quadrangular cartilage also tends to weaken the nasal support. A swing door procedure performed over the maxillary and anterior nasal spine (ANS) to correct a caudal septal deviation aggravates septal instability at the base. Most Asian rhinoplasty requires two dimensions of improvement: anteroposterior and cephalocaudal extension. When the whole tip is projected, the length of the nostril should also be increased [5, 6]. However, it is impossible to even worry about this in a secondary operation. Not only the lack of donor cartilage but also because of scar tissue, the nose is often impossible to be lengthened as much as desired. In the case of the author, short nose correction is performed using the following two methods. The SLEG method has various donor cartilage options, whereas the cantilever graft has no other method than the costal cartilage. Secondary short nose deformity can be reconstructed using allograft, but this concept is excluded because the author does not have enough evidence on it. The opinion on IHCC will be discussed in Chap. 13.

Septal L-Strut Extension Graft (SLEG)

SLEG is the method that the author prefers to create a septum-dependent tip [7].

- An appropriate amount of autologous cartilage should be prepared.
- In most secondary cases, there may be no longer existing septal and concha cartilages. The rib cartilage is the best and definitive source for septal reconstruction [8].
- The septal L-strut extension graft can be applied using folded cymba concha and folded cavum concha in most Asians (Fig. 11.4).

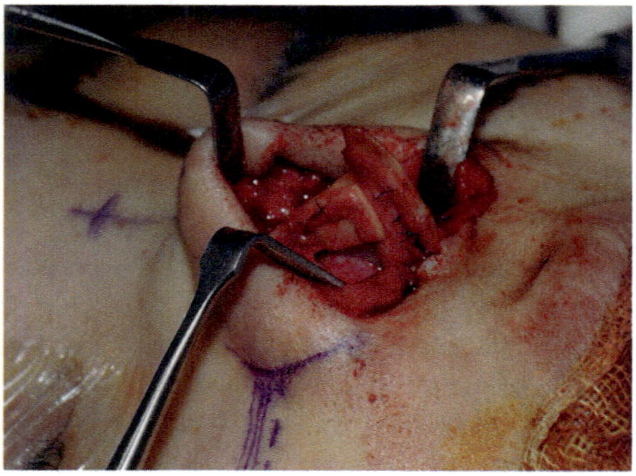

Fig. 11.4 The septal L-strut extension graft (SLEG) can be applied using folded cymba concha and folded cavum concha

- Dissecting the septum may be impossible in cases where the mucoperichondrium had been destroyed.
- There is severe destruction where the Medpor was applied at the septum as a spreader or septal extension graft.
- If there are severe destructions at the keystone area, stable fixation between the caudal nasal bone and the anterior grafts is needed after drill holes are made. The same principle applies to the ANS area.

11.3 Techniques of Septal L-Strut Extension Graft for Asians

Effective L-strut (anterocaudal) expansion requires various combinations of autologous cartilage. Sometimes the amount of septal cartilage is insufficient, making it impossible to perform effective L-strut extension. Cymba concha and cavum concha are required to perform L-strut extension. For patients with small ears, rib cartilage may be the primary option. The tongue-and-groove method also uses the septal cartilage for bilateral spreader implantation. In L-strut's caudal extension, rib cartilage provides the most source when the septal cartilage is lacking. It is most advantageous to use cymba cartilage in Asians who do not prefer tip stiffness. During the author's 20-year experience, cymba concha was used in the caudal septum for a modified tongue-in-groove technique and was useful in obtaining the tip's projection. Cymba concha, when folded, can produce 4–5 mm wide and 20 mm or longer (data in publishing, Aesthetic Surgery Journal) and are sufficient to support the medial and medial crura of the lower lateral cartilage of the Asian population (Fig. 11.5). In particular, by applying the tongue-in-groove method around ANS using a cymba concha for tip support loss after performing the caudal septum swing door technique, both projection and stability can be obtained. Additional support can be obtained by performing sutures so that the concave sides face each other during folding. It is essential to attach the cartilage mucoperichondrium of the cymba on the convex side to gain additional strength from the brittle tendency (Fig. 11.5).

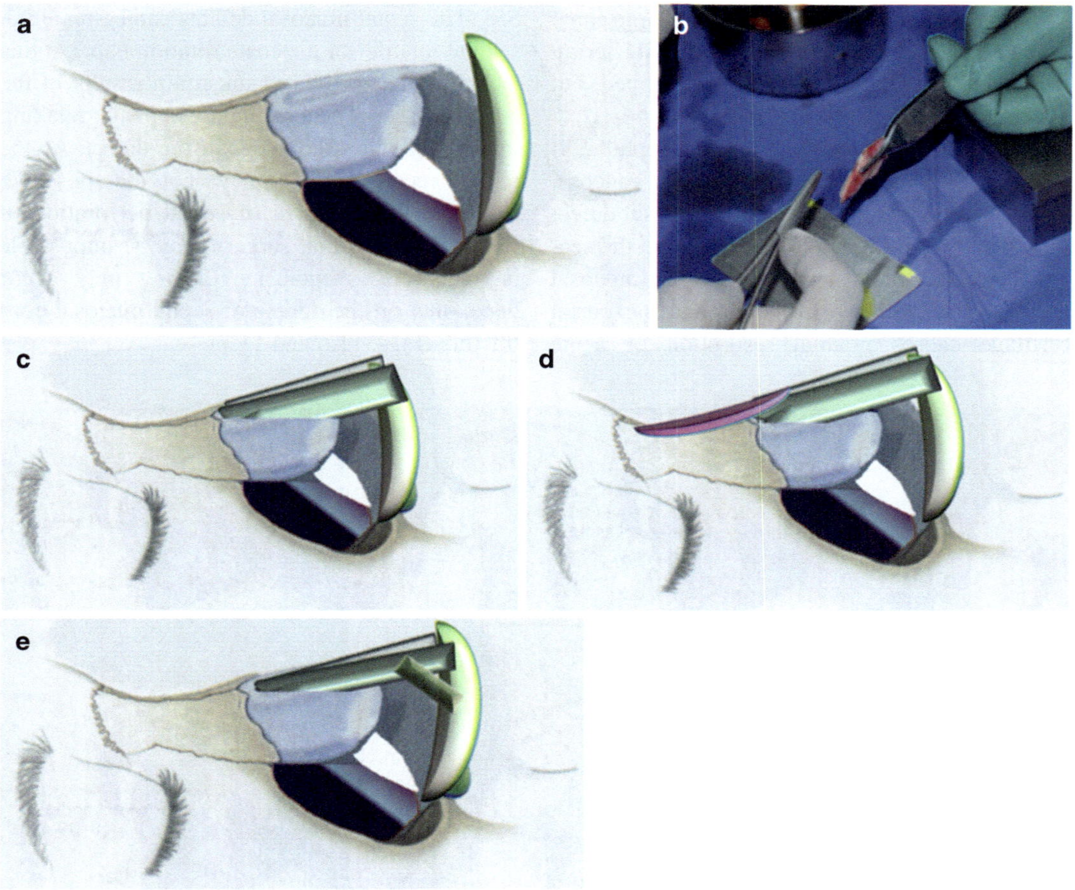

Fig. 11.5 Techniques of septal L-strut extension grafting. (**a**) Caudal SEG: folded cymba concha is sutured on both sides of the ANS for support and caudal extension, a modified tongue-in-groove technique. (**b**) Folded cymba concha: facing concave sides were sutured. Minimal continuity in the middle enhances strength. (**c**) Bilateral extended spreader graft: visible spreader grafts are applied anteriorly. (**d**) Radix graft: any type of soft tissue is grafted on the nasion to smooth the dorsum. (**e**) Rafting graft: small pieces of cartilage are applied between the anterior and caudal pillars. (Material from: Hwang and Dhong. Septal Extension Graft in Asian Rhinoplasty Facial Plastic Surgery of North America, 2018, Elsevier)

11.4 Extended Spreader Graft: Modified Tongue-and-Groove Graft

The septal cartilage is most suitable for L-strut's anterior extension. However, since most septal cartilage cannot be used in a secondary operation, conchal cartilage or costal cartilage is used. The anterior extension requires more width than other existing spreader grafts. In other words, this application can be described as a "visible spreader" graft. Simultaneously, this technique is the "modified tongue-and-groove technique" of Dr. Guyuron [9]. The anterior extension is possible from the keystone area to the tip, so the excessive anterior extension must be avoided since it leads to difficulties in obtaining a smooth line in the keystone area and requires more graft on the nasion. Multiple sutures are needed between the anterior margin of the existing septum and posterior margin of the inserted extended spreader graft (Fig. 11.5).

Case Study
A 37-year-old female patient has a history of removing late-onset inflammation after rhinoplasty using Medpor and silicone implants. She underwent septal reconstruction using sixth ribs.

Three months after the operation, discharge came out from the columella. After administering empirical antibiotics, the discharge stopped, but the volume of the tip lobule was lost.

The septal collapse caused by septal SSI causes irreversible contracture of septal mucosa. It is recommended to correct the mucosal defect first, then do the framework operation in the second stage. Cartilage exposure due to mucosal defects after framework operation using costal cartilage causes gradual resorption or acute SSI. The septal mucosal defects can be repaired, such as an inferior turbinate rotation flap, but this technique has produced uncertain results in the author's cases. The asymmetric cephalic relaxing incision can be used to repair the defect. As the septal reconstruction may not be possible, depending on the size of septal perforation, it should be noted that surgery may be impossible or incomplete septal lengthening may occur depending on the degree of septal mucosal contracture (Figs. 11.6 and 11.7).

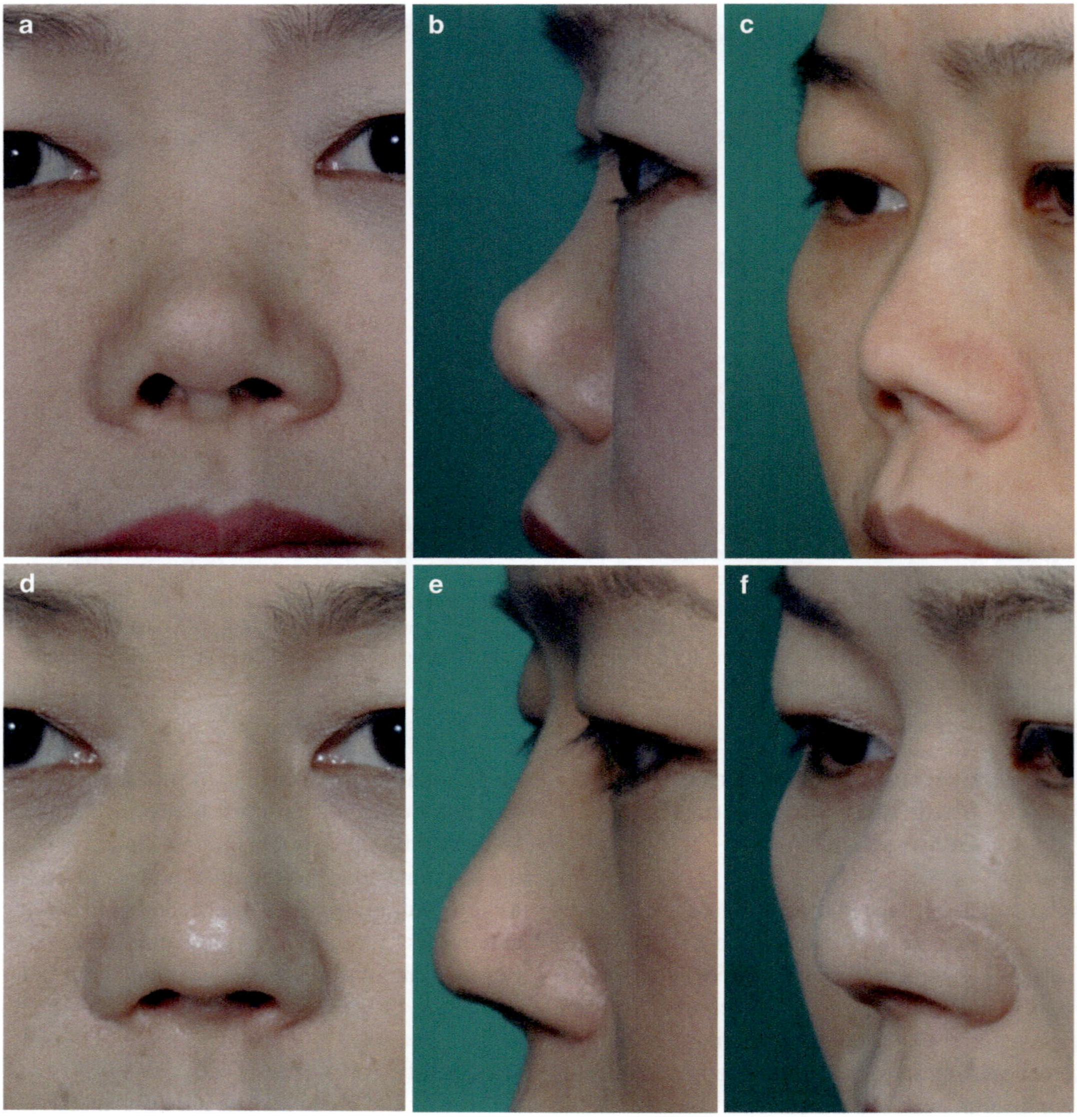

Fig. 11.6 The septal collapse caused by septal SSI causes severe contracture of septal mucosa. (**a–c**) Preoperative views. (**d–f**) Postoperative views after L-strut reconstruction

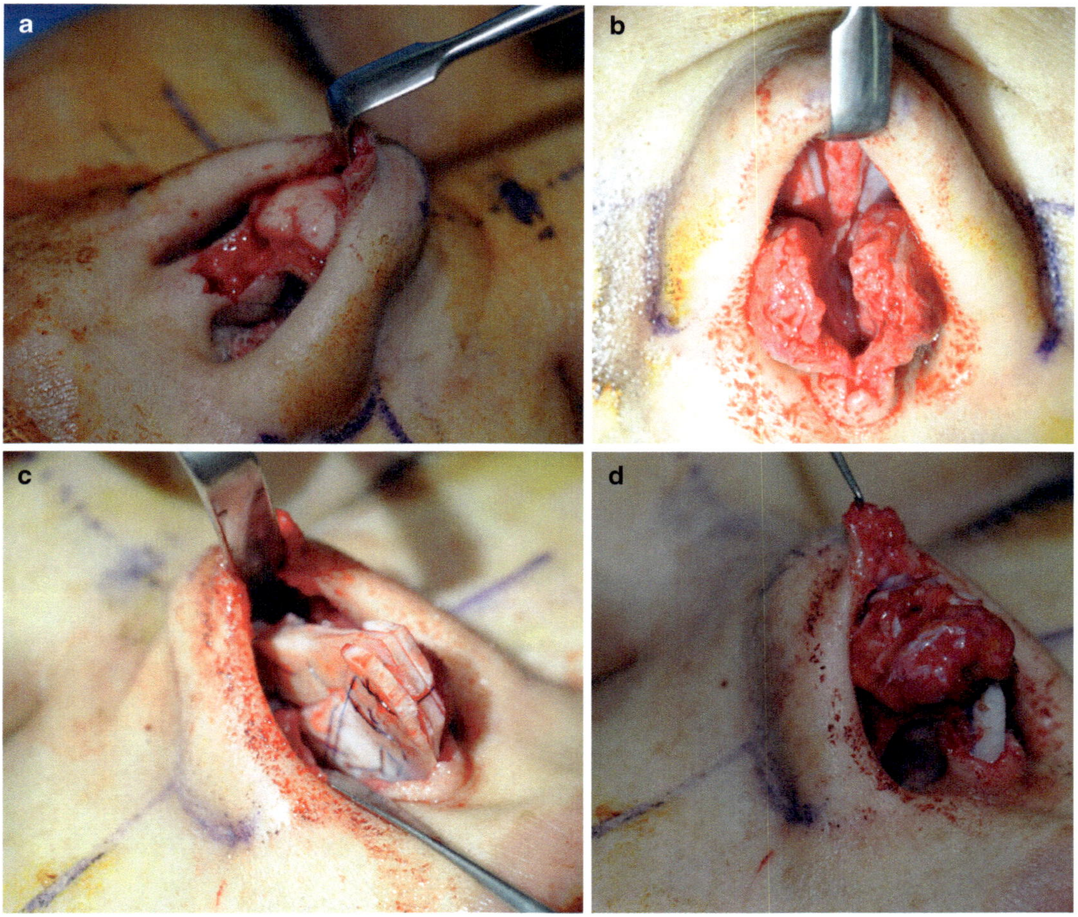

Fig. 11.7 Septal L-strut extension graft. (**a**) Intraoperative view. The vast cartilage destruction was identified under the tip allograft. (**b**) After resection of scar tissue, the nasal framework is almost lost. (**c**) Septal L-strut was reconstructed using costal cartilage. (**d**) Soft tissue was grafted on the tip

Cantilever Graft

Since long ago, rhinoplasty using rib cartilage has been performed. The cantilever graft consisting of dorsal onlay graft and columella segment was introduced 50 years ago to correct cleft lip and nose deformity in the Western operation. Surgery in a traditional cantilever graft that sustains the underlying tension, calvarial bone was introduced by nasal root integration. There are numerous reports on different techniques.

The author has also experienced secondary rhinoplasty forcibly stretching with the L framework made in this way, and it remains mostly a bad memory.

Case Study
A 22-year-old male patient visited the author to correct cleft lip and nose deformity after several previous surgeries. This patient was corrected by making an L-shaped cantilever graft using the sixth rib. The costal cartilage was carved by balanced cutting to prevent warping and waited for more than 1 hour in the saline at the time of surgery. A single K-wire was fixed on the nasal root for 7 days. After 4 months, a mild hump and a deformity of the s-shaped dorsal graft was found at the visit. After waiting for another 2 months, revision rhinoplasty underwent. The fixed L-graft was removed, and the healthy part was sliced into a small piece, and cymba concha was harvested

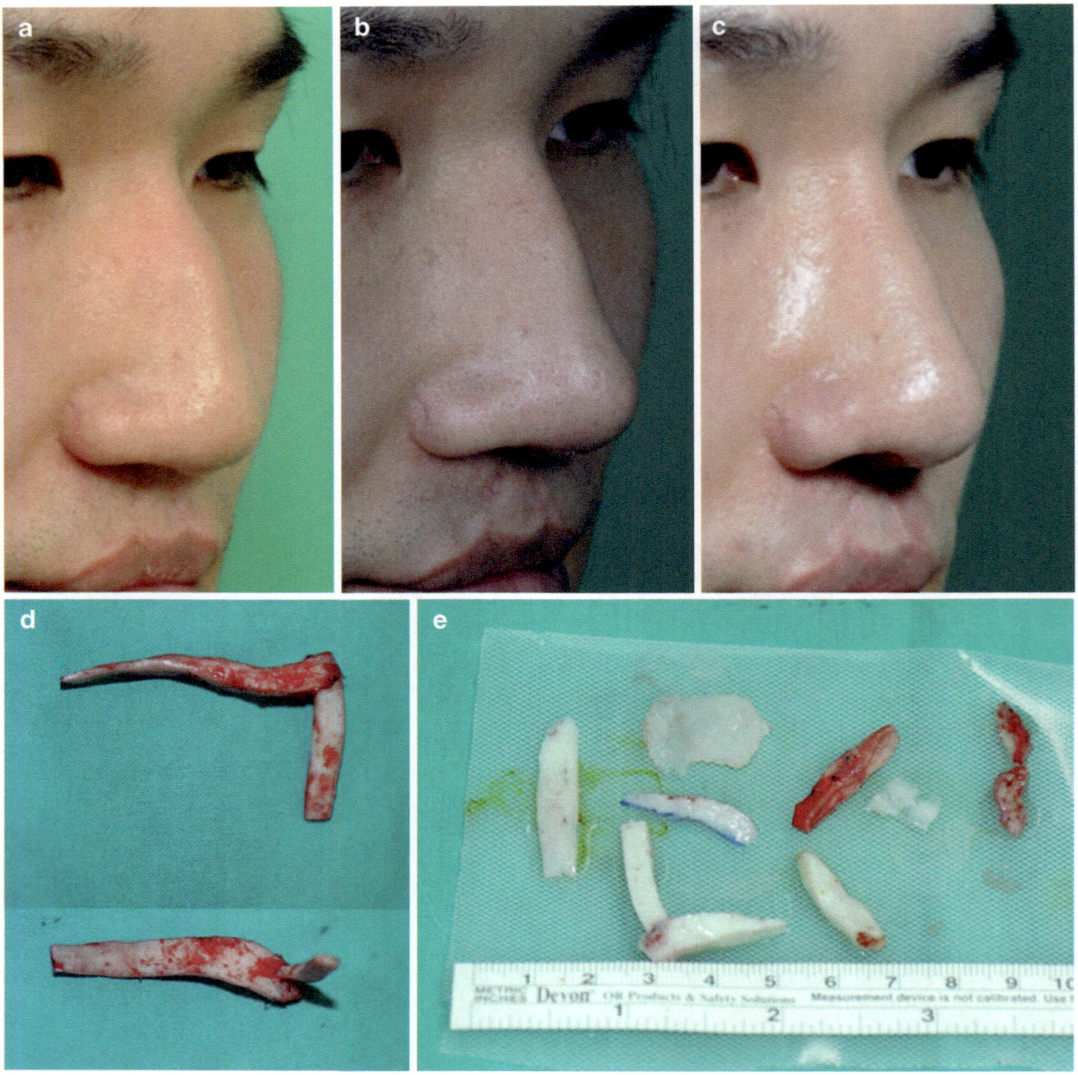

Fig. 11.8 Cantilever graft was removed because of the warping, then it was substituted by SLEG combining septal cartilage, cymba concha, and reused sliced costal cartilage. (**a**) Before the cantilever graft. (**b**) After the warping of the cantilever graft. (**c**) After the SLEG. (**d**) The warping of the costal cartilage. (**e**) Septal cartilage, cymba concha, and sliced costal cartilage

for caudal septal extension graft (CSEG). The septal surgery was performed to widen the right nasal cavity, and the posterior quadrangular cartilage dislocated to the right side was removed (Fig. 11.8 and Video 11.4).

The biggest problem with the cantilever graft is warping of the costal cartilage. In the surgery of secondary cleft lip and nose deformity, the cantilever graft can be considered first because many patients have a severe deviation of septum and vomer junction. However, the author prefers to make septum-dependent dorsum and tip with SLEG mentioned above, rather than the cantilever graft. For solid dorsal graft using rib cartilage, the author believes that Dr. Toriumi's method has the most scientific evidence. Although we have a different perspective on adipose-derived stromal cells, the author thinks the use of fatty tissue is an excellent method. This will be discussed in Chap. 13 [10].

References

1. Kim YK, Shin S, Kang NH, Kim JH. Contracted nose after silicone implantation: a new classification system and treatment algorithm. Arch Plast Surg. 2017;44(1):59–64.
2. Cottle MH, Weiss JA, Pottorff E, Herzon E. Hyaluronidase in rhinoplasty. Arch Otolaryngol. 1950;52(3):369–72.
3. Hwang SM, Lim O, Hwang MK, Kim MW, Lee JS. The clinical analysis of the nasal septal cartilage by measurement using computed tomography. Arch Craniofac Surg. 2016;17(3):140–5.
4. Kim J-S, Khan NA, Song HM, Jang YJ. Intraoperative measurements of harvestable septal cartilage in rhinoplasty. Ann Plast Surg. 2010;65(6):519–23.
5. Zelken J, Chang C-S, Chuang S-S, Yang J-Y, Hsiao Y-C. An economical approach to ethnic Asian rhinoplasty. Facial Plast Surg. 2016;32(1):95–104.
6. Dhong E-S, Kim Y-J, Suh MK. L-shaped columellar strut in East Asian nasal tip plasty. Arch Plast Surg. 2013;40(5):616–20.
7. Hwang N-H, Dhong E-S. Septal extension graft in Asian rhinoplasty. Facial Plast Surg Clin North Am. 2018;26(3):331–41.
8. Toriumi DM, Pero CD. Asian rhinoplasty. Clin Plast Surg. 2010;37(2):335–52.
9. Guyuron B, Varghai A. Lengthening the nose with a tongue-and-groove technique. Plast Reconstr Surg. 2003;111(4):1533–9; discussion 1540–1.
10. Toriumi DM. Dorsal augmentation using autologous costal cartilage or microfat-infused soft tissue augmentation. Facial Plast Surg. 2017;33(2):162–78.

Secondary Septal Surgery 12

Pearls

- Testing the hydrodissection while injecting local anesthetics into the septum is a definite method for identifying the dissectability. In case of easy infiltration, the mucoperichondrium remains, making the secondary septal dissection possible.
- If no dissection is possible, the area should be excluded from the scope of surgery. Unlike other areas, you can find a thin "no man's area."
- When the posterior septum is healthy and the deviation of the anterior septum is severe, the reverse swing door method can be applied for improving nasal function.
- Transverse K-wire fixation is helpful for the stability of the unsupported keystone area.
- Nasal bone after severe NEO fx, the decrease in intranasal cavity volume after septal collapse is expected.
- Septal collapse due to SSI in the septum after septorhinoplasty causes septal mucosal contracture. This short nose deformity is the most difficult to reconstruct.

12.1 The Previous SMR State: "No Man's Land"

From the author's current perspective, the first interview with the patient at an outpatient clinic starts with whether the patient has had a history of SMR or not. Nowadays, most reoperation patients are in a post-SMR state, septal status is the most critical factor in planning the central component's strategies [1]. If patients complain about the obstructive nose, the surgeon should consider reoperation, and the revisional septoplasties revealed promising results [2, 3].

The lumination of the endoscope and gentle press by a cotton tip can be used to check the thin mucosa or measure the amount of quadrangular cartilage harvested (Video 12.1).

- A definite method for identifying the dissectability is testing the hydrodissection, which can be observed while injecting the local anesthetics. In case of easy infiltration, cartilage remains, or the mucoperichondrium remains, making it easy for the hydrodissection.
- If the mucoperichondrium is lost, the septum will not be dissected easily (Video 12.2).
- If no dissection is possible, the area should be excluded from the scope of surgery. Unlike other areas, you can find a thin "no man's land" (Fig. 12.1).

Supplementary Information The online version of this chapter (https://doi.org/10.1007/978-981-16-0542-0_12) contains supplementary material, which is available to authorized users.

E.-S. Dhong, M.-W. Na, *Asian Septorhinoplasty*, https://doi.org/10.1007/978-981-16-0542-0_12

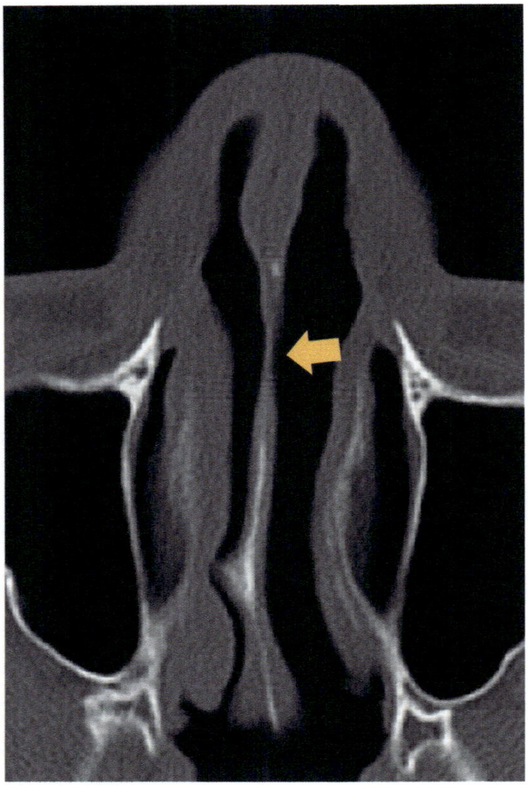

Fig. 12.1 No man's land; if the hydrodissection is not possible, do not dissect that area

12.2 The Revisional Septoplasty

Cause

The septal cartilage will grow again if mucoperichondrium is well preserved during harvesting. Adolescents with serious nasal malformation, including huge hump, have emotional problems. It is the reason for performing definitive rhinoplasty at that age. In patients who have not passed their growth period, the septal cartilage will grow again after primary septoplasty.

Anatomic Considerations

The cartilage of the previous SMR site can be harvested again. If the cartilage is regenerated, the dissection is possible. EPP can be harvested and used as a material by connecting the remaining quadrangular cartilage. Since reharvesting is insufficient, even a small piece of EPP can be useful in making the septum straight again. For the harvest of EPP, the author uses an oscillating saw and a small reciprocating saw.

Case Study

A 16-year-old male visited the author with hump nose deformity. The author persuaded the patient to delay the operation 2–3 years later, but the parents complained of a callus on his nose by self-compression due to stress and learning disabilities. Septorhinoplasty with humpectomy, medial, and lateral osteotomy was performed. Four years later, he revisited the author with septal deviation with reverse -c shape deformity. On inspection, convexity on the left side of the septum was found. The revision septoplasty was performed. After reharvesting of the septum, the spreader graft and rafter batten graft on the right side was reinforced to straighten it (Figs. 12.2 and 12.3).

12.3 Saddle Nose Deformity

Cause

- When an excessive amount of quadrangular cartilage is harvested, and the septal L-support is weak.
- When the support of the keystone area is weak.
- After the septal infection with the central contracture.
- After over-resection of the dorsal component.

Treatment

The method of camouflage with a cantilever graft is not a physiologic method. The author prefers septal reconstruction because there is an improvement in nasal physiology after surgery. Several methods of septal reconstruction according to the classification of the saddle nose have been introduced [4–6].

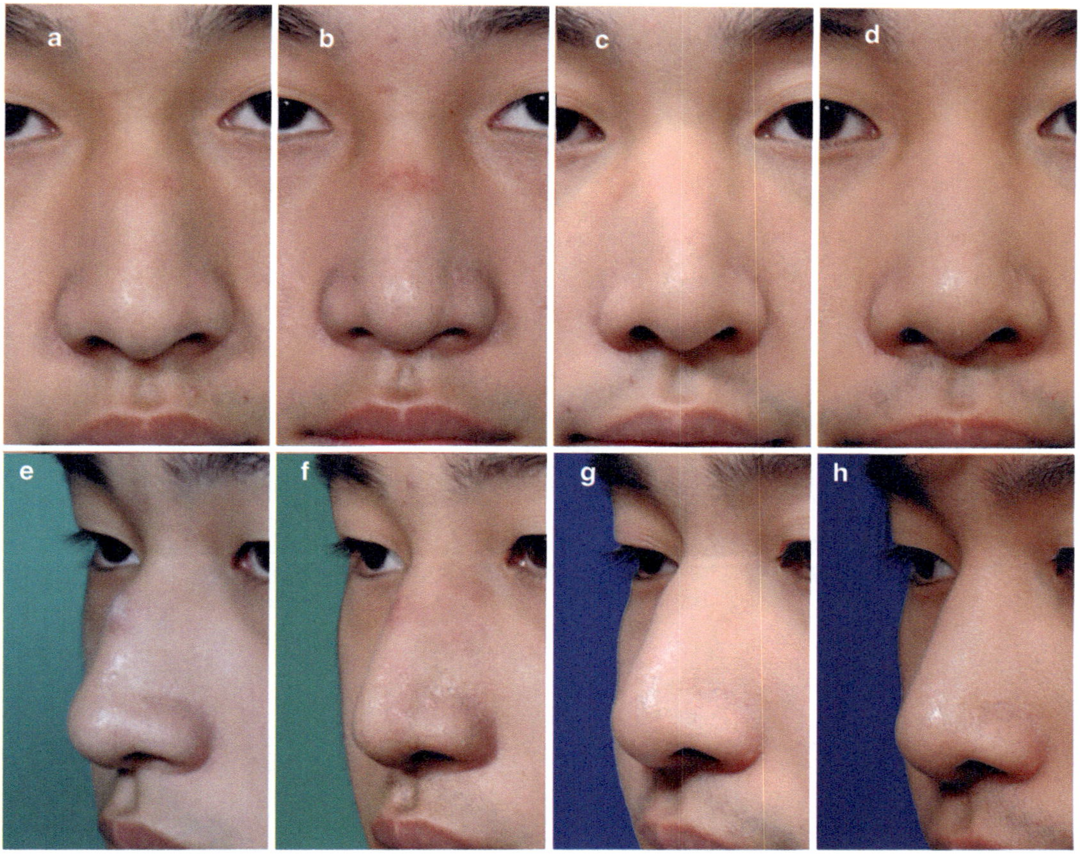

Fig. 12.2 Revisional septorhinoplasty due to the regrowth of the septal cartilage. (**a**, **e**) Preoperative view at age 16. (**b**, **f**) Postoperative view: hump reduction and septorhinoplasty. (**c**, **g**) Recurred hump and deviation at age 20. (**d**, **h**) Post-revisional septorhinoplasty

The reconstruction of the anterior septum is essential. There are only two types of donor cartilage, the costal cartilage, and the conchal cartilage. The presence of the remaining septum decides how high the extended spreader graft is to be performed anteriorly to correct the saddling. The spreader graft opens the internal valve and is an excellent way to correct the deviation of the lower two-third of the nose. It may be solved by performing a double or triple spreader graft on one side rather than a bilateral spreader graft in case of severe deviation. Of course, inferior turbinoplasty should be done considering the MCA of the internal valve on the other side. However, what is needed here is not the conventional spreader graft or the extended spreader graft for length extension, but the anteriorly extended spreader graft.

The Dorsal Margin of Anterior Extended Spreader Graft (AESG)

Should the ULC be lifted and sutured with AESG like the cartilaginous dorsum? Should the two anterior margins of the AESG directly form a cartilaginous dorsum? It is possible. Even after two margins pop out and ULC cannot catch them up, the skin is not demarcated with two lines after redraping in most Asians. However, in a female patient with a thin skin in Asians, to prevent a sharp dorsal demarcation, a layer of SMF can be

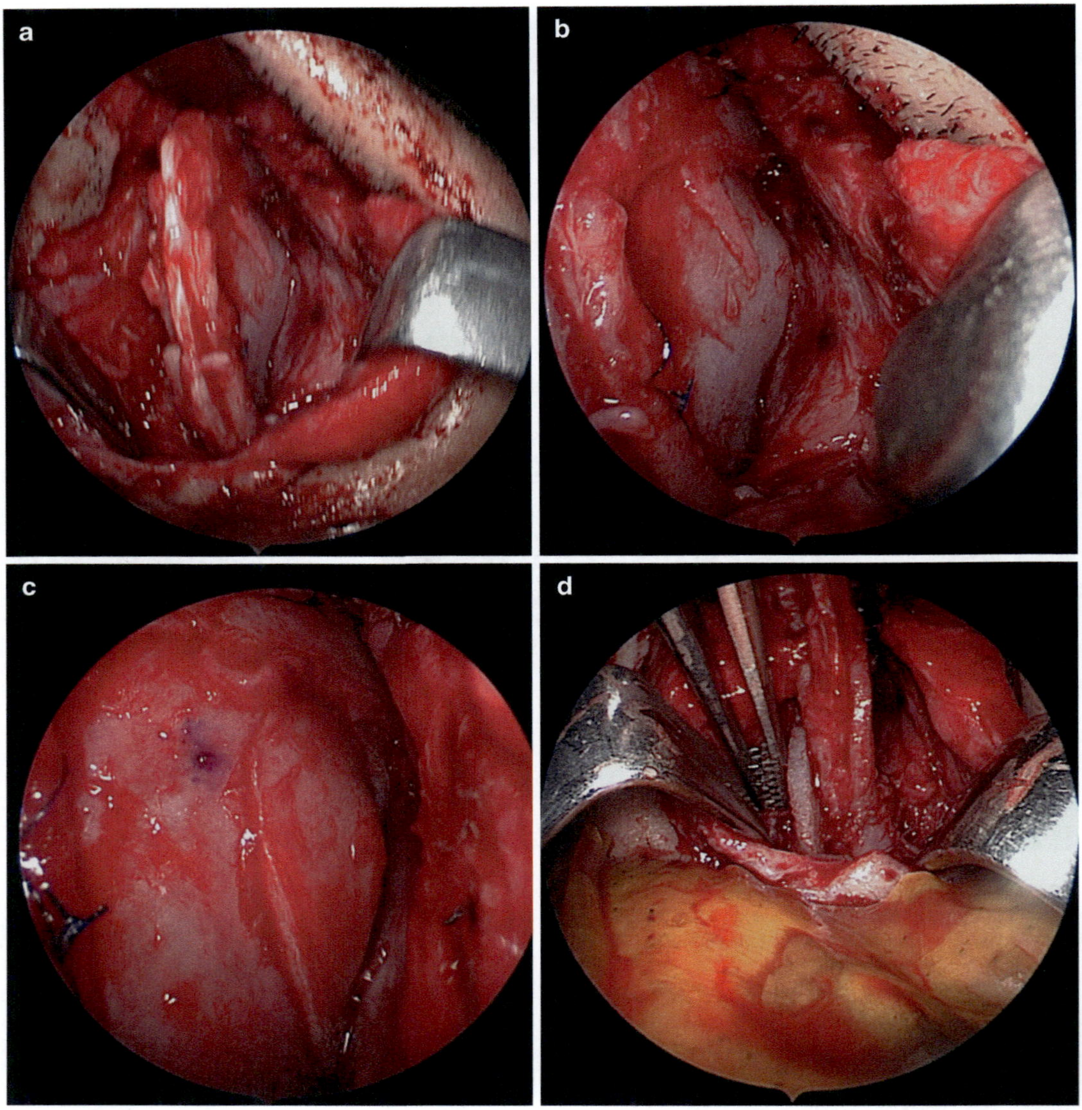

Fig. 12.3 Endoscopic views. (**a**) A previous caudal septal batten graft was found. (**b**) Left side convexity was found at the previous SMR site. (**c**) SMR has performed again. (**d**) A small piece of batten graft was applied to both sides of the caudal septum at ANS

applied to the dorsum for the smoothing of the dorsal line. If ULC does not follow, adding lateral dissection can recruit an extra length of ULC. The catch-up repair can be possible. There are obvious advantages and disadvantages to whether the donor cartilage is the concha or the costal cartilage.

Case Study 1: AESG by Conchal Cartilage
A 23-year-old male patient underwent septoplasty by an ENT doctor with a nasal septal deviation 4 years before the visit. The anterior margin and the caudal margin were found 8 mm in the surgical field. The cymba concha was used as a caudal septal extension graft, the cavum concha

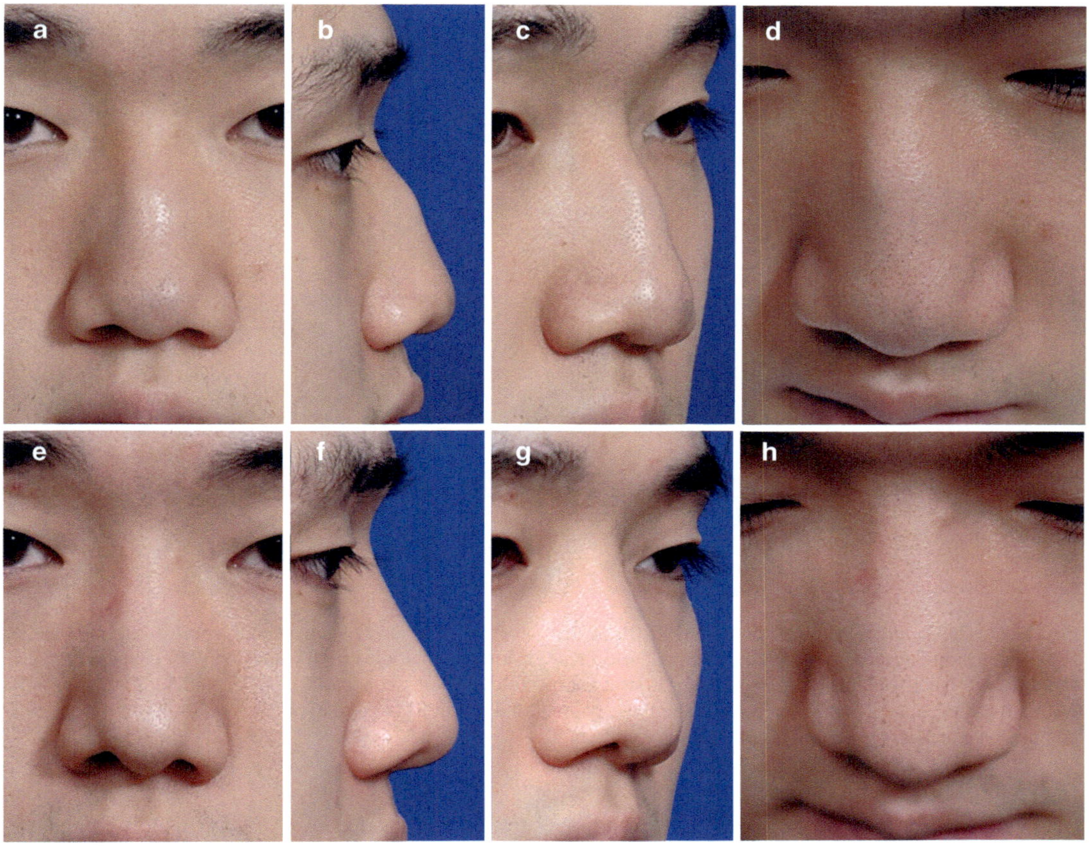

Fig. 12.4 Saddle nose was corrected by AESG using folded cavum concha. (**a**–**d**) Preoperative views. (**e**–**h**) Long-term postoperative views

was used as an anterior extended spreader graft, and a single layer of SMF was applied on the dorsum (Figs. 12.4 and 12.5).

Case Study 2: AESG by Conchal Cartilage
A 55-year-old man had a history of nasal bone fracture 20 years ago. He had been diagnosed with septal abscess 4 years ago, and I&D was done at an ENT clinic. The ear cartilages were used because he disagreed with postoperative tip hardness. One layer of SMF was implanted in the dorsum (Figs. 12.6 and 12.7, Videos 12.3 and 12.4).

12.4 Implant-Related Problems

The characteristic of Medpor and others is to destroy the septum. After removal, most of the contact site is found to be destroyed. Since the septal dissection must be performed, reconstruction after removal equals secondary septoplasty and please refer to Chap. 4 for details.

12.5 Collapsed Septum

It mainly causes the depression of the septum after trauma, such as Lefort fracture and nasoethmoid-orbital fracture (NEO fracture), and the collapse of EPP and nasal bone. Also, cartilaginous collapse occurs even when the entire septal support is lost due to SSI after septorhinoplasty.

Clinical Features

In the collapsed septum, the nasal cavity is narrowed. In most patients, if the narrowed cavity is

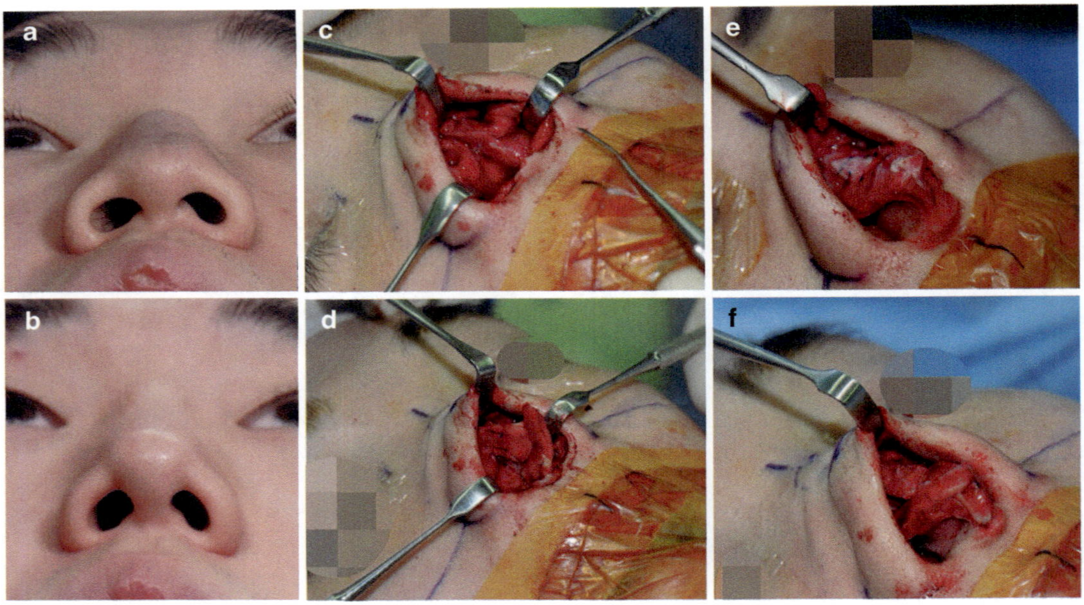

Fig. 12.5 The saddle nose with hump after SMR. (**a**, **b**) Pre- and postoperative basal views. (**c**) The anterocaudal septum was destroyed, and the remaining L-strut was weak. (**d**) After septal L-strut was reconstructed by cavum and cymba conchas. (**e**) Lateral crural spanning graft and for the long axis of the lateral crural divergence angle. Moreover, middle crural extension graft using the applied folded cymba conchal tip. (**f**) The shield graft, cap graft, and dorsal SMF were applied

not widened, there is no improvement in symptoms. In addition to doing a dorsal graft to improve the shape, it is necessary to return the depressed nasal bone to its original position to improve function. An effort may be required to return the damaged nasal bone to its original position. In severe depression of NEO fracture, reducing the nasal bone may not be possible if the bone fragment is too small or the fracture is complex. When the septum collapses, the nose's length is shortened, and the shortened soft tissue causes contracture.

Strategy

The "Key Factor": The Keystone Area

The critical role is in the keystone area. It is no exaggeration to say that the success or failure to reconstruct a collapsed septum depends on how strong a keystone area is reconstructed. In the absence of stability of the left and right nasal bones, the stability can be maintained with the transverse nasal k-wire [7]. At this time, the nasal bone's posterior sinking does not occur if the left and right sides have stability connected to the maxilla. Recently, TCC suture, which is useful for fixing the extended spreader graft near the keystone, is also useful [8]. However, the stability of the nasal bone must be premised. If this fixation becomes impossible, it is sometimes better to reshape the malunion bone by rasping and leave it in place for stability. The K-wires are retained for more extended periods, helping bone union more, but they are usually removed when skin lesions develop. If there is no stability in bilateral keystone areas, a longer spreader graft should be used. If this is not possible, cantilever graft is the answer.

The Reverse Swing Door Concept

If the collapse of the nasal pyramid is due to the impact from the front, the forceful tension of the quadrangular cartilage is applied anterior to posteriorly. The physical energy dispersed by microfracture or dislocation of the posterior

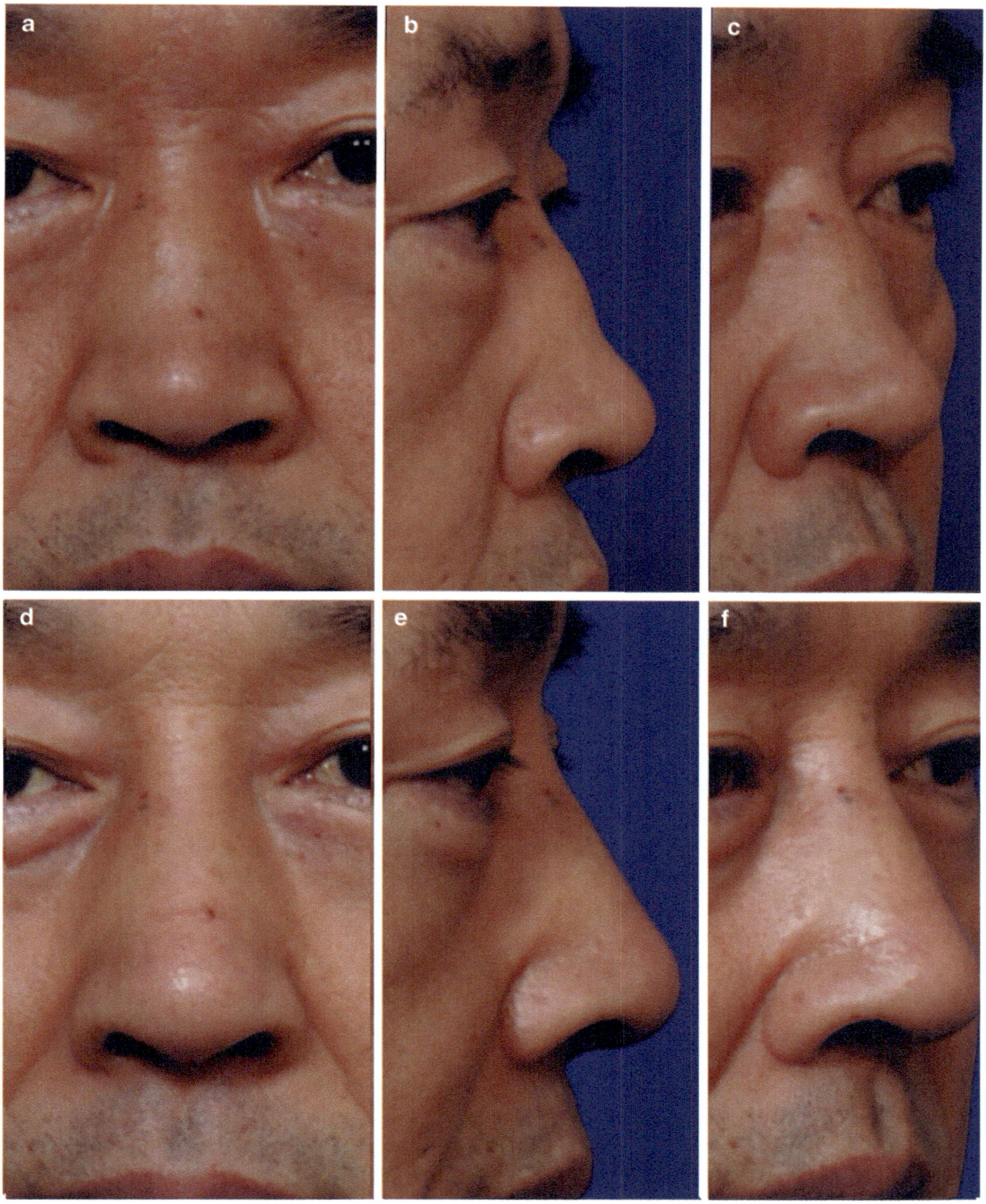

Fig. 12.6 The saddle nose after septal infection. (**a**–**c**) Preoperative views. (**d**–**f**) Postoperative views

quadrangular cartilage. As a result, septal deviation proceeds by the overgrowth of microfractures quadrangular cartilage. Most deviation corrections are performed toward preserving or straightening the anterior portion of the septum.

The concept of a "swing door" procedure that releases the posterior septum tension while preserving the entire septum requires a solid premise of a keystone area's stability. In other words, all these swing door procedures are possible

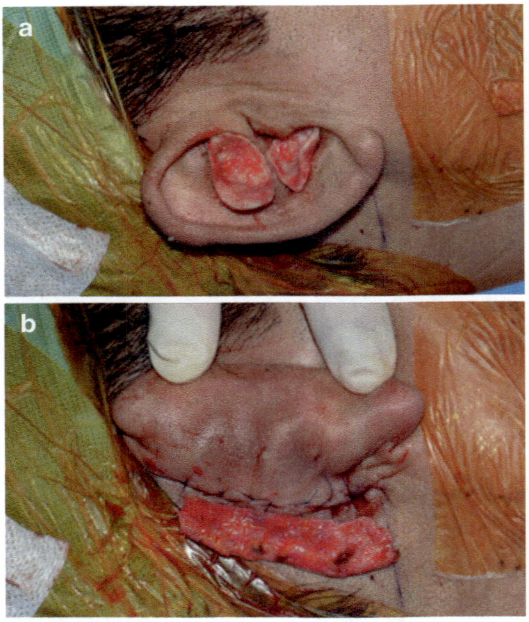

Fig. 12.7 The graft materials: Two conchas and superficial mastoid fascia. (**a**) Cymba and cavum conchas. (**b**) SMF

only when the keystone area is in good condition. Conversely, if there is no deviation of the posterior septum or if the posterior septum is sound, but the keystone area is collapsed, of course, this is very rare. The high septal deviation can be corrected by the "reverse swing door" procedure [9]. The author does not use this method for routine septal deviation correction. However, if the EPP and the septum-vomer junction are well preserved, the opposite tension release is possible using the "reverse swing door" concept [10].

Case Study 1: Old Nasal Bone Fracture
A 44-year-old man visited with an old nasal bone fracture and a nasal obstruction on the right. The camouflage method was explained, but the primary purpose was to resolve the nasal obstruction, so an operation was planned to return the nasal framework to its original shape. Relifting the depressed nasal bone was planned with the reverse swing door method of the collapsed septum. The stability of the keystone was maintained with a K-wire fixation to the right-side nasal bone, which was stable. The nasal function recovered (Figs. 12.8 and 12.9, Video 12.5).

Case Study 2: NEO Fracture
A 25-year-old woman showed septal collapse after reduction as a NEO fracture that occurred with severe laceration by in-car traffic accident. The nasal cavity was narrowed due to severe shrinkage, but the lowered nasal bone could not be advanced anteriorly. If the bony malunion was returned to its original position, too many bone defects occurred, so only the anterocaudal extension of the septum was focused after the partial reverse swing door procedure, and the rectus fascia onlay graft camouflaged the very low bony dorsum from the nasion (Figs. 12.10, 12.11, and 12.12, Video 12.6).

12.6 The Infected Nose

Unlike trauma, the collapse by infection is more complicated. The septum is sometimes preserved in the contracted nose. However, the septum is collapsed when SSI is accompanied by septal infection after SRP. The lengthening can be performed with 2–3 reoperations, but the amount is limited. The most challenging part in short nose correction is septal mucosa contracture, and in some patients, it is not possible to extend the length of the desired length. Even if the external L-framework is operated in the cantilever method, an extra composite graft may be required to correct the retracted nostril and columella. Transposition flaps from the inferior turbinate or nasolabial fold can cover the mucosal defects; however, the author does not recommend this method to young doctors who are starting their practices. The first choice should be a composite graft.

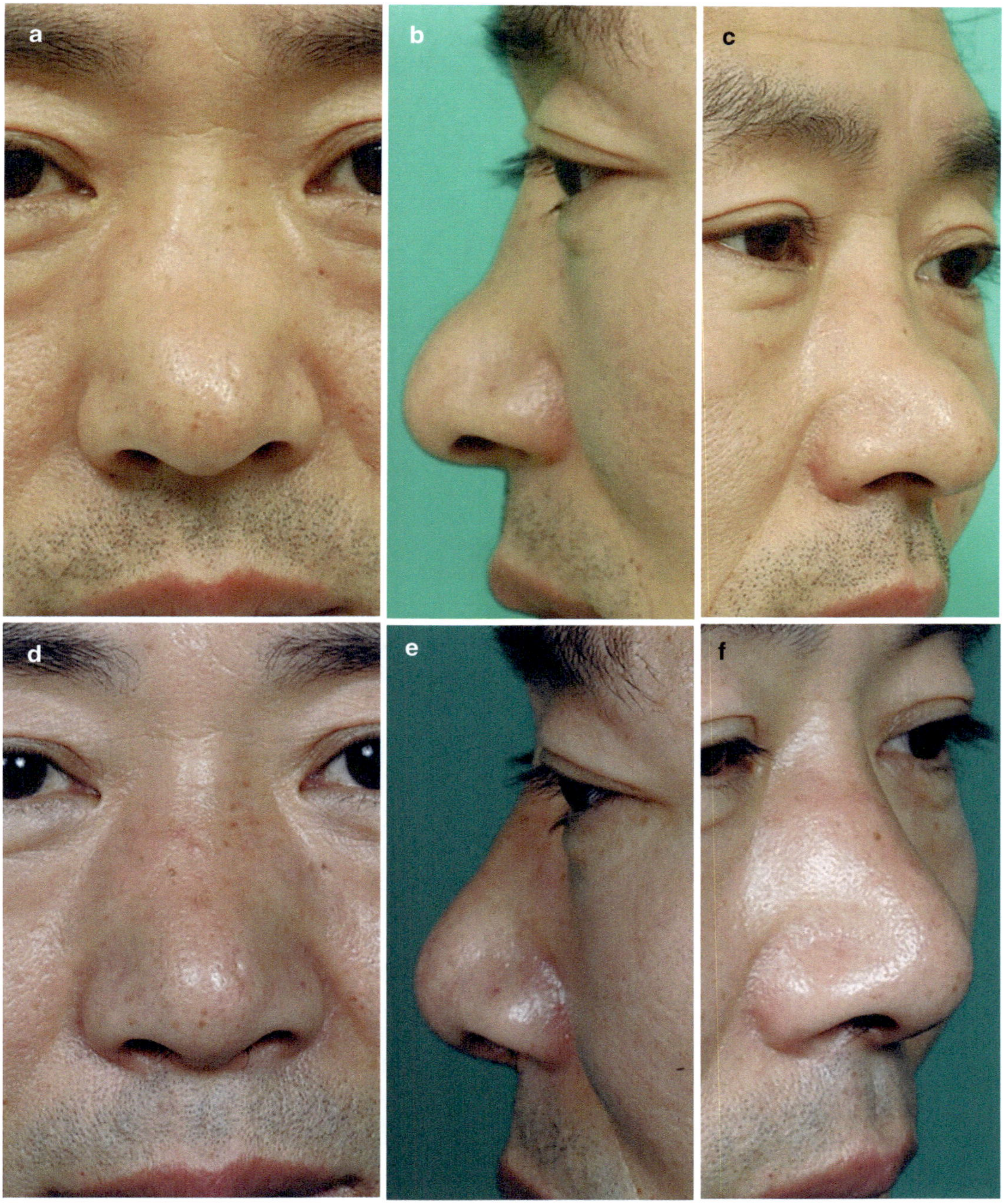

Fig. 12.8 Old nasal bone fracture was corrected by bone repositioning with the reverse swing door procedure. (**a**–**c**) Preoperative views. (**d**–**f**) Postoperative view

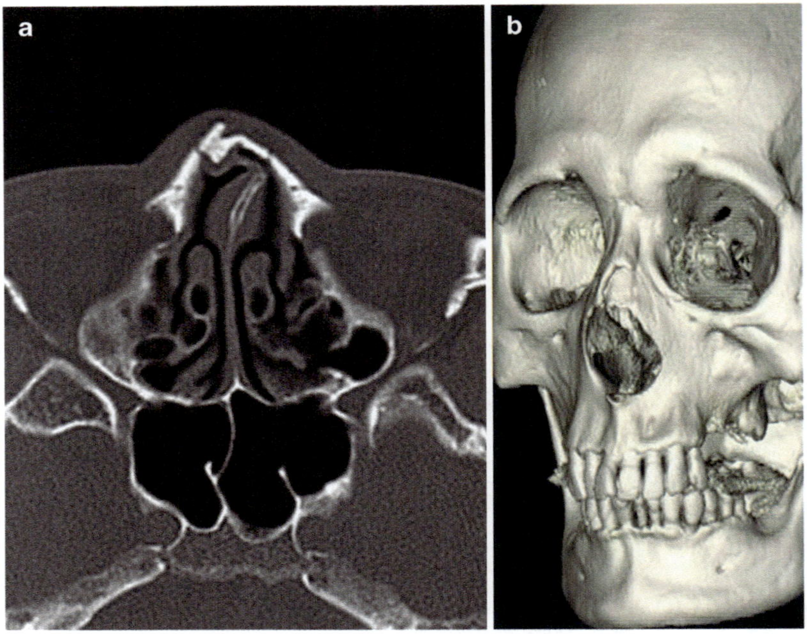

Fig. 12.9 Preoperative CT scan. (**a**, **b**) Lt. nasal bone was depressed with severe deformity at the high septum. However, the posterior septum was relatively sound

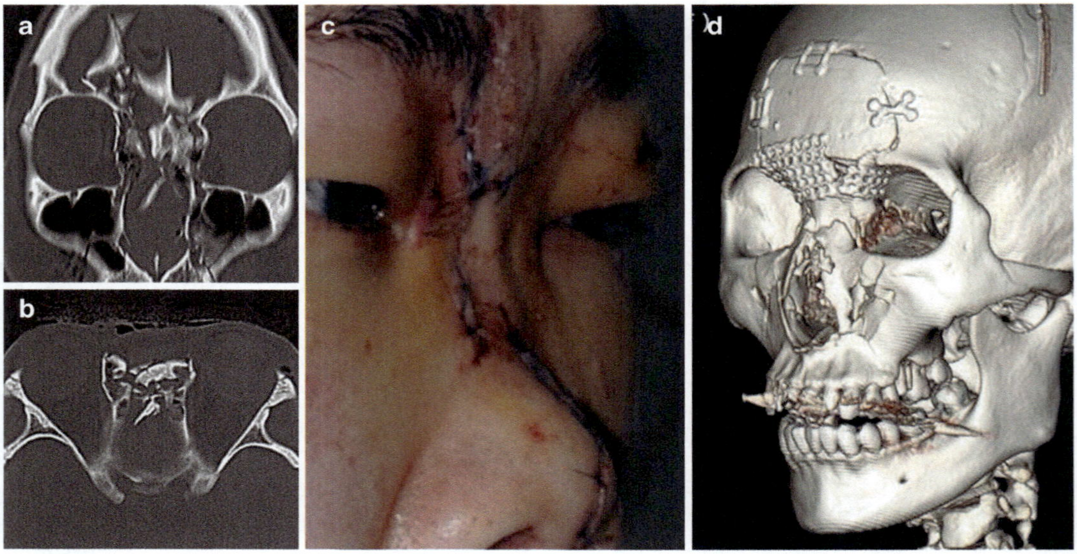

Fig. 12.10 Severe NOE fracture (**a**, **b**) Preoperative coronal and axial views. (**c**) After the key suture was done, the bony dorsum was found collapsed. (**d**) After reduction with cranialization of the frontal sinus

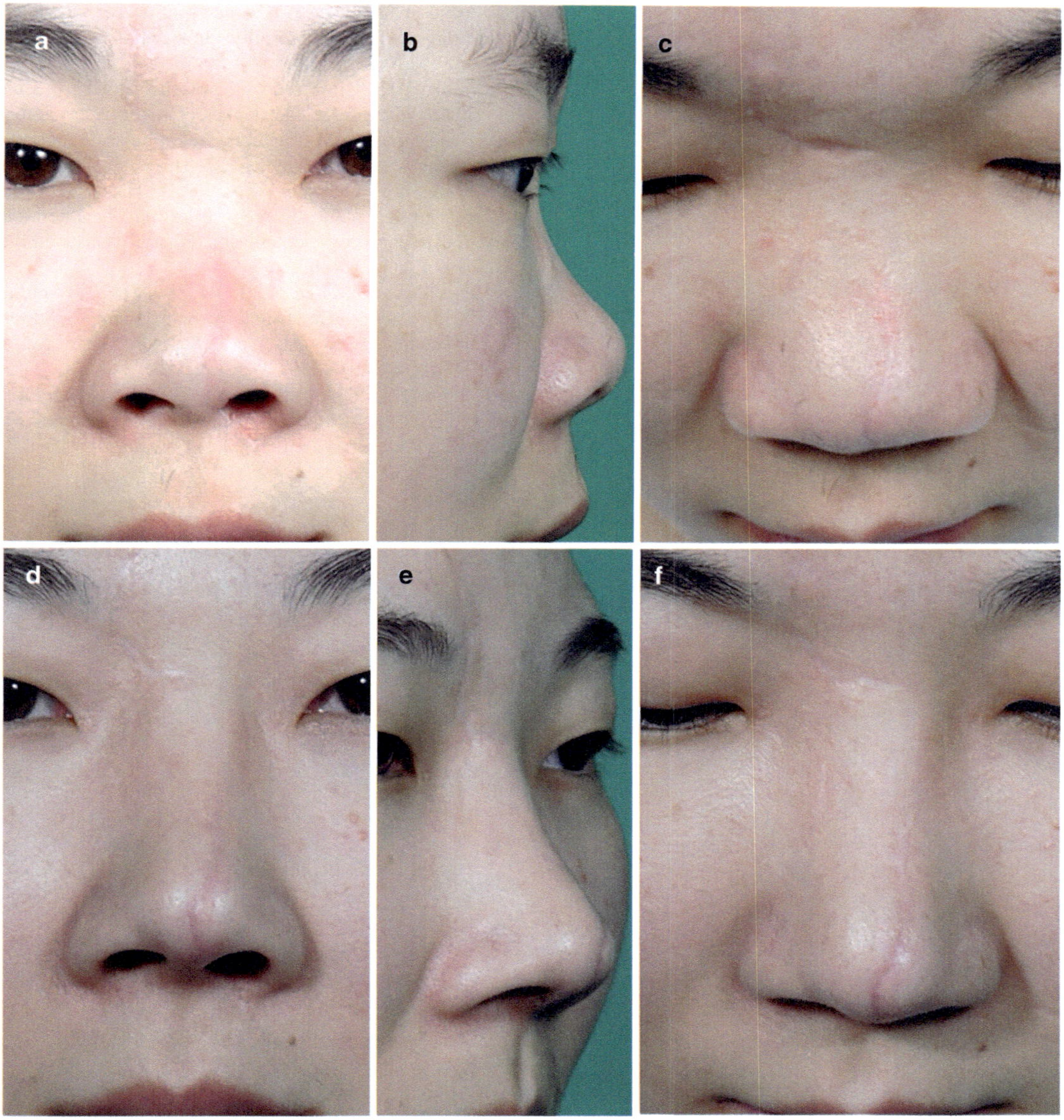

Fig. 12.11 Septal L-strut reconstruction using costal cartilage after the partial reverse swing door procedure. (**a**–**c**) Preoperative views. (**d**–**f**) Long-term postoperative views

Fig. 12.12 Intraoperative view before closure: shield graft, lobule graft using morselized costal cartilage

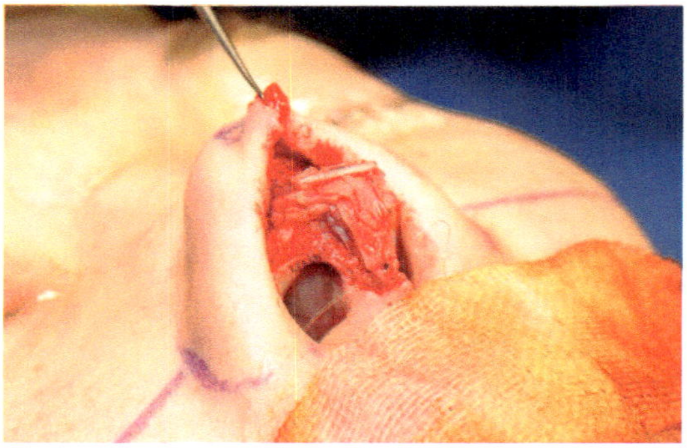

References

1. Sillers MJ, Cox AJ 3rd, Kulbersh B. Revision septoplasty. Otolaryngol Clin N Am. 2009;42(2):261–78, viii
2. Becker SS, Dobratz EJ, Stowell N, Barker D, Park SS. Revision septoplasty: review of sources of persistent nasal obstruction. Am J Rhinol. 2008;22(4):440–4.
3. Gillman GS, Egloff AM, Rivera-Serrano CM. Revision septoplasty: a prospective disease-specific outcome study. Laryngoscope. 2014;124(6):1290–5.
4. Daniel RK. Rhinoplasty: septal saddle nose deformity and composite reconstruction. Plast Reconstr Surg. 2007;119(3):1029–43.
5. Cakmak O, Emre IE, Ozkurt FE. Identifying septal support reconstructions for saddle nose deformity: the Cakmak algorithm. JAMA Facial Plast Surg. 2015;17(6):433–9.
6. Pribitkin EA, Ezzat WH. Classification and treatment of the saddle nose deformity. Otolaryngol Clin N Am. 2009;42(3):437–61.
7. Wadley JK. "How I do it"—plastic surgery practical suggestions on facial plastic surgery: correction of unstable nasal fractures by intranasal support. Laryngoscope. 1979;89(2):327–31.
8. Rezaeian F, Gubisch W, Janku D, Haack S. New suturing techniques to reconstruct the keystone area in extracorporeal septoplasty. Plast Reconstr Surg. 2016;138(2):374–82.
9. Choi JY, Lee JS, Kim JJ, Ha BJ, Shin MS. Correction of deviated nose using reverse swinging door procedure. J Korean Soc Plast Reconstr Surg. 1999;26(6):1107–11.
10. Dhong ES. Septorhinoplasty: endoscopic approach and reinforcement of nasal support line. J Korean Soc Aesth Plast Surg. 2010;16(3):111–6.

13 Think Inside the Box: Absorbable Plate, IHCC, and the Stem Cells

Pearls

- When making a framework with absorbable mesh alone, there is insufficient evidence that it can function as a long-term nasal framework only with fibrous tissue generated in the pores present therein.
- The larger or thicker the absorbable material is, the longer it takes for absorption. Therefore, there are also many tissue reactions.
- Any absorbable material is not free from infection or immune reaction.
- The adoption of PDS foil and PDS plate is relatively beneficial with the evidence and results from many rhinoplasty surgeons.
- IHCC is a nonviable biological material.
- IHCC use is not recommended as a tension-bearing frame.
- In IHCC, resorption can occur in the form of fracture, so it cannot be asserted that there is no late-onset immune reaction at all.
- The efficacy of IHCC may vary from manufacturer to manufacturer.
- It is reasonable to view IHCC as a nonviable material, which has no tissue integrity.
- However, IHCC does not form a capsule due to its biological aspect.
- Since it is applied at the last stage of Asian rhinoplasty, complications take on a more complex aspect, requiring autologous costal cartilage.
- Free fatty tissue is beneficial for soft tissue enhancement in the secondary nose.
- Also, contained preadipocytes can induce recipient-dependent neo adipogenesis.
- However, there is little evidence that SVF contains cytokines that reduce soft tissue contracture in the contracted nose or soften the contracture.
- Do not get confused, administering SVF, and administering ASCs. ASCs are the passaged plated cells.
- ASCs can also be differentiated to myofibroblast, like HDF does, depending on the surrounding wound environment, and can be the source cells of contracture.
- There is no biological in vitro evidence that neither SVF nor hASCs can improve soft tissue contracture caused by inflammation.

13.1 Absorbable Materials

The Fate of Absorbable Plate

Among the commercially available absorbable materials, there are polyglycolic acid (PGA), polylactic acid (PLA), polydioxanone (PDO/PDS), polycaprolactone (PCL), or combinations of these materials. Currently, ready-made plates for rhinoplasty include PCL mesh (TnR mesh; T&R Biofab Co., Ltd., Siheung, Korea) and PDS plate (Ethicon Inc., Johnson & Johnson, Somerville, NJ). Polymers of PLA or PGA or polymers of poly-L-lactic acid (PLLA)/hydroxy-

E.-S. Dhong, M.-W. Na, *Asian Septorhinoplasty*, https://doi.org/10.1007/978-981-16-0542-0_13

apatite (HA) are widely used in craniomaxillofacial surgery. According to the manufacturer's information, the PDS plate resorbs within 25 weeks, and its stability is maintained for 10 weeks. The biodegradation process depends on contact with body fluids, temperature, motion, molecular weight, the crystalline form and geometry of the material, and the implanted tissue [1, 2]. The absorption of PLA/PGA products is eliminated by hydrolysis and metabolism, and macrophages and giant cells absorb particles that cannot be hydrolyzed. PCL performs the same process and is decomposed into CO_2 and H_2O and absorbed. Usually, when hydrolysis occurs beyond the range of metabolism, it is said that the inflammatory reaction becomes more active [3]. The author believes that the degree of absorption varies depending on the recipient, the plate was found as particles even after 2 years postoperatively. About the complication, immune reactions have been reported, and low-grade inflammation occurred even within a few months of application. Prolonged swelling resulted in nasal obstruction, especially when applied to the septum. However, absorbable plates have been used in craniofacial surgery, and there is no lack of evidence for absorption. The belief that absorbable plates can be used for rhinoplasty is that if alloplastic materials are absorbed and disappeared eventually, there will be no problems in the long term. However, a greater belief is that the scaffold disappears, and cartilage or fibrous tissue grows into the pores, filling the pores and eventually being substituted for autologous tissue. Reports of inflammatory reactions lead to unwanted discharge, leading to an adverse immune reaction in the intraseptal or surgical pocket [4]. Also, the follow-up period was short, and there is insufficient evidence for reporting inflammatory reactions and comparative reports of infection rates [5].

All alloplastic materials have physical and chemical properties. In addition to the abovementioned chemical properties, thick materials may cause tissue damage due to physical properties depending on the application site. There is already a lot of evidence of craniofacial surgery showing temporary compression of the bone surface (Fig. 13.1).

Two Different Concepts in Adopting Absorbable Plates

Temporary Support

PDS foil or PDS plate can be used as a cartilage stabilizer by molding fragmented cartilage on a flat plate. Many studies report that the PDS plate used with cartilage is advantageous in terms of material usage [6].

The author often uses it for flattening the tortuous ear cartilages. The author's method is to apply a chondrotomy to eliminate curvature

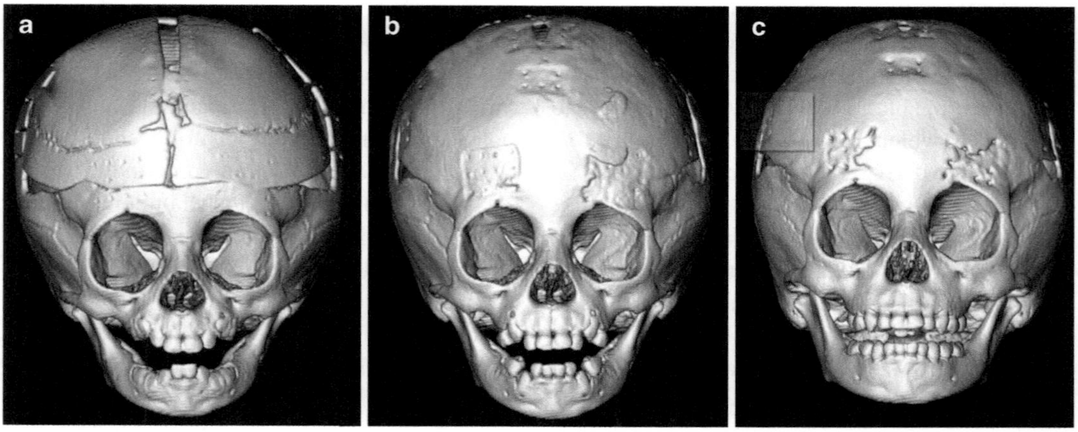

Fig. 13.1 Bone depression where the absorbable plate was applied. (**a**) Postoperative 6-month view. (**b**) Postoperative 12 months. (**c**) Even a postoperative 30-month's view shows bone depression where the absorbable plate was fixed

when folding conchal cartilage. As the number of chondrotomy increases, the cartilage's integrity decreases, and stability is lost, so it is used as the concept of the internal splint. If possible, the author tries to place the plate inside the cartilage and prohibit the PDS plate's direct exposure. The PDS plate is always used with cartilages.

Scaffold Recruiting Cartilage

The PCL mesh plate is introduced to be used for nose surgery independently. Pros explained that 50% of the absorbable mesh is made up of pores, so fibrous tissue or cartilage grows into the pores. The fibrous tissue is proliferated, and this tissue can constitute the framework. However, considering the physical properties, the evidence is needed to determine whether fibrous tissue can sustain the physical properties as a nasal framework. What is more problematic is the mechanical surface property of the plate itself. It can be predicted that multiple micropores eventually form a rough surface, and this surface can easily cause erosion to the fragile septal mucosa.

Two Different Techniques

Combining with Cartilage

Most thin PDS foils or PDS plates are introduced as a method of using cartilage, and a plate is used to mold the pieces into a big one. Eventually, cartilage fragments' survival is expected to play a supportive role by healing with neighboring cartilage fragments. If mucoperichondrium is preserved and cartilage is regenerated in the septal pocket, survival can be expected more.

Absorbable Materials Only

Below are several types of commercialized methods. The author has no experience with the three methods. The author is operating on patients with problems using the below methods.

SEG

A method for applying a PCL mesh instead of a cartilage framework for a septal extension by itself has recently emerged [5]. The plate is too thick to integrate the cartilage. Only the PCL mesh plate without attaching cartilage is used as the septal extension graft.

Tip Plasty: Soft Ball

For tip plasty, PCL in ball shape was introduced for onlaying at the tip.

Thread Tip Plasty

There are various thread names for counter-rotating the nasal tip or projecting the tip using a PDO thread cog so-called noninvasive rhinoplasty. This is a tip plasty using absorbable thread, which is the same concept as face-lift by a thread.

13.2 Pitfalls of the "Myth"

- There is a lack of evidence that the fibrous tissue generated in the pores in the absorbable mesh can function as a long-term nasal framework.
- The larger or thicker the absorbable material is, the longer it takes for absorption. Therefore, there are also many tissue reactions.
- There is no evidence that the use of absorbable materials that are not self-organized has a permanent effect. Any material is not free from infection or immune reaction.
- The adoption of PDS foil and PDS plate with evidence and results of many rhinoplasty surgeons is a relatively useful cartilage salvage method.

13.3 IHCC (Irradiated Homologous Costal Cartilage)

Is it a Viable Material?

There is only one reason to use IIHCC. Autologous material should be used, but there is a burden on the harvest.

- IHCC is considered a nonviable biologic material.

There are many reports on IHCC, and it is undeniably a convenient and useful material in that it is a material that can be useful in situations where secondary rhinoplasty or sudden cartilage is required. Compared with autologous costal cartilage, some studies show less warping and the same performance in all respects [7]. In a previous study, the author reported a resorption and fracture rate of approximately 2% in IHCC and reported a safe material. However, as experience increases, IHCC draws closer to the pessimistic conclusion that IHCC is a nonviable biological material, "a dead graft."

There is a limit to growing new cartilage, so IHCC cannot be regarded as a viable graft.

- It is not recommended to use for tension-bearing frames.
- The reason why resorption can occur in the form of fracture and viability declines over time is why it cannot be asserted that there is no immune reaction.
- The efficacy may vary from manufacturer to manufacturer.
- It is reasonable to view it as an alloplastic material that is nonviable and has no tissue integrity. However, it does not form a capsule due to its biological aspect.

Since it is often applied at the last stage of Asian rhinoplasty, complications take on a more complex aspect, which in turn requires autologous costal cartilage. When the remaining capsule from the previous silicone is not removed, the capsular contracture occurred in the later applied IHCC. Also, it is not completely free from late-onset inflammation. The reason is that it is not a viable graft. As the number of patients undergoing surgery increases, many causes are often combined. In other words, it is challenging to determine the cause of the contracture that occurred later in the case of applying IHCC as a septal extension graft.

Pitfalls of the "Myth"

- Surgery with IHCC forms no neocartilage in the long term, and tissue integration does not occur like autograft.
- IHCC is only a nonviable biologic graft and can be considered an alloplastic implant in some sense.

13.4 Human Adipose-Derived Stromal (Stem) Cells: hASCs

The author has been conducting basic research on human adipose stromal cells' biology for over 15 years and is still conducting basic research on ASCs and soft tissue contracture [8–14].

The author believes that fat graft is a useful ancillary procedure for rhinoplasty with the perspective of biological tissue recruitment. The fat graft literally injects fatty tissue directly into the tissue, so the author thinks it is a beneficial soft tissue management method. There are several reports on delivery modality, but the author thinks that direct injection or tissue-integrated graft are all excellent methods. What the author wants to discuss in this chapter is to report the harm of direct-to-consumer advertising of "the myth of stemness" [15].

- It is an act of harassing a complicated patient again. It is about stem cell treatment, which is conducted by directly charging the high cost of treatment but still lacks evidence.
- This chapter criticizes the early adoption of fatty tissue derivatives that do not benefit patients.

13.5 Direct-to-Consumer Portrayal of Stem Cell Medicine

A few decades ago, there have been pros and cons about the clinical application of new technologies. However, in-depth regulation is indeed necessary for the direct clinical application of stem cells. Although this may vary from country to country, the risk may be larger than the benefit relevantly in common [16].

Several studies have already given direct IV doses of adipose-derived stem cells [17] and even administering SVF directly as IV doses [18]. Although 10 years have passed, clinically significant effects have been reported, but no established treatment methods have appeared. There have already been reports of problems in the plastic surgery field regarding these problems [19]. A bigger problem is the reality that the high cost of treatment is charged along with this irrelevance and that this cost becomes a burden for previous surgeons. As a fellow plastic surgeon, the author feels exhausted from demanding evidence for an unscientific procedure. It is true that research reports are limited because it is illegal to inject cultured cells directly in some countries. There have been reports of sound effects by injecting stem cells into Asian contracted noses, but if you carefully read the description of stem cells, you can see that the scientific basis is insufficient [20].

The following summarizes the superficial contents of the current knowledge and the problems of early adoption of hASCs while the author has been conducting basic research on hASCs. Bench to bedside translational research requires a lot of persistence and precise in vitro data, and in vivo data must also be objective.

Counterpoints of Injecting "Adipose-Derived Stem Cells(?)" into the Contracted Nose

Contracture is one of the most severe complications after silicone-based rhinoplasty. It manifests as rigidity or hardening of the scar, deformity, asymmetry, displacement, and foreshortened nose. The causes of capsular contracture are still unclear because of the various factors contributing to it, such as hematomas, seroma, and infections. Myofibroblast displays one of the predominant cells in the capsule, and 25% of it originates from bone marrow during the inflammatory phase. Various inflammatory cytokines are responsible for the differentiation of myofibroblasts. Transforming growth factor-beta (TGF-β) plays a crucial role in differentiation, but this single factor cannot thoroughly explain differentiation. Recent studies show that interleukin-3 (IL-3) and granulocyte-macrophage colony-stimulating factor (GM-CSF) are inflammatory cytokines that contribute to the accumulation of myofibroblast-like cells, differentiation of stem cells, and stimulation of TGF-β expression. Both IL-3 and GM-CSF are produced in acute and chronic lesions within the wound and stimulate fibrosis and induce granulation tissue. Zafirlukast and montelukast are uniquely effective medicines based on clinical evidence for improving contracture, which are leukotriene receptor antagonists (LTRA) and interfere with eosinophil survival-enhancing activity (ESEA). Cysteinyl-leukotriene antagonists can inhibit dose-dependently the release of Th2 cytokines: IL-3, IL-4, and GM-CSF. In breast capsular contracture, implantation into the subglandular area, which contains a large amount of adipose tissue, often leads to a more severe degree of inflammation resulting in capsular contracture than insertion into the submuscular area, which possesses less adipose tissue. Recent studies show that human adipose-derived stem cells (hASCs) can differentiate into myofibroblasts. The hypothesis insisting that fibroblast, with hASCs, may play an essential role in capsular contracture has relevant proofs.

Human Adipose-Derived Stem (Stromal) Cells Differ from Stromal Vascular Fraction

The human adipose-derived stem (stromal) cells are different from the stromal vascular fraction. Why is it said to give stem cells while using SVF? The processed lipoaspirate (PLA) obtained by centrifuging lipoaspirate is dissolved in collagenase and then centrifuged again to obtain the stromal vascular fraction (SVF). Currently, many countries are clinically available in using SVF so far. The cells that grew by plating this SVF attached to the floor are called ASC. There is a predetermined promise for ASCs. Cells that are $CD73^+$, $CD90^+$, $CD105^+$, and simultaneously, $CD45^-$, $CD34^-$ should have been characterized [21]. If these CD markers are different, it should not be called ASC. The standard may change after the writing of this chapter, but the rules for cells' characteristics, especially the multipotent differentiation, should be kept. In the case of the sialomucin family, CD34, the representative ones that show positivity are BMSCs, hematopoietic stem cells, skeletal muscle satellite cells, keratinocyte stem cells, hair follicle stem cells, and adipogenic precursors. There was a theory that ASC was of $CD34^-$ pericyte origin [22], and there was a claim of $CD34^+$ pericyte after, but $CD34^-CD105+$ is the current consensus [23]. Later $CD106^-$, $CD36^+$ were added [24].

- A stromal cell is $CD34^+$, and a passaged ASC is $CD34^-$.
- The aqueous form of SVF is a combination of pericytes, preadipocytes, hematopoietic cells, endothelial progenitor cells, endothelial cells, and stromal cells, which are CD 34^+ $CD105^-$. Of course, SVF secretes VEGF, HGF, and bFGF, which play an essential role in wounds, and TGF-β, which will be critical in this chapter, and research on this is active.
- Many substances are involved in wound contracture in the cytokine contained in SVF.

13.6 Can ASCs Be Administered to Treat Contractures?

The causes of contracture are fibroblast and myofibroblast. In the cell's cytoplasmic skeleton, the level of expression of alpha SMA, SM 22α, or calponin can be indirectly determined. The most critical cytokine for contracture is activation of TGF. Of course, numerous cytokines are involved in contracture. Fibroblasts present in the wound are activated and transformed into myofibroblasts, as well as all types of cells (mesothelium, endothelium, epithelium) may occur metaplasia into myofibroblasts by surrounding inflammatory reactions. Related here is the inflammatory cytokine, the most important of which is TGFβ. The same mechanism works for ASCs. In other words, under the same circumstances, ASCs in chronic wounds are enough to cause tissue contracture [10]. Even ASCs' conditioned media did not antagonize the action of TGFβ, and there is no evidence to prevent myofibroblast differentiation [25]. The author is not against applying free fatty tissue graft. In a situation in which passaged ASCs can act like fibroblasts, and the role of anti-myofibroblast differentiation among the paracrine cytokines has not been proven, direct injection to the patient does not provide any evidence for prevention or treatment of contracture. The myth should be discarded.

- ASCs also show characteristics of myofibroblasts in inflammatory conditions like human dermal fibroblasts (HDF) (Fig. 13.2).
- There is no evidence that the paracrine action of ASCs prevents differentiation into myofibroblasts.

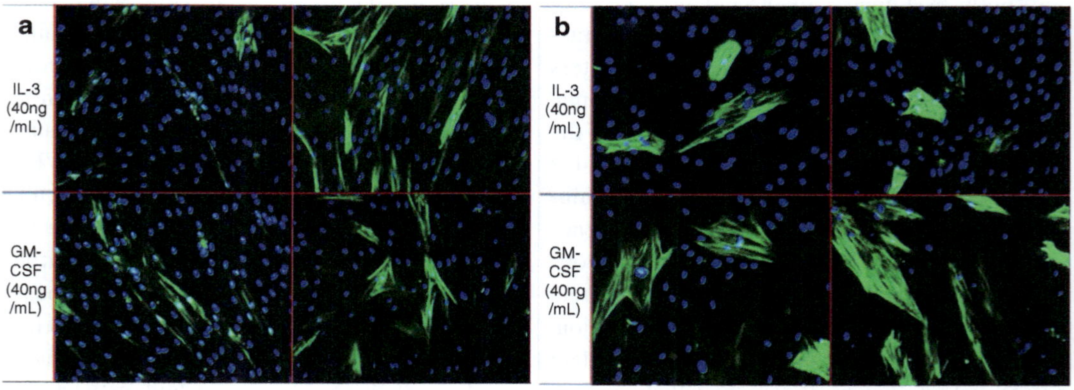

Fig. 13.2 The expression of α SMA when treated with IL-3/GM-CSF (40 ng/mL) ×400 magnification. (**a**) Human dermal fibroblast (HDF). (**b**) Human adipose-derived stromal cells (hASCs)

Pitfalls of the "Myth"

- Free fatty tissue causes soft tissue enhancement. Also, contained preadipocytes can induce recipient-dependent neo adipogenesis.
- However, there is little evidence that SVF can soften the contracted nose or relieve the contraction because it contains cytokines that cause soft tissue contracture.
- Do not assume that you are administering ASCs while administering SVF.
- ASCs can also be differentiated into myofibroblast-like HDF depending on the surrounding wound environment and can be source cells of contracture.
- There is no biological in vitro evidence that neither SVF nor hASCs can improve soft tissue contracture caused by inflammation.

References

1. Park Y-W. Bioabsorbable osteofixation for orthognathic surgery. Maxillofac Plast Reconstr Surg. 2015;37(1):6.
2. Bali RK, Sharma P, Jindal S, Gaba S. To evaluate the efficacy of biodegradable plating system for fixation of maxillofacial fractures: a prospective study. Natl J Maxillofac Surg. 2013;4(2):167–72.
3. Landes CA, Ballon A, Roth C. In-patient versus in vitro degradation of P (L/DL) LA and PLGA. J Biomed Mater Res B Appl Biomater. 2006;76(2):403–11.
4. Wang LL, Frankel AS, Friedman O. Complications of Polydioxanone foil use in nasal surgery: a case series. Facial Plast Surg. 2018;34(3):312–7.
5. Park YJ, Cha JH, Bang SI, Kim SY. Clinical application of three-dimensionally printed biomaterial Polycaprolactone (PCL) in augmentation rhinoplasty. Aesthet Plast Surg. 2019;43(2):437–46.
6. Boenisch M, Nolst Trenité GJ. Reconstruction of the nasal septum using polydioxanone plate. Arch Facial Plast Surg. 2010;12(1):4–10.
7. Alhussain OH, Alhussain GO, Rajkhan AA, Suhluli AJ, Alharbi SJ, Sherwani AA, et al. Efficacy of autologous vs. homologous costal cartilage grafts in dorsal augmentation rhinoplasty: a systematic review and meta-analysis. Ann Med Health Sci Res [Internet]. 2020;10(5). https://www.amhsr.org/articles/efficacy-of-autologous-vs-homologous-costal-cartilagegrafts-in-dorsal-augmentation-rhinoplasty-asystematic-review-and-me.pdf.
8. Moon K-C, Lee H-S, Son S-T, Lee J-S, Dhong E-S, Jeong S-H, et al. Effects of granulocyte-macrophage Colony-stimulating factor on neuronal senescence in ultraviolet irradiated skin. J Craniofac Surg. 2019;30(3):930–5.
9. Namgoong S, Lee H, Lee J-S, Jeong SH, Han S-K, Dhong E-S. Comparative biological effects of human amnion and chorion membrane extracts on human adipose-derived stromal cells. J Craniofac Surg. 2019;30(3):947–54.
10. Lee J-S, Tae S-S, Kim D-Y, Han S-K, Kim W-K, Dhong E-S. Do IL-3/GM-CSF effect on the myofibroblastic differentiation of human adipose derived stromal cells? Exp Cell Res. 2017;355(2):67–82.
11. Moon K-C, Lee J-S, Han S-K, Lee H-W, Dhong E-S. Effects of human umbilical cord blood-derived mesenchymal stromal cells and dermal fibroblasts on diabetic wound healing. Cytotherapy. 2017;19(7):821–8.
12. Gu JH, Lee JS, Kim D-W, Yoon E-S, Dhong E-S. Neovascular potential of adipose-derived stromal cells (ASCs) from diabetic patients. Wound Repair Regen. 2012;20(2):243–52.
13. Dhong E-S, Hwang N-H, Kim D-W, Rajashekhar G, Johnstone BH, March KL. Morphologic changes in photodamaged organotypic human skin culture after treatment of autologous adipose-derived stromal cells. J Craniofac Surg. 2012;23(3):805–11.
14. Hwang N-H, Jung J-E, Lee J-S, Jeong S-H, Dhong E-S, Han S-K. Effects of granulocyte macrophage Colony-stimulating factor inhibition on the skin/nerve cell model in vitro. J Craniofac Surg. 2020;31(5):1483–7.
15. Gilbody S. Benefits and harms of direct to consumer advertising: a systematic review [Internet]. Quality and safety in health care, vol 14. 2005. p. 246–50. https://doi.org/10.1136/qshc.2004.012781.
16. Ogbogu U, Rachul C, Caulfield T. Reassessing direct-to-consumer portrayals of unproven stem cell therapies: is it getting better? Regen Med. 2013;8(3):361–9.
17. Fang B, Song Y, Lin Q, Zhang Y, Cao Y, Zhao RC, et al. Human adipose tissue-derived mesenchymal stromal cells as salvage therapy for treatment of severe refractory acute graft-vs.-host disease in two children. Pediatr Transplant. 2007;11(7):814–7.
18. Riordan NH, Ichim TE, Min W-P, Wang H, Solano F, Lara F, et al. Non-expanded adipose stromal vascular fraction cell therapy for multiple sclerosis. J Transl Med. 2009;7:29.
19. Gir P, Oni G, Brown SA, Mojallal A, Rohrich RJ. Human adipose stem cells: current clinical applications. Plast Reconstr Surg. 2012;129(6):1277–90.
20. Oh YH, Seo JW, Oh SJ, Oum IT, Kim G, Kim J, et al. Correction of severely contracted nose. Plast Reconstr Surg. 2016;138(3):571–82.
21. Dominici M, Le Blanc K, Mueller I, Slaper-Cortenbach I, Marini F, Krause D, et al. Minimal criteria for defining multipotent mesenchymal stromal cells. The International Society for Cellular Therapy position statement. Cytotherapy. 2006;8(4):315–7.
22. Crisan M, Casteilla L, Lehr L, Carmona M, Paoloni-Giacobino A, Yap S, et al. A reservoir of brown adipocyte progenitors in human skeletal muscle. Stem Cells. 2008;26(9):2425–33.

23. Traktuev DO, Merfeld-Clauss S, Li J, Kolonin M, Arap W, Pasqualini R, et al. A population of multipotent CD34-positive adipose stromal cells share pericyte and mesenchymal surface markers, reside in a periendothelial location, and stabilize endothelial networks. Circ Res. 2008;102(1):77–85.
24. Bourin P, Bunnell BA, Casteilla L, Dominici M, Katz AJ, March KL, et al. Stromal cells from the adipose tissue-derived stromal vascular fraction and culture expanded adipose tissue-derived stromal/stem cells: a joint statement of the International Federation for Adipose Therapeutics and Science (IFATS) and the International Society for Cellular Therapy (ISCT). Cytotherapy. 2013;15(6):641–8.
25. Liguori TTA, Liguori GR, Moreira LFP, Harmsen MC. Fibroblast growth factor-2, but not the adipose tissue-derived stromal cells secretome, inhibits TGF-β1-induced differentiation of human cardiac fibroblasts into myofibroblasts [Internet]. Sci Rep. 2018;8. https://doi.org/10.1038/s41598-018-34747-3.

14 Pus Draining Status After Complicated Septorhinoplasty: When to Do the Secondary Rhinoplasty?

14.1 Background of Choosing this Case

When the author encounters a patient who is draining pus in an outpatient clinic, the first thought may be, "Why did the patient come to this hospital instead of where he/she has been operated?" However, the patient came to visit in a desperate condition. The doctor who performed the surgery previously might send the patient because he could not solve it. Choosing the best way to do it is to salvage both the patient and doctor in trouble. After septorhinoplasty became popular, septal extension grafts after SMR and alloplastic implants use simultaneously resulted in SSI after surgery, leaving the most severe sequelae. The pus-drainage will not improve unless alloplastic material and infected cartilage are removed. If the alloplastic implant and cartilage in the nasal framework on the undersurface are removed, will the nose's shape be maintained? Because of this fear, cartilage cannot be removed quickly, and only empirical antibiotics are used in various situations, resulting in irreversible consequences.

Pearls

- Patients with septal extension graft and alloplastic implants at the same time should be aware that it is a very urgent situation if SSI occurs after surgery.
- It is essential to be aware of any problems that may arise after removing the implant in the nose by setting the surgery's timing well.
- Once the pus is drained, all nonviable grafts must be removed. The viable graft can also be checked with the naked eye and left behind.
- SSI is a situation in which the infected tissue must be surgically removed, but it is a unique situation that requires medical control.
- Choosing the appropriate antibiotic using multiple nasal or discharge cultures is the way to succeed.
- The degree of cellulitis of columellar and dorsal skin is the criterion for determining the surgical timing. Even if the pus is drained, if the redness of the pocket skin and surrounding swelling is low, and the amount of pus in the prescribed antibiotics suddenly begins to decrease, surgery using autogenous graft may be considered. Mostly, late-onset inflammation is regarded as a low-grade infection.

Supplementary Information The online version of this chapter (https://doi.org/10.1007/978-981-16-0542-0_14) contains supplementary material, which is available to authorized users.

E.-S. Dhong, M.-W. Na, *Asian Septorhinoplasty*, https://doi.org/10.1007/978-981-16-0542-0_14

- However, if SSI has occurred, active I&D should be performed first, and the flap should be monitored well. If flap swelling and rubor are severe, any graft to make the shape is not recommended.
- The framework reconstruction can be considered if the cellulitis is not severe. As it may cause more severe contracture if the framework is not considered for fear of repeated SSI.

14.2 Case Study

History

Three months before visiting the author, he underwent septorhinoplasty with a hump correction and dorsal Gore-tex implantation. SSI occurred 10 days after surgery, and the culture result was MRSA. After SSI was discovered, the wound was irrigated several times. After that, vancomycin was administered IV for 1 month at the same ENT clinic. Then, he was transferred to another university hospital. It was the fifth week postoperatively. The Gore-tex tip was partially removed, and the infected materials were removed by curettage and irrigated. However, the columella drained pus continuously after the removal, and columellar retraction was noted. He was referred to the author in the 10th week after the primary surgery.

Physical Exam and Diagnostic Findings

The first visit: A small opening was seen in the columella, and discharge was continuously drained. Vancomycin was cut, and mupirocin ointment was applied. Oral clindamycin was administered because MRSE was rediscovered in the culture performed just before the visit.

A culture study was conducted, and surgery was recommended even if there was no pus drained.

The second visit: the first visit culture was negative, and the discharge decreased after Clindamycin administration. The author recommended immediate surgery but wanted surgery after a month due to the patient's circumstances. LFT increased in liver function test.

Operation; Three weeks after the first referral to the author, surgery was performed. A total of 13 weeks postoperatively, the tertiary operation was performed.

Endoscopic Findings

Central flopping was found at the SMR status, but there was no pus pocket or perforation in the nasal septum.

A puncture confined to the columellar was found. Also, bulging of the columella on the right side was found (Fig. 14.1).

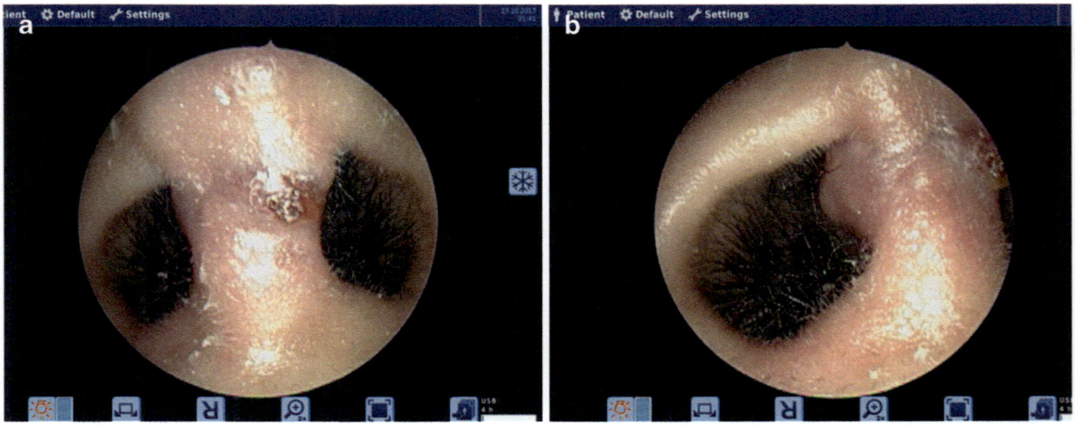

Fig. 14.1 The pus-draining anterior columellar lesion. (**a**, **b**) Close-up views

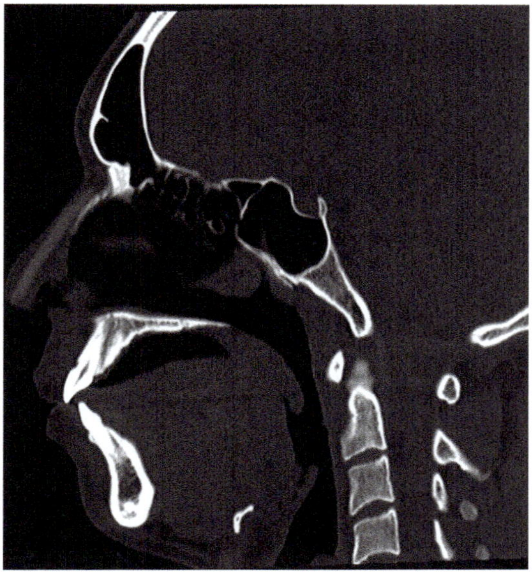

Fig. 14.2 Sagittal CT scan shows a long dorsal implant and impending protrusion

CT Scan

The alloplastic material presumed to be a long Gore-tex was up to the nasal tip, and the skin thickness of the tip was thin enough to suspect impending protrusion (Videos 14.1 and 14.2, Fig. 14.2).

Culture Study and Antibiotics

- 1st culture: no bacterial.
- 2nd culture (2 weeks after the 1st visit): Paenibacillus polymyxa (moderately).
  - Clindamycin resistant Oxacillin resistant Penicillin resistant.
  - Levofloxacin sensitive Vancomycin sensitive.
- 3rd culture (operation day): no bacterial.

Choice of antibiotics: Tarivid ointment for 7 days preoperatively and postoperatively

IV Vancomycin for 5 days peri- and postoperatively

Preoperative Surgical Planning

- The cartilage destruction of the columella is judged to be severe, which is the pus pocket.
- Since cellulitis is not severe, it was decided to reconstruct the nasal framework using a cartilage graft to solve the retracted columellar.
- The caudal septal extension will be performed first, then the extended septal extension graft will follow according to the anterior septum condition.
- The loss of dorsal height that occurs after implant removal will be reconstructed with SDF.

Intraoperative Findings

There were still unhealed columellar lesions, and incisions were made using this area. The left nasal cavity was narrower than the right side, and the lower edge of the implant was observed on the ceiling of the right nasal cavity (Video 14.3).

A mucocele-like pocket was found under the dorsal Gore-tex, showing a late-onset inflammation pattern with mucin collected (Video 14.4 and Figs.14.3 and 14.4). As a result of the lower anterior septum's dissection after removing the entire

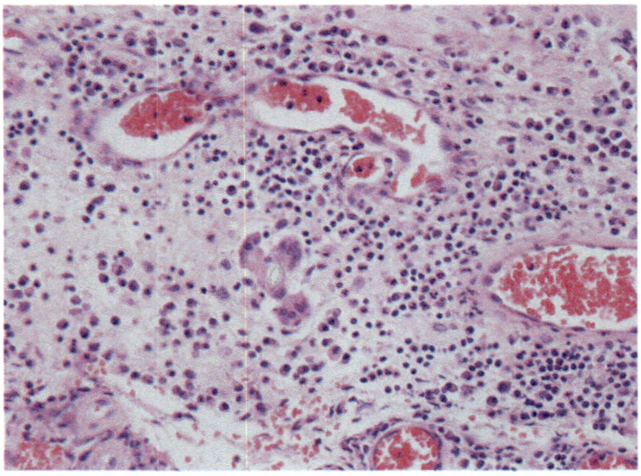

Fig. 14.3 Chronic active inflammation with granulation tissue: aggregation of inflammatory cells. (×400 H&E)

pocket, the spreader grafts on both sides, which were presumed to have been applied in surgery, were found (Video 14.5). It was decided to curettage some and leave the rest for anterior septal support. There was no history of using silicone implants in the past, but it was found that capsules were formed around Gore-tex. The caudal septum almost disappeared, but the anterior septum retained the spreader's shape, and bleeding was also found during the scrape, so it was decided to leave it after careful curettage.

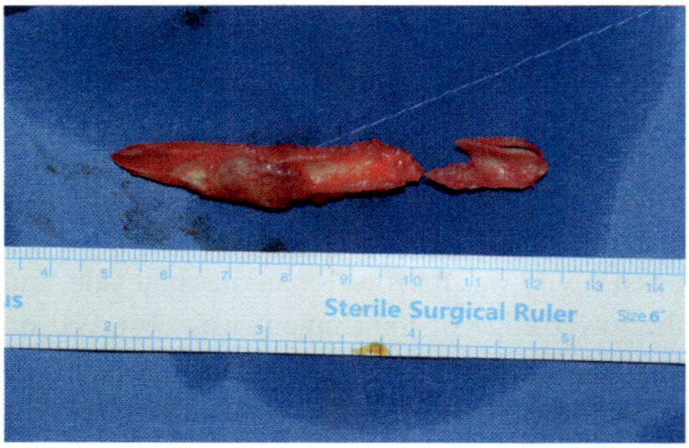

Fig. 14.4 Explanted Gore-tex and dirty capsules

14.3 Operative Strategies

- For caudal septal support, folded cymba cartilage was applied to the caudal septum (Video 14.6).
- The lateral crural spanning graft was performed on the LLC's upper part to prevent counter-clockwise rotation of the tip and increase tip support.
- The missing dorsal volume was filled with SDF.
- Operative Strategies.
- For caudal septal support, folded cymba cartilage was applied to the caudal septum.

Postoperative Results

Even though SSI appears to be well controlled with antibiotics, it can cause ongoing inflammation. Within such a short period, a typical late-onset mucin-producing pocket could be found. Since the patient did not have pus-drainage at the time of surgery, the nasal framework using a cartilage graft was possible, and the columellar retraction could be resolved (Figs. 14.5 and 14.6).

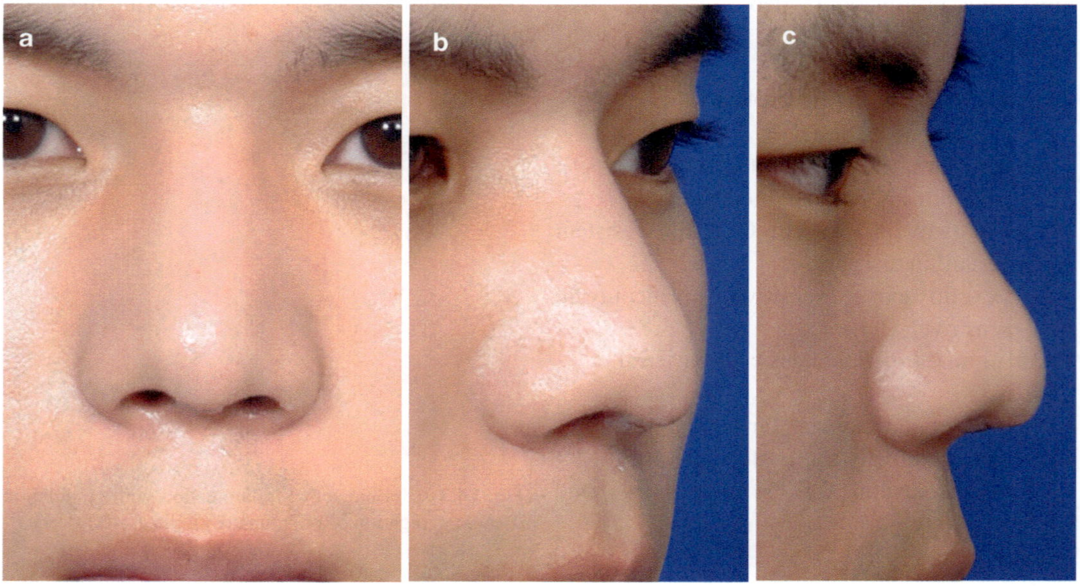

Fig. 14.5 Pre- and postoperative views. (**a**–**c**) Preoperative views. (**d**–**f**) Postoperative 2 months views

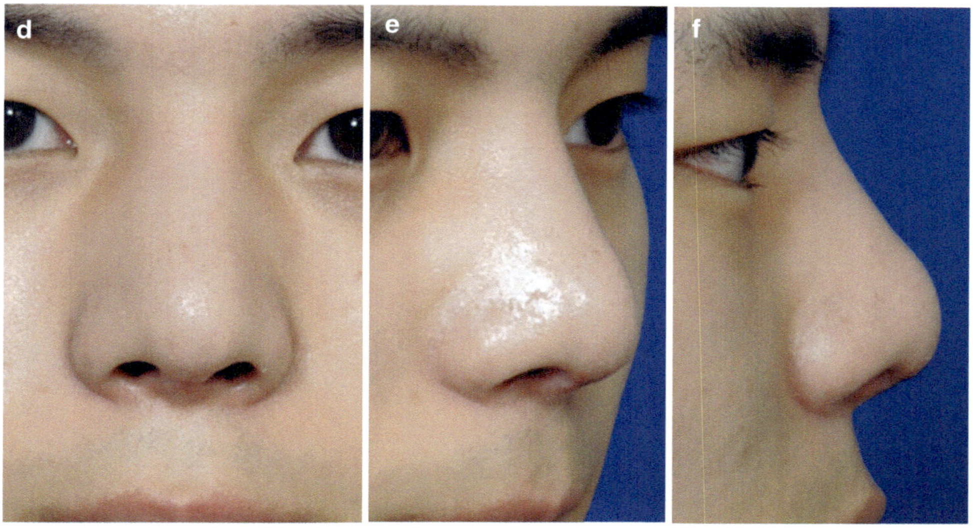

Fig. 14.5 (continued)

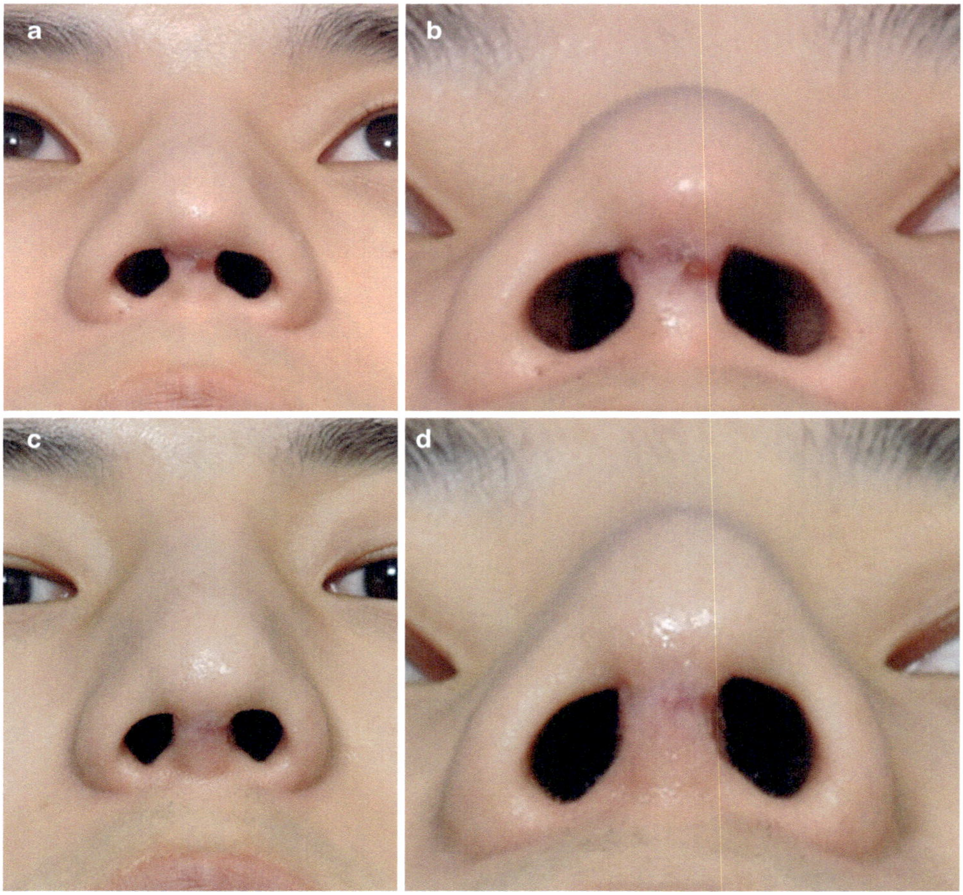

Fig. 14.6 The basal views and the columellar lesion. (**a**, **b**) Preoperative views. (**c**, **d**) Postoperative 2 months views

Nasal Tip Necrosis: The Midline Forehead Flap Should Be the Last Choice

15

15.1 Background of Choosing this Case

As the number of surgeries increases, the circulation to the nasal tip suffers. The author has experienced a few patients transferred to the author with columella necrosis after cosmetic surgery. The author also saw a patient who underwent the six different doctors' rhinoplasties, but the author thinks there is a particular reason for columellar necrosis. Vascular compromise can occur when a nonspecific mechanical trauma is applied to the tip skin or soft tissue around the LLC is not properly stretched, and excessive tension is applied. Both patients suffering from columella necrosis and surgeons are facing enormous stress and those cases become legal complaint cases. In fact, in Korea, midline forehead flaps were applied to the patients, which had become significant social issues with bad results. The problem is that the midline forehead flap is not an improper operation, but applied to a patient who has undergone nose surgery for cosmetic purposes can develop into a case that adversely affects the whole plastic surgeons or plastic surgeries in general. For recruiting soft tissue less than 0.5 × 1 cm, making a midline forehead scars ten times longer is harsh. The authors have even experienced a patient with the hair-growing columella. We have to try the most straightforward method first, and we need to share the wisdom to make sure this method does not fail, so the author has selected these patients in this chapter.

Pearls

- The midline forehead flap is a useful surgery, but it should not be chosen as the first modality of columellar necrosis caused as the complication of esthetic rhinoplasty.
- In composite graft from the ear, integral skin portion and cartilage must be attached, and perichondrium must be preserved to increase survival.
- The surgeon should know how to increase the survival rate of composite grafts.

15.2 Case Study

History

A 37-year-old male patient with a bulbous nose and low nasal dorsum underwent septorhinoplasty using silicone in a private clinic.

- Four months after surgery, a silicone change was made at the same hospital, and columellar revision was made.

Supplementary Information The online version of this chapter (https://doi.org/10.1007/978-981-16-0542-0_15) contains supplementary material, which is available to authorized users.

E.-S. Dhong, M.-W. Na, *Asian Septorhinoplasty*, https://doi.org/10.1007/978-981-16-0542-0_15

- After 3 months, the silicone was changed again, and the columellar was revised using the conchal cartilage.
- Columellar necrosis occurred within 5 days after surgery.

First Choice by the Author: Composite Graft

Physical Exam and Diagnostic Findings

There was necrosis of the entire layer of columella and infratip lobule, and the wound was not open and sat down. There was no evidence of cellulitis in the skin around the necrosis (Fig. 15.1). The CT scan showed dorsal silicone and columellar alloplastic material with a white shadow (Video 15.1).

Preoperative Surgical Goals

The author chose a composite graft using conchal cartilage and attached skin as a salvaging method. Dorsal silicone was left as it is, and only the columella was reconstructed. The nasolabial perforator flap was the second choice if the composite graft was not taken, and the midline forehead flap was planned as the third option. The reason was that the patient's skin was very thick, and the forehead was relatively narrow.

Strategy for Composite Graft

- The cartilage covers the middle crura on both sides to the medial crura like the shape of the shield graft.
- The perichondrium attached to the cartilage is preserved so that the surrounding blood supply can go to the skin more smoothly.
- Hyperbaric O_2 therapy will be performed.

Intraoperative Findings

Immediately after removing the necrotic skin, discolored cartilage was seen and removed. This piece was IHCC; however, no information could be obtained (Fig. 15.2).

Most of the caudal portion of the middle crus and medial crus disappeared and after debridement. The defect became more extensive than the primary lesion.

Operation Method

- The cartilage that is larger than the range of the skin is designed (Fig. 15.3).
- As designed, it was harvested from the posterior surface of the cavum (Fig. 15.4).
- After removing the necrotic skin, the surrounding margin was debrided to make it sharper.

Result

The entire graft survived.

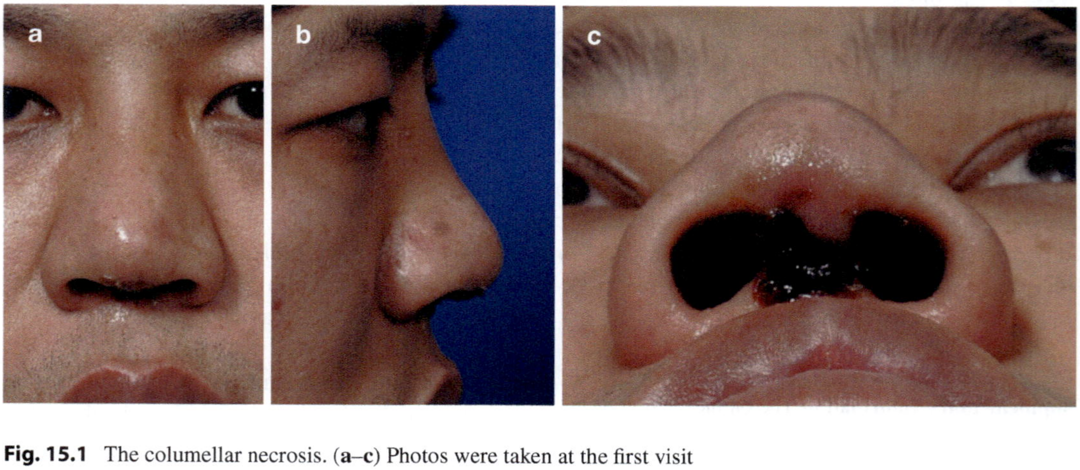

Fig. 15.1 The columellar necrosis. (**a**–**c**) Photos were taken at the first visit

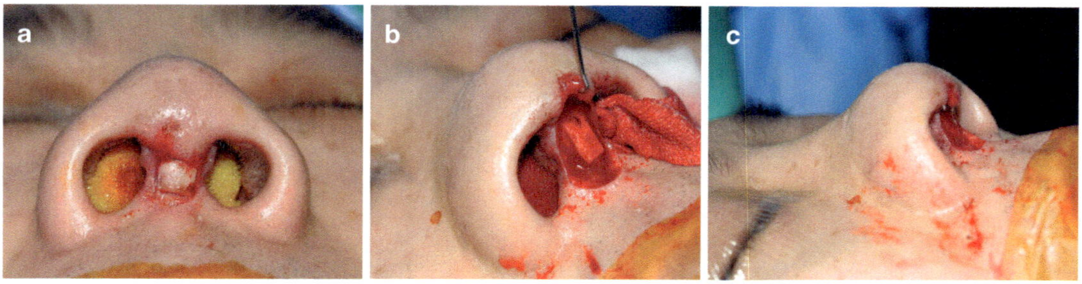

Fig. 15.2 Debridement to make a clean skin margin. (**a**) IHCC was found after removing the necrotic columella. (**b**) Margin debridement and removal of IHCC. (**c**) Wide defect remained

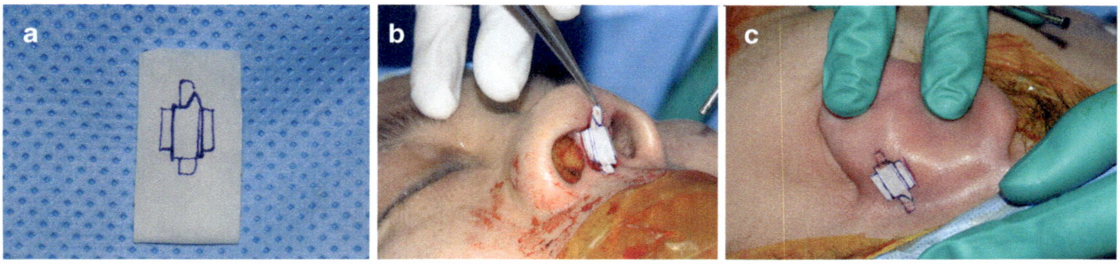

Fig. 15.3 Schematic of the composite graft. (**a**, **b**) The design and the application at the lesion. (**c**) The posterior auricular circus at the cavum concha was harvested

Secondary Operation: SRP

Physical Exam and Diagnostic Findings

Definite septorhinoplasty was performed 18 months after the last surgery.

The dorsal silicone was found, and the rigid scar tissue over the nasal tip was removed. The tip was like one big scar. Septorhinoplasty using sixth costal cartilage was planned. An L-sturt extension graft was applied for nasal lengthening. The nasal tip plasty was focused on reducing the bulbosity and creating the supra-alar groove.

Strategy for SRP

- He had a very thick skin, so costal cartilage was harvested, and a profound extension against tension was planned.
- The projection was increased at the dorsum by diced costal cartilage to be wrapped in the rectus fascia.

Intraoperative Findings

The 3.5 mm silicone was removed from the dorsum, and the very thick capsule and surrounding contracture had to be removed. The caudal septum remained, but very weak. The loss of the caudal margin of the LLC's middle crus and medial crus existed as in the first surgery, but the shield graft applied in the composite graft was integrated to form a caudal margin. This cartilage was used as the medial crura.

Operation Method

- An incision was applied using the scar on the bottom of the composite graft.
- Since it was SMR state, it was difficult to maintain the length of the nose with the remaining L-strut, so a long extended spreader graft (9 × 20 mm) was applied using a slice of the sixth rib, and a caudal septal extension graft using a slice of the costal cartilage was applied to the caudal portion (5 × 18 mm) (Fig. 15.5).

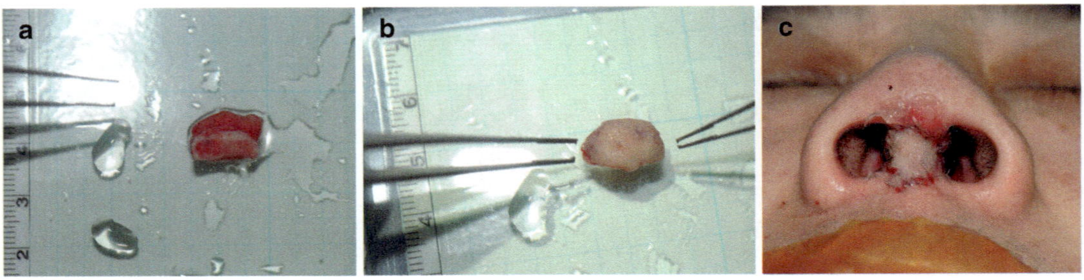

Fig. 15.4 Composite graft. (**a**, **b**) The perichondrium attached to the cartilage was preserved so that the surrounding blood supply can go to the skin more smoothly. (**c**) After the repair. The open dressing was done

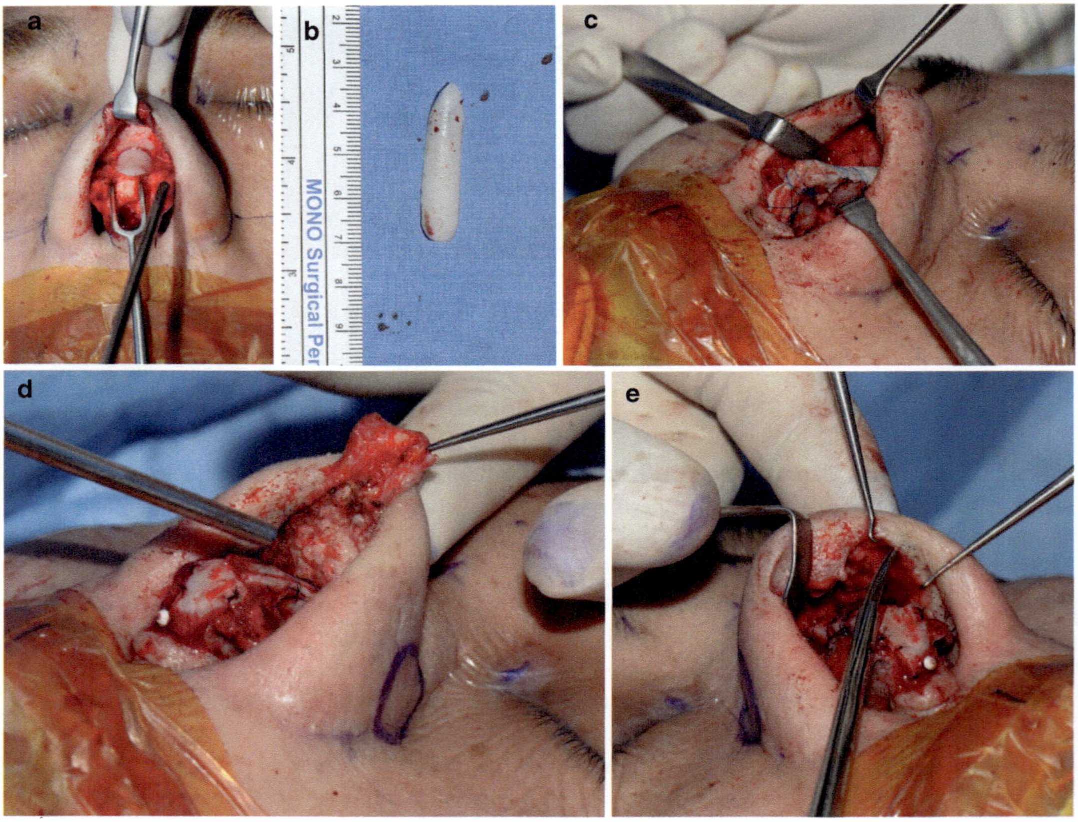

Fig. 15.5 Septal reconstruction using SLEG. (**a**, **b**) Intraoperative silicone implant. (**c**) Septal L-strut extension graft. (**d**, **e**) Sleeve down technique of dorsal skin envelope

- The loss of the caudal margin of the LLC's middle crus and medial crus existed as in the first surgery, but the shield graft applied in the composite graft was integrated to form a caudal margin. This cartilage was used as the medial crura.
- For the creation of the supra-alar groove, the LLSAN deep in the dermis and a portion of the fat layer were removed.

Result

- There was no skin loss of the composite graft.
- The overall retraction of the nose was improved, and the profile was improved.
- The columellar retraction was improved, and supratip soft tissue removal and supra-alar groove shape improvement were obtained (Figs. 15.6 and 15.7).

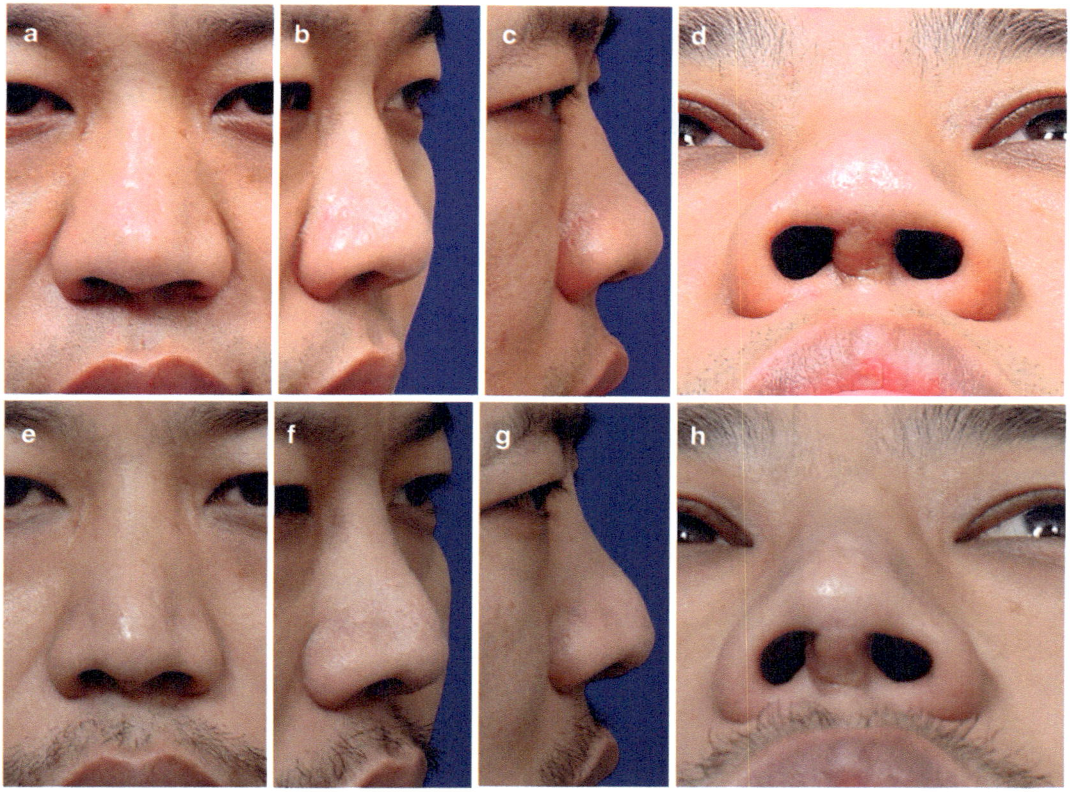

Fig. 15.6 Septorhinoplasty using costal cartilage was performed 18 months after the composite graft (**a**–**d**) Preoperative views. (**e**–**h**) Long-term postoperative views

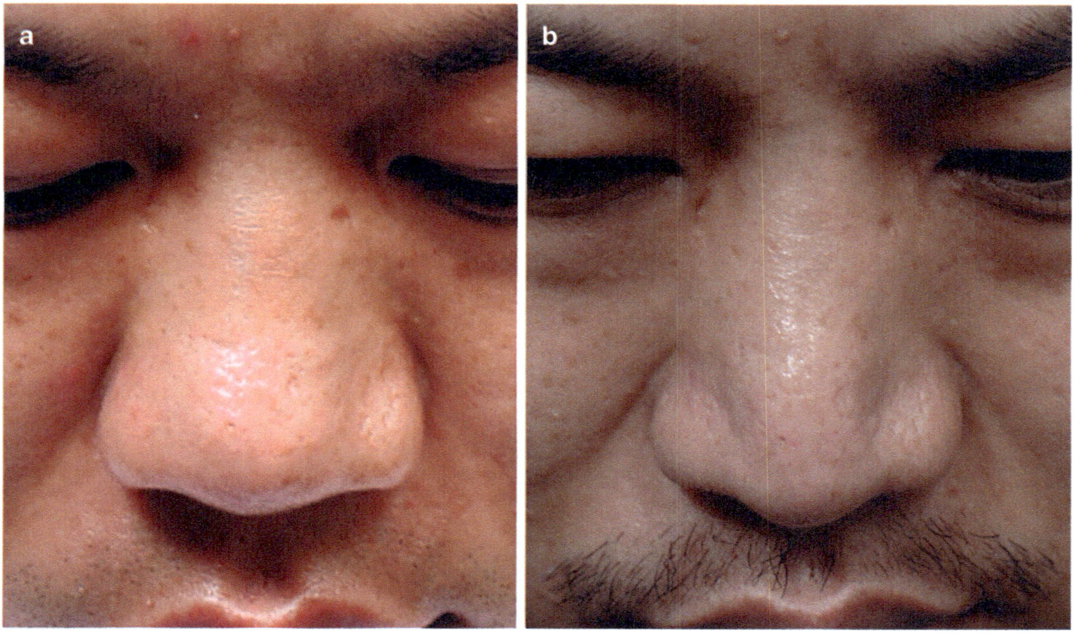

Fig. 15.7 Comparative views. (**a**, **c**) Pre- and postoperative bird's eye view. (**b**, **d**) Before the composite graft and the long-term result

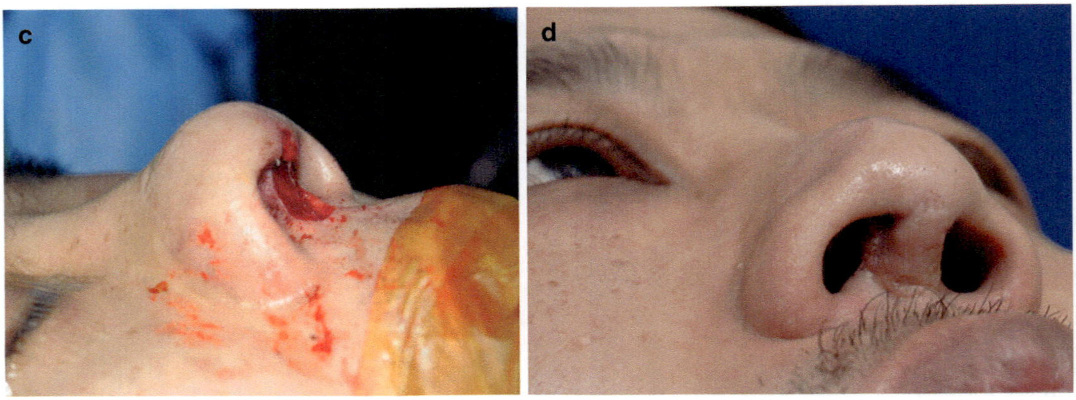

Fig. 15.7 (continued)

When You Encounter Very Small Septal Cartilage

16

16.1 Background

A common problem in Asians is that the nasal septal cartilage is collected less than expected. In old age, the amount of quadrangular cartilage decreases. It is relatively more ossified, and the amount of cartilage harvested is small. If the nose is small, or there is a history of fractures, it is possible to predict that flat quadrangular cartilage will be small. However, many Asians have a small volume of quadrangular cartilage attainable even in younger patients than the standard without any trauma history. Ossification can be detected in a CT scan in advance, but all slices of scan cannot be contained.

This patient was selected to know how to collect quadrangular cartilage wisely in an unpredicted situation.

Pearls

- When encountering unexpectedly small quadrangular cartilage, the EPP cartilage junction must be well protected.
- If the EPP-quadrangular junction is well connected, a more extended graft is available.
- EPP harvest should be performed according to a planned osteotomy.
- Osteotomy can be performed with the freer elevator, but a saw can be the alternative if it does not work well.
- A reciprocating saw and an oscillating saw should be provided.
- Efforts are made to prevent damaging the mucosal pocket.

16.2 Case Study

History

A 39-year-old man complained of nasal stuffiness on his right side and wanted to correct a reverse C-shape deformity. He had no history of trauma.

Physical Exam and Diagnostic Findings

There was no particular abnormality on physical examination.

The patient had severe nasal obstruction with a NOSE scale of 16/20.

Supplementary Information The online version of this chapter (https://doi.org/10.1007/978-981-16-0542-0_16) contains supplementary material, which is available to authorized users.

E.-S. Dhong, M.-W. Na, *Asian Septorhinoplasty*, https://doi.org/10.1007/978-981-16-0542-0_16

Endoscopic Findings

There was a protrusion suspicious of septal dislocation in the right nasal crest. Attenuation of the nasal mucosa at the nasal crest was observed. It could be suspected that lacerations existed along the maxillary crest.

The right nasal cavity looked narrower than the left, but the left EPP was also convex (Video 16.1 and Fig. 16.1).

Acoustic Rhinometry

The right MCA (minimal cross-sectional area) was measured to be 0.55, and the right nasal cavity was more obstructed (Fig. 16.2).

Preoperative Surgical Planning

- A spreader graft was planned on the patient's right anterior septum with septal cartilage.
- For the mild hump correction, only the left nasal dorsum would be rasped to obtain a straight line.

Intraoperative Findings

After the L-strut of 11 mm-width was preserved, a very small quadrangular cartilage was found.

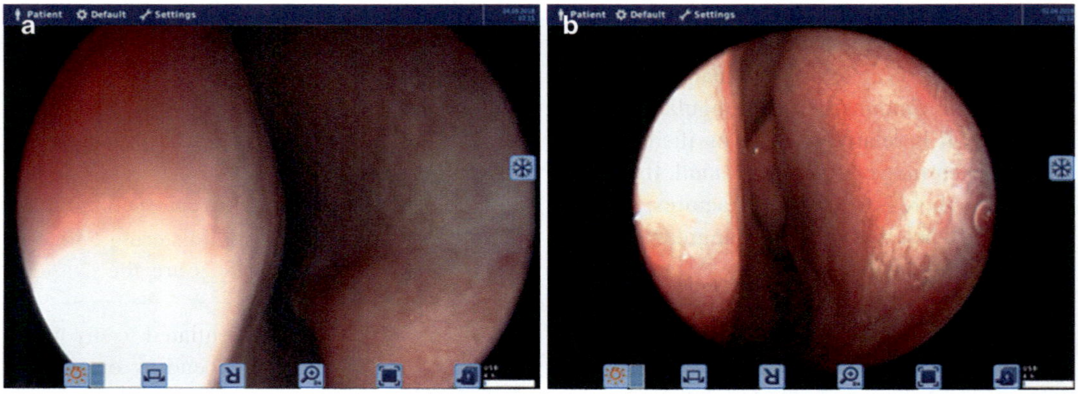

Fig. 16.1 Endoscopic views. (**a**) The right nasal cavity: septal concavity and protruded septal cartilage on the maxillary crest and vomer. (**b**) The left nasal cavity: convexity of EPP

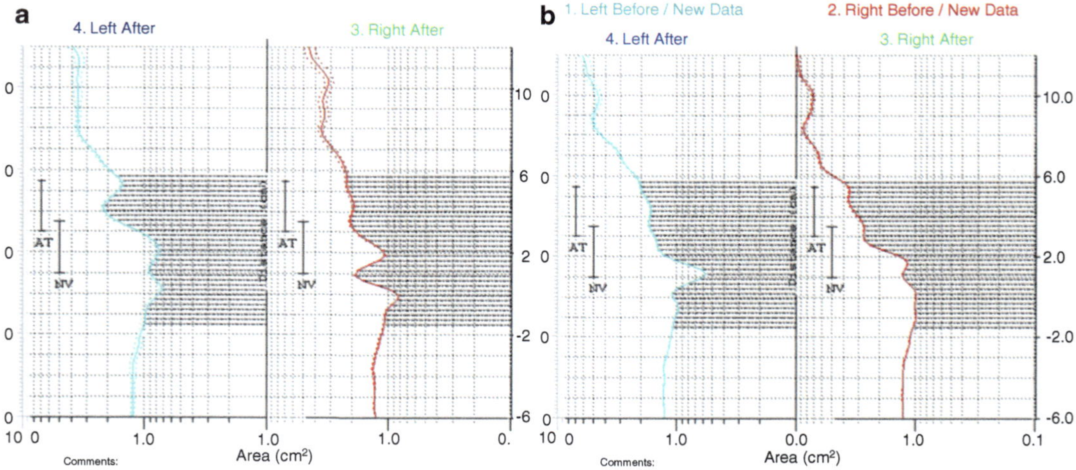

Fig. 16.2 Acoustic rhinometry. (**a**) Preoperative AR showed right MCA is located anteriorly and smaller. (**b**) Postoperatively the right curve improved. The patient NOSE score improved from 16/20 to 8/20

16.3 Operative Strategies

- Quadrangular cartilage attached with EPP (20 × 29 mm) was harvested (Fig. 16.3).
- More EPP (7 × 16 mm) was harvested and used for stabilizing the caudal septum.
- Bilateral spreader graft (9 × 26 mm) was applied (Fig. 16.4).
- A PDS plate obtained stability to integrate the anterior extended spreader graft and caudal septum (Video 16.2).
- For the correction of convexity, a mattress suture was applied to the left lateral crus (Video 16.3).
- Small columellar strut, columelloseptal suture, and tip cartilage shield graft were applied for the ideal LLC shaping (Video 16.4 and Fig. 16.5).
- Bilateral out fracture of inferior turbinate was performed (Video 16.5).
- Bilateral coblation of inferior turbinate was performed (Video 16.6).

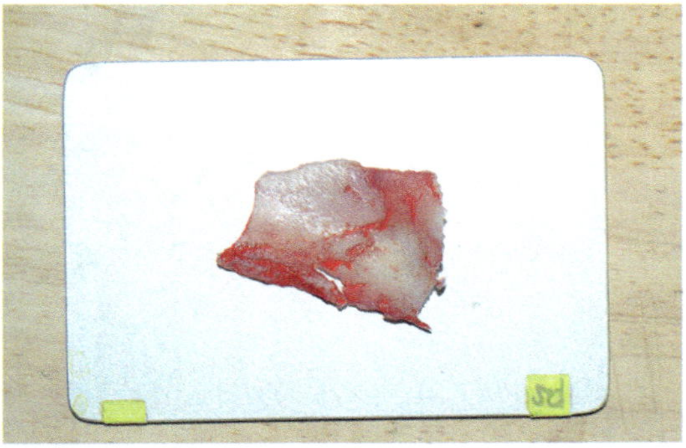

Fig. 16.3 Harvested septal cartilage (20 × 29 mm). This was cut into two spreader grafts

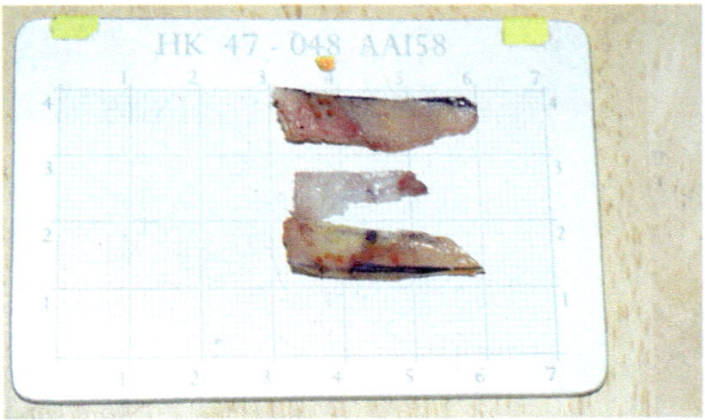

Fig. 16.4 Cartilage with bone segment was ready for the bilateral spreader graft. Multiple drill holes were made for the suture. (center) A bone piece harvested from EPP (7 × 16 mm) was prepared for the small caudal batten graft

Postoperative Results

- The NOSE scale decreased from 16 points to 8 points.
- The curve on the AR on the Rt side improved (Fig. 16.2).
- The stuffy nose disappeared. He smells better and sleeps better (Video 16.7).
- The reverse C-shape deviation was corrected (Figs. 16.6 and 16.7).

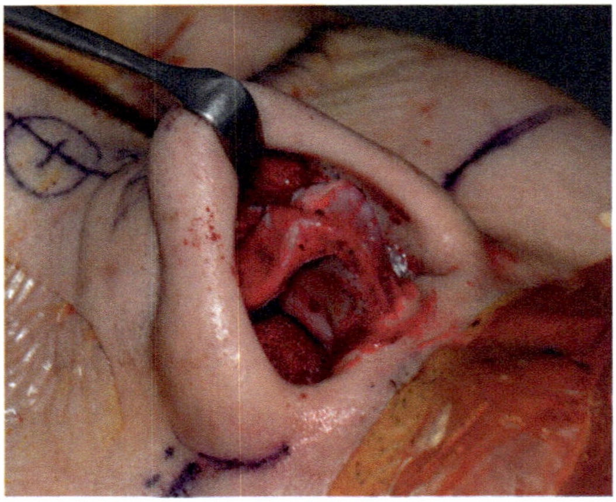

Fig. 16.5 The feature of the LLCs: Small columellar strut graft and short shield graft

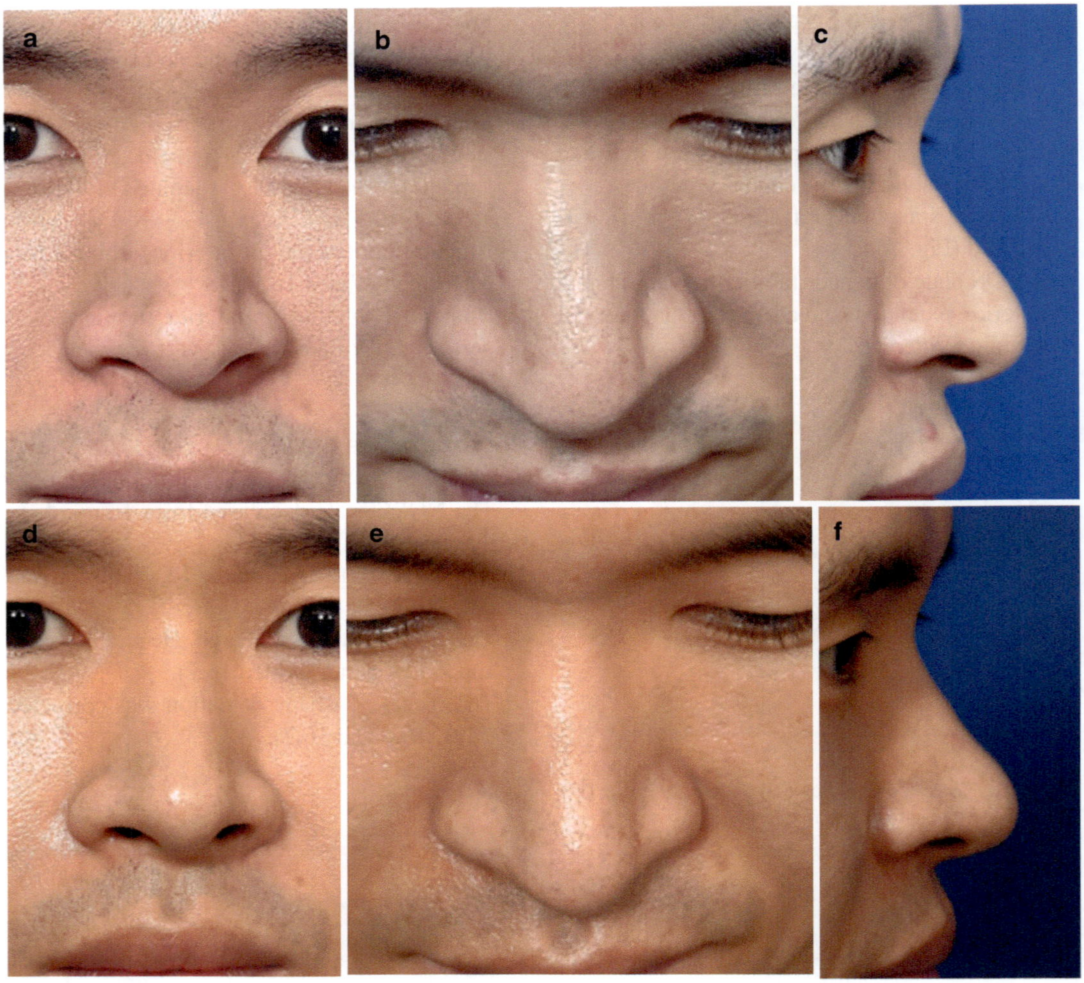

Fig. 16.6 Pre- and postoperative views. (**a**–**c**) Preoperative views. (**d**–**f**) Long-term postoperative views

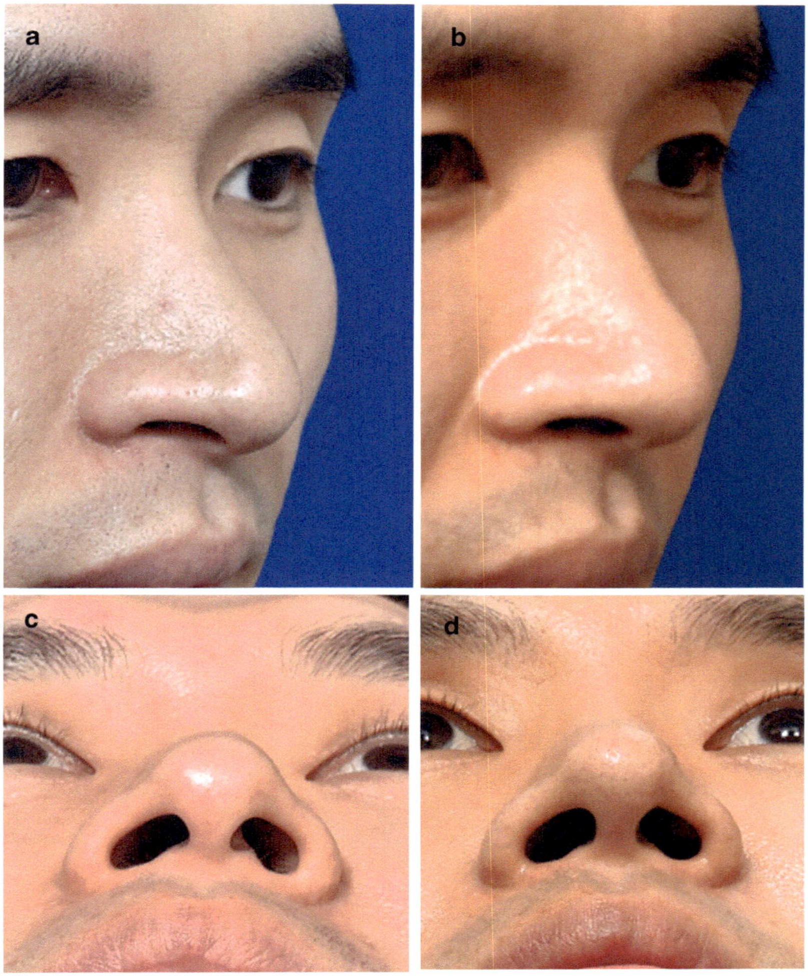

Fig. 16.7 Pre- and postoperative views. (**a**, **c**) Preoperative views. (**b**, **d**) Long-term postoperative views

17 Hypoplastic Lower Two-Third Nose: Camouflage Vs. Reconstruct the Framework

17.1 Background of Selecting this Patient

This feature accounts for many patients of Asian rhinoplasty. The bony dorsum is appropriately projected, whereas the height of the cartilaginous dorsum is relatively low. Whether the clinical manifestation is a saddle nose or a hypoplastic lower two-third nose without a saddle, there is likely a septal deviation or septal depression. If there is a deviation or tilt of the septum or a defect, the cartilaginous dorsum is usually very low. In these patients, choosing a dorsal alloplastic implant is not a good option. Dead space will be created in the lower part of the implant, even though it fits the nasion. Conversely, many surgeons do resect the bony dorsum to fit the upper one-third nose. The author prefers to perform only by increasing the lower two-third nose. This method can express the dorsum and tip as septum-dependently. In the author's choices, costal cartilage is the last resort of choice. The costal cartilage has already been introduced as a novel technique several times, and the author agrees that there is no better way than that. However, the author prefers septal reconstruction to solid costal cartilage onlay graft. If septal surgery is not possible, the camouflage method will be a second strategy. The author disagrees with the notion that patients complain of discomfort with the stiff nasal tip, which other Asian surgeons are concerned about. However, various Asian problematic noses can only be reconstructed by costal cartilage. If some membranous septum is left, the nasal tip can be movable on a long term. The autologous costal cartilage is the last scone of the rhinoplasty surgeon and is a treasure trove that allows multiple surgeons.

Pearls

- If the lower two-third of the nose is hypotrophied, the upper one-third of the nose may look rather large. In this situation, the right plan will be only enhancing the hypoplastic portion. Surgeons should imagine the original state of the nose.
- The long extended spreader graft's success in the correction of the over-resected nose is the stability of the rhinion region.
- The soundness of the anterocaudal margin of the lateral nasal bone plays an important role in the success of the surgery.
- Anterior projection of more than 3 mm is not easy by applying separate L-strut extension graft using conchal cartilage.
- More projection is possible only by costal cartilage.

Supplementary Information The online version of this chapter (https://doi.org/10.1007/978-981-16-0542-0_17) contains supplementary material, which is available to authorized users.

E.-S. Dhong, M.-W. Na, *Asian Septorhinoplasty*, https://doi.org/10.1007/978-981-16-0542-0_17

17.2 Case Study

History

First Operation

A 26-year-old female patient with a hump nose and deviation underwent septorhinoplasty with corrective osteotomy and SMR, dorsal graft with alloderm, and IHCC at a private clinic. After that, the dorsum was too high, and the deviation recurred.

Revision at the Private Clinic

Alloderm removed and first fat injection 3 months after surgery. Two months later, she received the second fat injection. Another month later, she received third fat injection.

Tertiary Operation at a Different Clinic

Three months later, IHCC was removed at another private clinic through cosmetic dissatisfaction such as tip asymmetry, and secondary rhinoplasty was performed using bilateral conchal carriage and SDF. After 2 days of operation, SDF was removed due to inflammation. After the last operation, a severe saddle nose occurred, and she visited the author 1 year and 3 months later.

Physical Exam and Diagnostic Findings

At the first examination, the tip felt hard, and there was no movement at all. The dorsal skin adhered to the underneath tissue. After a three-month follow-up, she took Zafirlukast and continuously massaged the nose. The skin, including the tip and dorsum, was observed to become soft (Video 17.1).

17.3 Nasal Swab Study

Zafirlukast was prescribed, and culture studies were conducted periodically during the follow-up period. Follow-up every 2 weeks and six culture studies were conducted. When MRSA was first identified, mupirocin ointment was applied, and then it was not identified. MRSE was cultured in the last culture before surgery. Tarivid ointment was applied to the nasal cavity for 1 week before surgery. Ciprofloxacin was selected and used for 4 days from the day of surgery, and the culture performed immediately before surgery was negative. Antibiotics were continuously used without changing.

Endoscopic Findings and CT Scan

The ceiling of the nasal cavity was found low from external nares to INV. She did not complain of a stuffy nose. A CT scan showed over-resected dorsum and showed deformity in which the open roof was not closed at all (Video 17.2).

17.4 Acoustic Rhinometry

From the entrance to INV, it did not show a sudden MCA. Nose score was 7/20.

Preoperative Surgical Goals

- The anterior septum was reconstructed with a thin slice of costal cartilage. With this spreader graft, the cartilaginous dorsum was projected.
- Bone fixation was attempted to fix the weak rhinion area.

Strategy for the Operation

- The skin was very thin. The solid dorsal graft would cause excessive tension in the nasal tip skin.
- A solid dorsal graft was not required because she did not want the projection of the nasion area.
- However, considering the overall dorsal line, it was judged that the augmentation of 2 mm of the bony dorsum was necessary.
- More than two suitable ear cartilages were left, but a long spreader graft was needed, so

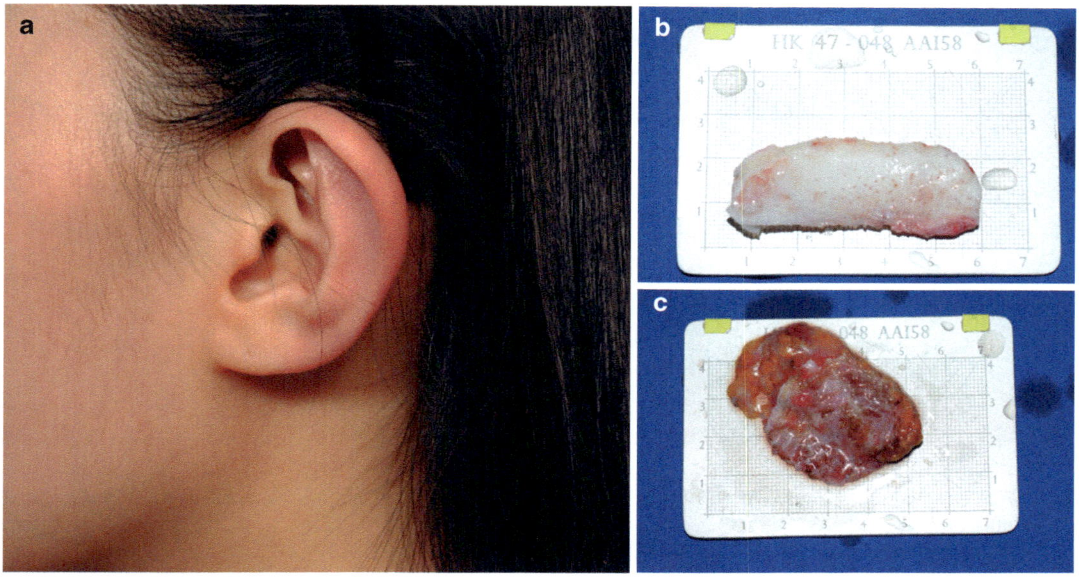

Fig. 17.1 The materials of the operation. (**a**) The ear cartilage was already harvested from the left cymba and cavum concha. (**b**) Sixth costal cartilage. (**c**) The rectus fascia

the author decided to use costal cartilage (Fig. 17.1).
- A long extended spreader graft was required to improve the inverted V deformity.
- The lateral wall of the nasal bone was relatively palpated, but the lateral osteotomy would not be performed.

Intraoperative Findings

- The ossification of costal cartilage was found.
- Although the anterior septum was almost lost, detachment of the left and right mucoperichondrium was possible successfully.
- The lateral nasal bone in the rhinion site was partially destroyed.

17.5 Operation Method

- Extended spreader graft was performed using costal cartilage of long slices (9 × 25 mm).
- Two layers of caudal septal extension graft were also applied to the caudal septum (6 × 18 mm).
- To prevent warping, coaptation was performed using multiple sutures.
- Except for the two 5.0 nonabsorbable sutures, only PDS 4.0 and 5.0 were used.
- For a smooth dorsal line, partially rolled rectus fascia was grafted onlay to the dorsum (Video 17.3). The bony dorsum area over the nasion, the fascia was rolled, but the lower two-third area was not rolled.

17.6 Result

- After surgery, inverted V deformity disappeared, but some deformity reappeared after the dorsal resorption.
- But the saddle nose deformity was improved.
- She did not appeal for nasal obstruction after septal reconstruction.
- Vast resorption of dorsal rolled rectus fascia occurred.
- The author persuaded secondary insertion of dorsal onlay graft, but she did not want a revision. The dorsal esthetic line was agreeable with the patient.
- Severe warping has not occurred (Figs. 17.2, 17.3, 17.4, 17.5, and 17.6).

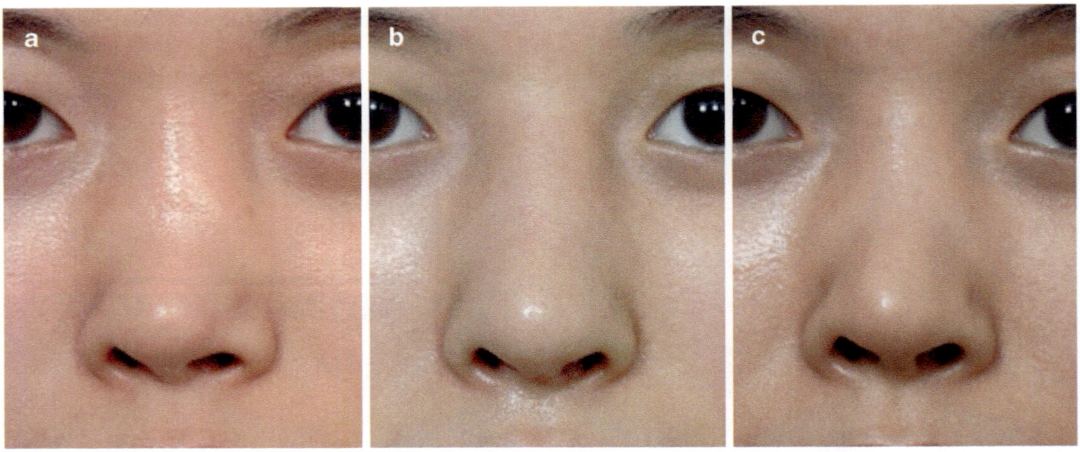

Fig. 17.2 Pre- and postoperative AP views. (**a**) Preoperative view. (**b**) Postoperative 6 months view. (**c**) Postoperative 18 months view

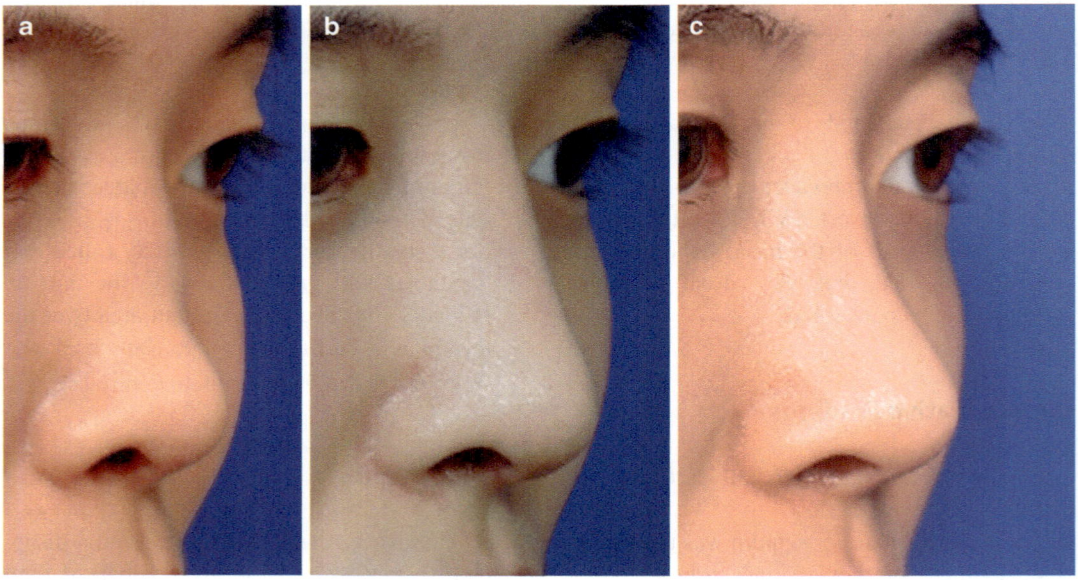

Fig. 17.3 Pre- and postoperative quarter views. (**a**) Preoperative view. (**b**) Postoperative 6 months view. (**c**) Postoperative 18 months view

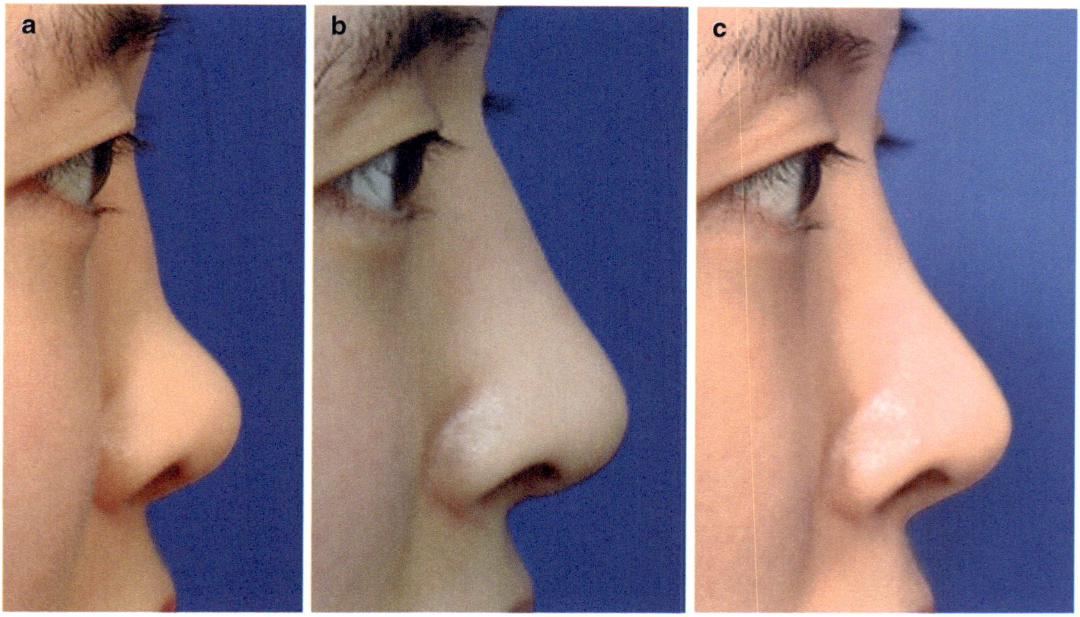

Fig. 17.4 Pre- and postoperative lateral views. (**a**) Preoperative view. (**b**) Postoperative 6 months view. (**c**) Postoperative 18 months view

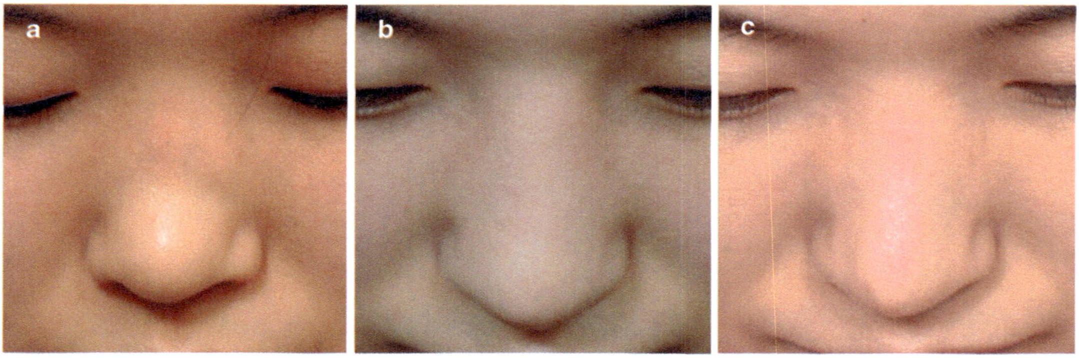

Fig. 17.5 Pre- and postoperative bird's eye views. (**a**) Preoperative view. (**b**) Postoperative 6 months view. (**c**) Postoperative 18 months view

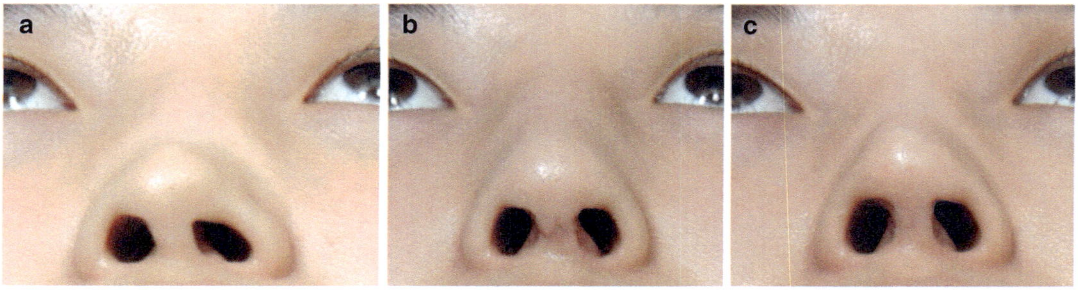

Fig. 17.6 Pre- and postoperative worm's eye views. (**a**) Preoperative view. (**b**) Postoperative 6 months view. (**c**) Postoperative 18 months view

Correction to: Controlling Asian Tip: Facet and Supra-Alar Groove

Correction to:
Chapter 9 in: E.-S. Dhong, M.-W. Na, *Asian Septorhinoplasty*,
https://doi.org/10.1007/978-981-16-0542-0_9

In chapter 9, Figures 9.6, 9.7, 9.8, 9.10, and 9.11 were incorrectly published. This has now been corrected by replacing them with the correct figures.

The corrected figures and their captions are printed below:

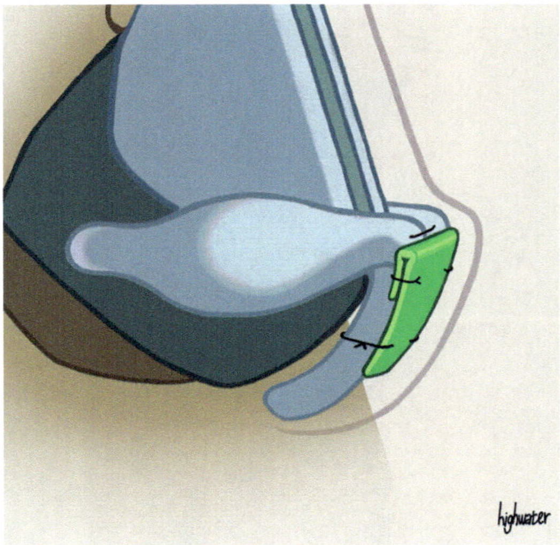

Fig. 9.6 Shield graft, the figure expresses the double-layered graft at the upper side. It is common to apply one layer

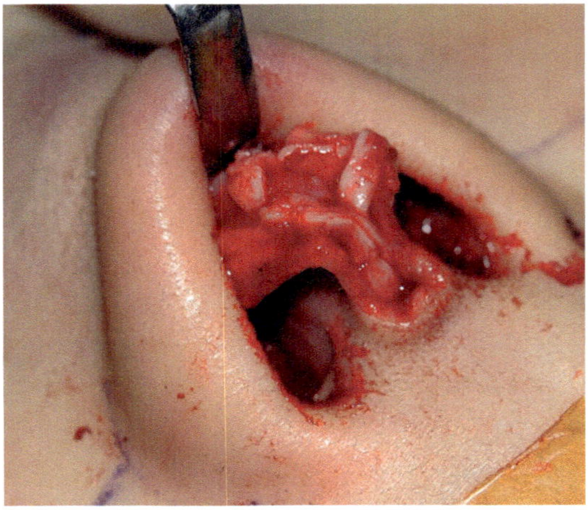

Fig. 9.7 Midcrural extension graft: Middle small rim of double conchal cartilage

The updated version of this chapter can be found at https://doi.org/10.1007/978-981-16-0542-0_9

E.-S. Dhong, M.-W. Na, *Asian Septorhinoplasty*, https://doi.org/10.1007/978-981-16-0542-0_18

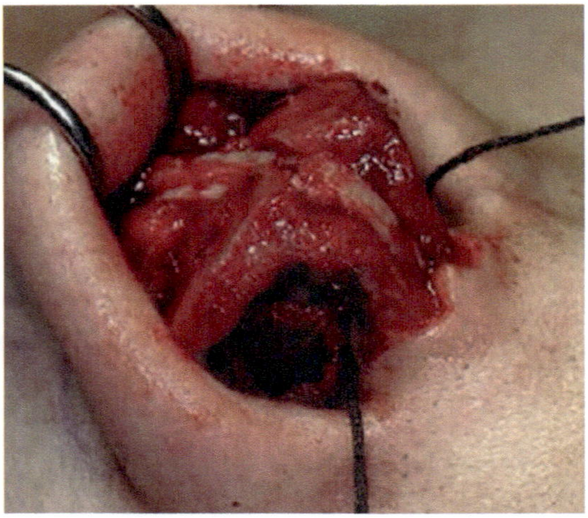

Fig. 9.8 Septal extension graft reaches to the middle crura modifying the tip-lobular angle

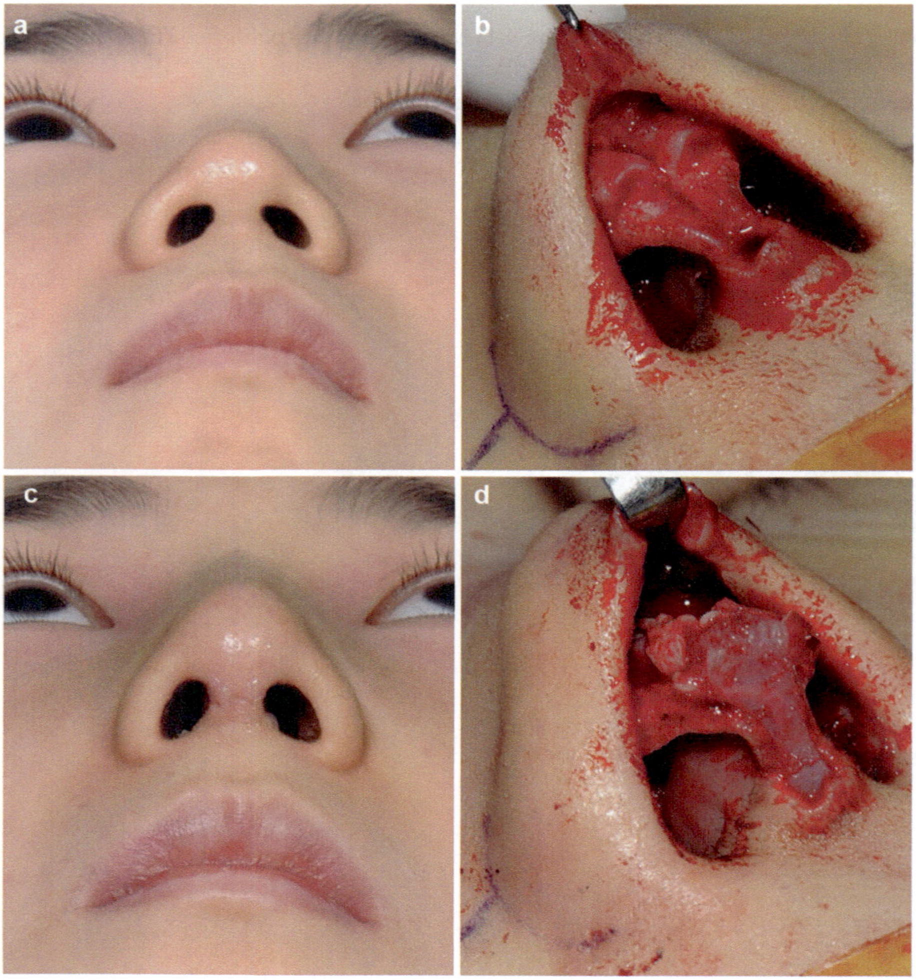

Fig. 9.10 Underdeveloped middle crura in primary rhinoplasty: reconstructed with midcrural extension graft and a shield graft. (**a**) Preoperative view. (**b**) Before the grafts. (**c**) Postoperative view. (**d**) Before closure

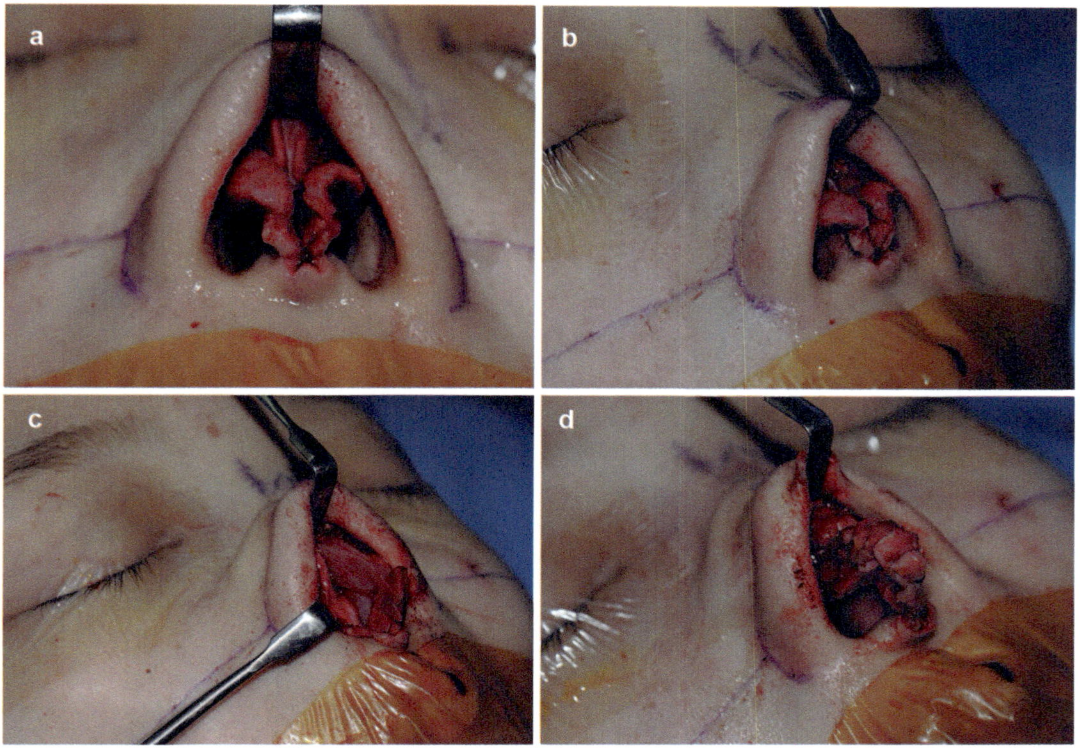

Fig. 9.11 Tortuous middle crura in primary rhinoplasty: Septal L-strut extension graft, shield graft, and a tip onlay graft using SMF (**a**, **b**) Intraoperative view before the grafts. (**c**) Septal L-strut extension graft. (**d**) Tip onlay graft

GPSR Compliance

The European Union's (EU) General Product Safety Regulation (GPSR) is a set of rules that requires consumer products to be safe and our obligations to ensure this.

If you have any concerns about our products, you can contact us on ProductSafety@springernature.com

In case Publisher is established outside the EU, the EU authorized representative is:

Springer Nature Customer Service Center GmbH
Europaplatz 3
69115 Heidelberg, Germany

Batch number: 10732801

Printed by Printforce, the Netherlands